ELEMENTARY PHYSICAL EDUCATION

A DEVELOPMENTAL APPROACH

ELEMENTARY PHYSICAL EDUCATION

A DEVELOPMENTAL APPROACH

Daniel D. Arnheim, D.P.E.

Professor, Physical Education, and Director,
Infant/Toddler Development Program,
California State University at Long Beach

Robert A. Pestolesi, Ph.D.

Professor and Chairman, Physical Education,
California State University at Long Beach

SECOND EDITION

with **540** illustrations

The C. V. Mosby Company

Saint Louis   1978

Cover photographs courtesy of Bob Bishop,
Visual Innovations, Inc.

SECOND EDITION

Copyright © 1978 by The C. V. Mosby Company

Previous edition copyrighted 1973

Printed in the United States of America

The C. V. Mosby Company
11830 Westline Industrial Drive, St. Louis, Missouri 63141

Library of Congress Cataloging in Publication Data

Arnheim, Daniel D
    Elementary physical education.

    First ed. published in 1973 under title:
Developing motor behavior in children.
    Bibliography: p.
    Includes index.
    1.   Physical education for children. 2.   Motor
ability. 3.   Child development. 4.   Physical
education for children—Curricula.   I.   Pestolesi,
Robert A., joint author. II.   Title.
GV443.A735   1978   372.8'6   77-26214
ISBN 0-8016-0326-9

CB/CB/B   9   8   7   6   5   4   3   2   1

My efforts in this book are dedicated to my Lord, Jesus Christ, whose strength has carried me through a most difficult period, and to my wife, Helene, whose constant encouragement and support have been a true blessing.

D. D. A.

To my wife, Marillyn, and the many teachers who have enriched children's lives through creative instruction in movement activities.

R. A. P.

Preface

Elementary Physical Education: A Developmental Approach is the second edition of the text *Developing Motor Behavior in Children: A Balanced Approach to Elementary Physical Education.* This name change was made to more clearly describe the content of the second edition and the current philosophy of the authors.

This text is especially written for the college student studying elementary physical education, the physical education specialist in the field, and the classroom teacher. It is also designed to serve as a guide and resource for professionals in disciplines other than physical education, such as, psychology, recreation, health care, child development, or special education. We have attempted to provide the reader with as complete and comprehensive a text as possible. The who, what, when, where, how, and why of elementary physical education have been presented in as much detail as possible with specific consideration given to the major concept that all physical education should be developmentally based. In this text, we have tried to clearly set forth our personal beliefs on key issues related to elementary physical education. These are:

1. Education of the physical being starts before birth.
2. Every child should participate in physical activity on a daily basis.
3. Every child should be given rich experiences in movement appropriate to his or her individual developmental capabilities.
4. Physical education is essential to a child's total physical, emotional, social and cognitive development.
5. Physical fitness must be considered one of the most important aspects of physical education and should be included in the curriculum for even the very young child.
6. Both indirect and direct teaching methods should be employed by the teacher, depending on the particular characteristics of the activity.
7. The physical education curriculum is educationally sound and should receive strong administrative support.

More specifically, this text is organized into four major sections: The Focus, The Developing Child, Instructional Foundations, and Introduction to Activities. The Appendixes, respectively, contain source materials and norms for the AAHPER Physical Fitness Test.

Part One, The Focus, introduces to the reader the importance of physical education and the importance of understanding the complexities of motor behavior as it relates to total human development. Aims, goals, and the primary objectives of elementary physical education and its relevance to the whole school curriculum are discussed. Also presented is an in-depth discussion of the teacher's role in planning and carrying out a program along with suggestions for the practical application of techniques on teaching and administering a highly successful program of elementary physical education.

Part Two, The Developing Child, gives selected information on human development from the time of conception through late childhood, with special emphasis on the importance of movement behavior. Part Two is concerned with the major concepts that movement is an integral part of a child's total development and that it is extremely important that a teacher should present physical activities that are appropriate for each child's maturational level.

Part Three, Instructional Foundations, provides detailed discussion of concepts, teaching methods, and approaches that are found in varying degrees in modern elementary physical education. It affords both theoretical and practical information in the highly important areas of basic body management through perceptual-motor training, movement education, physical fitness, integrated learning and classroom activities, and the exceptional child.

Part Four, Introduction to Activities, has been organized under level 1, level 2, level 3, and level 4. Introductory comments precede the activity chapters, explaining how Part Four can best be utilized by the teacher. Level 1, Beginning, covers the first 2 years of life, with selected activities and experiences based on the approximate maturational age in months. Level 2, Building; Level 3, Expanding; and Level 4, Refining, are organized and presented according to the types of activities that the child will perform. We have attempted to present the most current and developmentally sound activities possible. Activities are specifically chosen for their developmental value. Each activity area is presented in sequence from simple to complex. Each activity is presented with its behavioral objective, developmental goal, space and equipment needed, and relationship to basic motor ability evaluation.

To the many persons who assisted in the critical reading and typing of the manuscript, we extend our sincere gratitude. A special appreciation is extended to Helene Arnheim and Marillyn Pestolesi for their many hours of assistance and to Dennis Roberson for his creative suggestions on the organization of Part Four.

Daniel D. Arnheim
Robert A. Pestolesi

Contents

10 Physical fitness and movement efficiency, 211

11 Integrated learning and classroom activities, 236

12 The exceptional child: from the limited to the gifted, 259

PART FOUR

INTRODUCTION TO ACTIVITIES—FROM DISCOVERY TO COMMAND

13 Level 1: Beginning, 277

14 Level 2: Building, 294

15 Level 3: Expanding, 337

THE FOCUS

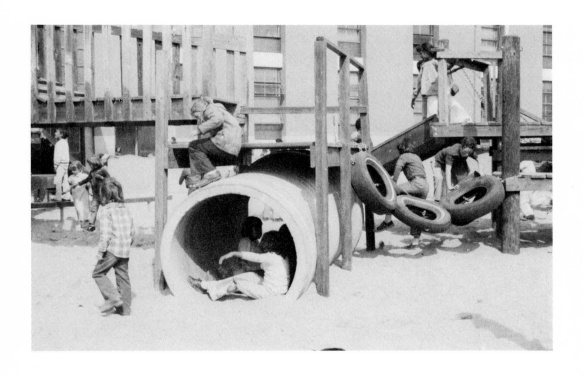

Part One presents a philosophy of developmental elementary physical education. Focus is on program aims, goals, and objectives; the role of the teacher; and effective program management.

1

Prepare for action

What more exciting experience can children have than that of learning to move their bodies effectively in space? Add to this the ability to successfully perform a variety of motor tasks and they will be engulfed with personal enjoyment, pride, and favorable self-image. This concept is certainly not new, since history reveals that the idea of physical education is as old as the human species. In the beginning, primitive man utilized effective motor skills for the sole purpose of survival. The motor skills of running, throwing, and striking were needed to effect the kill and accomplish a successful hunt. Since life itself was dependent on the successful execution of the hunt, man found it necessary to create better and more efficient methods to accomplish the kill (Fig. 1-1). Man soon discovered that the better-skilled hunters had the most success and were emulated by other hunters in their technique. Trial and error revealed that hunting could become more effective when an implement was introduced into the action. This brought about a greater demand for coordinating the hand and eye to successfully strike the intended object. These basic survival skills were passed down from father to son and perfected as new techniques were discovered. Tribesmen began to challenge each other to contests as each tried to gain the recognition and respect that was a by-product of physical superiority.

Today, as in the past, skilled movement commands respect. Whether it is the skill of a professional athlete or the motor prowess of an elementary school child, the successful accomplishment of motor activities is personally rewarding and highly regarded by all.

WHY PHYSICAL EDUCATION?

Children love to move and run for sheer enjoyment. Their endless reserves of energy during play constantly amaze adults. The desire for favorable recognition achieved through successful motor performance is basic to the innate urge to communicate, experiment, and express oneself through movement. Participating

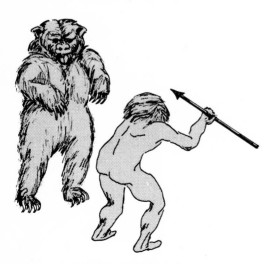

Fig. 1-1. Primitive hunter.

3

in a well-planned, progressive, sequential program of physical activities is one of the most satisfying experiences a child can have.

Humans are designed for a variety of motor responses utilizing both large and small muscles; consequently, they must become aware at an early age of the values and satisfactions that can be derived from physical activity. All learning is expressed in some form of motor response. Although the need for primitive survival skills has greatly diminished and modern medicine has done much to prolong our lives, the need for physical education is greater today than ever before. In this age of large urban centers, automated conveniences, and mass transportation, opportunities for the natural development of motor skills has been greatly limited. The contemporary child has little or no opportunity to climb a big oak tree, skip stones across a river, or challenge a friend to a balancing contest on a rail.

The New Physical Education must provide an environment of varied social and psychomotor experiences for all children. Traditional programs involving a few games and dances along with spontaneous play activity no longer meet the developmental needs of children in our changing sociological structure. Educators must view physical education as a major component of the school curriculum. Participation in physical activity should not be looked upon as a frill but as a necessary segment of the total learning experience. The psychomotor component often aids children in successfully accomplishing required school work.

Physical education is concerned with growth, development, and proper physical maintenance throughout life. This can be accomplished only through a program of physical activities designed systematically to meet the objectives of physical education for purposes of realizing socially acceptable individual outcomes. Physical education plays an increasingly important role in today's automated society and is a valid and important phase of education. Since its values are important to all students at all levels, it is a necessary part of general education and should be required of every child. The blending of mind and body into a well-rounded individual is best accomplished through specialized programs presented by professional teachers in facilities planned for movement.

A quality elementary physical education program is basic to the emergence of the complete child. Children who possess a realistic awareness of their movement potential and can organize these movement patterns into successful motor performances will experience an enjoyment made available through no other medium. On the playing field originate the significant forms of creative movement that are the foundations for healthful living and the maximum development of physical, social, and psychological human potential.

In recent times, because of research and concern for the underachiever, there has been a revitalization of bringing together the goals and objectives of the classroom with those of physical education. The physical education program that is conceived, planned, and carried out effectively can aid a child in reaching the optimal levels of the cognitive, affective, and physical domains. Children gain motoric sophistication by engaging in a great variety of movement experiences. They are increasingly identified as having perceptual-motor or neurological dysfunctions caused by being deprived of gross and/or fine motor opportunities.

Although there is conflicting evidence relating success in physical activities to success in the classroom, some literature indicates that motor development programs encompassing a variety of perceptual-motor activities can serve to help overcome some classroom readiness deficiencies. There is a strong indication based on subjective information from the

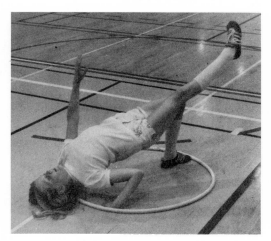

Fig. 1-3. Exploring movement capabilities within limited space.

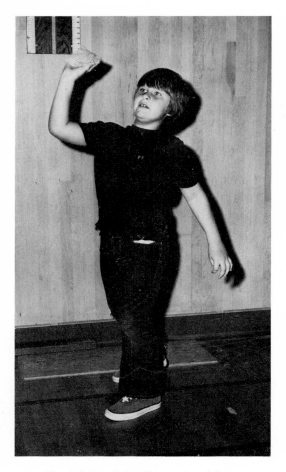

Fig. 1-2. Practicing the overhand throw.

Institute for Sensory Motor Development conducted at the California State University–Long Beach that confidence achieved on the playing field does much to alleviate fear and frustration in the classroom. A child having perceptual-motor deprivation during the early developmental growth stages will often be encumbered throughout life with emotional and motor as well as cognitive problems. Elementary physical education generally should allow for children to manage their total bodies and the objects with which they come in contact (Fig. 1-2). In addition to this, physical education should also provide opportunities for the development of healthy social relationships

and emotional stability so much needed for living a full and successful life in today's world.

Within individual capabilities and limitations, each child should have the opportunity for optimum growth physically, mentally, and emotionally. A sound physical education program offers activities geared to the child's maturational and readiness levels as well as providing a wide variety of positive attributes for the individual involved. Some of the attributes derived are motor pattern development, mechanical and postural efficiency, temporal and spacial awareness, body awareness, organic efficiency (which includes physical power, muscular and cardiorespiratory endurance, and flexibility), basic play skills, perceptual motor efficiency, coordination, and agility (Fig. 1-3). Since not all children learn at the same rate or in the same manner, programs involving these factors must be developed on an individual basis (Fig. 1-4). Periodic motor evaluations should be made to assess the maturational level at which each child is functioning. From this information, the teacher can properly select activities suited to the individual child's level of maturity. Other concomi-

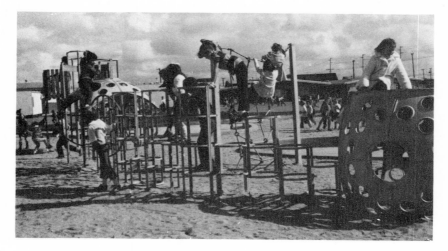

Fig. 1-4. Children exploring movement on playground equipment.

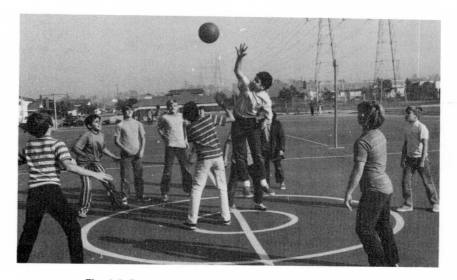

Fig. 1-5. Developing teamwork through group activities.

tants realized from a well-developed physical education program are self-confidence, safe use of apparatus and playground equipment, self-control, psychosocial development, learning to follow rules, and release from emotional stress.

Development of an aim

Prior to developing a well-organized physical education program, each teacher of physical education must thoroughly understand the proposed aims and desired objectives of physical education. The curriculum in physical education should be evaluated in line with the aims and objectives established for the realization of desired behavioral outcomes. Only in this manner can the activities presented in a balanced program meet the needs of all children at all levels.

An aim is usually defined as a generalized philosophical statement of purpose. It serves as a guide to the development

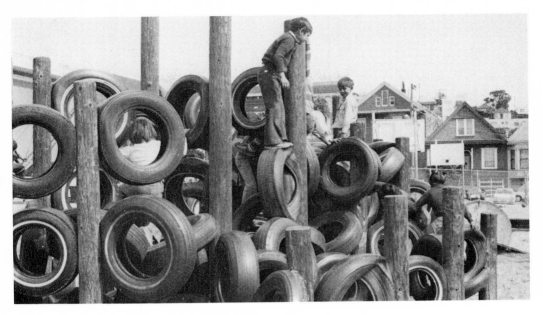

Fig. 1-6. Developing movement potential.

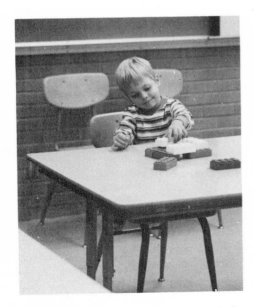

Fig. 1-7. Developing fine motor skill through finger control.

and selection of general and specific objectives that are more readily attainable. The aim of any discipline is first in the hierarchy of purposes that describe specific subject areas in the total school cur- riculum. In 1918 the Educational Policies Commission reiterated the purposes of education in American democracy. Of the seven objectives described in educational references,[6] physical education contributed directly to three: health, worthy use of leisure, and ethical character. More recently, the central purposes of education were reduced to four main objectives: self-realization, civic responsibility, economic efficiency, and human relations.[2] Although one might claim that physical education can contribute in varying degrees to all four, the areas of self-realization and human relations appear to be the most appropriate. The opportunities afforded children through the physical education program allow them to fully realize their personal capabilities as moving beings. It is important that elementary school children understand their strengths and weaknesses in order to develop a positive and accurate self-image. The physical education curriculum also provides for a variety of socially oriented activities. Children learn to interact in group situations in a

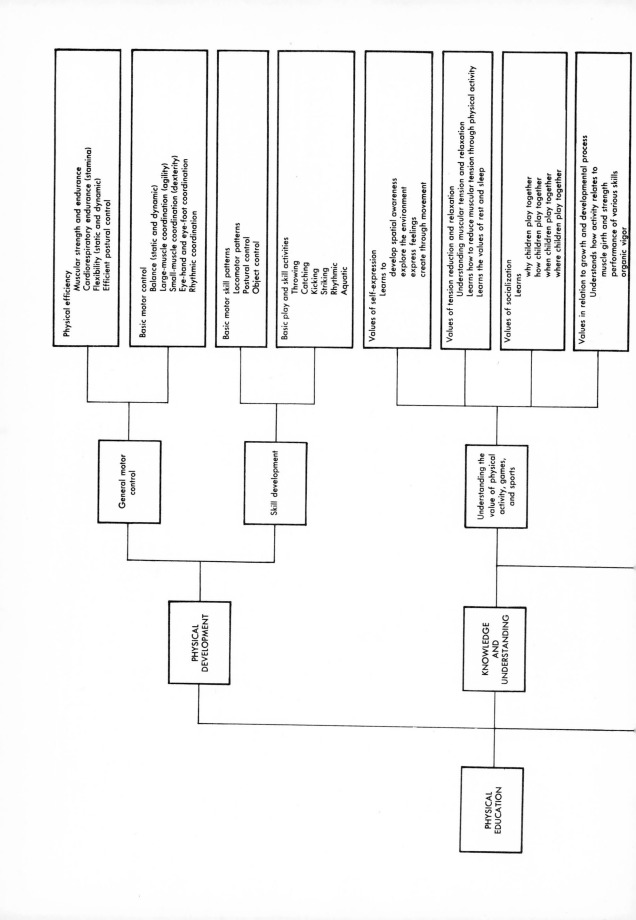

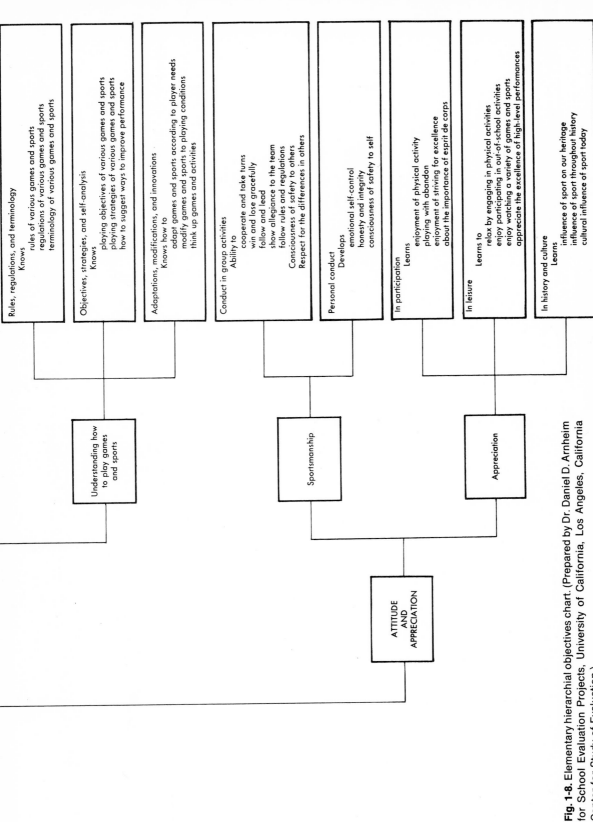

Fig. 1-8. Elementary hierarchial objectives chart. (Prepared by Dr. Daniel D. Arnheim for School Evaluation Projects, University of California, Los Angeles, California Center for Study of Evaluation.)

socially acceptable manner. Playing with others in activities in which added stress factors are introduced into the action prepares them for the dynamic world in which they live (Fig. 1-5).

Through the years many professional physical educators have expressed the aim of physical education in a variety of ways; the interpretations of their statements have always shown a great deal of similarity. Nixon and associates state that organized physical education should aim to make the maximum contribution to the optimum development of the individual's potentialities in all phases of life, by placing him in an environment as favorable as possible to the promotion of such muscular and related responses or activities that will best contribute to this purpose (Fig. 1-6).[5] LaPorte relates that the ultimate aim of physical education may well be to so develop and educate the individual through the medium of wholesome and interesting physical activities that he or she will realize his or her maximum capacities, both physically and mentally, and will learn to use those powers intelligently and cooperatively as a good citizen even under violent emotional stress.[4] Williams determined that physical education should aim to provide skilled leadership and adequate facilities that will afford an opportunity for the individual or group to act in situations that are physically wholesome, mentally stimulating and satisfying, and socially sound.[7] Hetherington states that physical education is that phase of education that is concerned, first, with the organization and leadership of children in big-muscle activities, to gain the development and adjustment inherent in the activities according to social standards, and second, with the control of health and growth conditions naturally associated with the leadership of the activities, so that the educational process may go on with or without handicaps (Fig. 1-7).[3] Bookwalter states that an aim of physical education is the optimum development, integration,

and adjustment physically, mentally, and socially of the individual through guided instruction and participation in selected total-body sports and in rhythmic and gymnastic activities conducted according to social and hygienic standards.[1]

We propose that the aim of physical education is to *facilitate the optimum growth and development of each individual through sequential, guided instruction and participation in sports and games, rhythms, and individual activities presented in a balanced manner leading toward the fulfillment of those physical, emotional, and social needs acceptable in today's society.*

The objectives of physical education

An objective might well be defined as a statement of purpose that is more immediate and specific in nature and that is in harmony with the established aim and more likely to be attained. We have described general objectives as including three major areas of physical education: physical development, knowledge and understanding, and attitude and appreciation. Fig. 1-8 is a model for a balanced approach to physical education. Each general objective has been divided into two subcategories that are listed as intermediate objectives of physical education.

Physical development. The general objective of physical development has been divided into the intermediate objectives of general motor control and skill development.

General motor control. The objective of general motor control has been further categorized into two specific objectives, one of which is *physical efficiency.* In order to fulfill the program requirements of this objective, activities must be offered that develop muscular strength and endurance, cardiorespiratory endurance, joint flexibility, and efficient postural control (Fig. 1-9). Each child should have the opportunity to become physically effi-

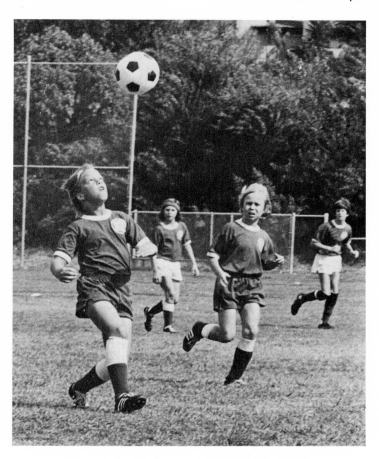

Fig. 1-9. Developing cardiorespiratory endurance.

cient so as not to deter the learning process involved in more refined activities.

The second objective is that of *basic motor control.* Children need to develop balance, large-muscle coordination, small-muscle coordination, eye-hand coordination, eye-foot coordination, and rhythmical coordination (Fig. 1-10). The development of these basic motor controls enables the child to successfully participate in sports and game activities. The child who has learned and developed basic motor control has the foundation necessary to learn motor skill patterns necessary for the successful accomplishment and enjoyment of more sophisticated game activities.

Skill development. The intermediate objective of skill development has been divided into the specific objectives of basic motor skill patterns and basic play skills. *Basic motor skill patterns* that should be developed are the various modes of locomotion such as walking, jumping, hopping, skipping, crawling, climbing, rolling, and sliding. The child should also learn adequate postural control for proper stature in a variety of positions.

Children not only must be able to control their own personal movements, but also should be able to develop this control to include objects in activities of throwing, catching, kicking, striking, pulling, pushing, stopping, and carrying (Fig. 1-11).

The accomplishment of basic motor skill patterns will enable the child then to

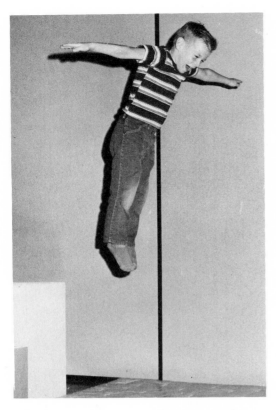

Fig. 1-10. Jumping with confidence in a balanced position.

successfully participate in *basic play skills* involving throwing, catching, kicking, striking, rhythmic, and aquatic activities.

Knowledge and understanding. Understanding the value of physical activity, games, and sports and understanding how to play games and sports are two more intermediate objectives of physical education.

Understanding the value of physical activity, games, and sports. Values of physical activity, games, and sports can be divided into the values of (1) self-expression, (2) tension reduction and relaxation, (3) socialization, and (4) physical activity in growth and development of the individual. In the area of *values of self-expression,* children should learn to develop spacial awareness in physical activity. Children should have the opportunity to explore the environment and learn to express their feelings through creative movement. In developing *values of tension reduction and relaxation,* children should become aware of how to reduce muscular tension through physical activity and should be made aware of the values of rest and sleep. Children should recognize why children play together,

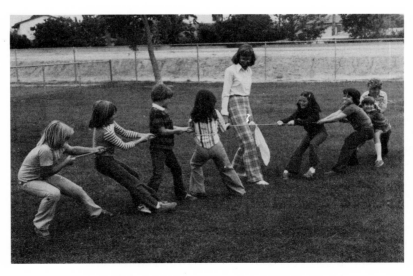

Fig. 1-11. Controlling the body through a pulling activity.

how they play together, when they play together, and where they play together. In developing an understanding of these *values of socialization,* children can better accept the variety of programs offered in the elementary school in relation to time and place of participation in each. Every child must understand the *values of physical activity* in relation to the growth and developmental process and must understand how activity relates to muscle girth and strength, to performance of various skills, and to organic vigor. As these values are presented to the children, activities involving games and sports should take on a new meaning through better understanding of the reasons for play.

Understanding how to play games and sports. Understanding how to play games and sports is divided into the following specific objectives: (1) rules, regulations, and terminology, (2) objectives, strategies, and self-analysis, and (3) adaptations, modifications, and innovations. Children should have a thorough understanding of the *rules* of the various games and sports presented. Specific *regulations* in game activities and the *terminology* used in the various games and sports will aid in a more thorough understanding and appreciation of the activities presented. Each child should be made aware of the playing *objectives* of the activity presented, and should acquire the playing *strategies* needed to experience a successful performance. This process aids in the development of the cognitive aspect of the individual. Children should also be taught how to objectively analyze their performances and suggest ways to improve the level of their participation. To complete the understanding of how to play games and sports, children should be taught how to adapt games and sports according to player needs and should be taught that certain games can be modified in relation to playing conditions and available facilities. Children should also be able to develop their creative ability

by designing new games and activities by drawing on their previous experiences. They should be encouraged to investigate their individual motor capabilities and to seek to create new movement activities.

Attitude and appreciation. Children learn to enjoy physical activity through successful performance in a variety of game situations (Fig. 1-12). The child also learns to play with complete, "carefree" abandon, realizing the full value of physical activity. Children enjoy striving for excellence in physical activities that are within their own capabilities. Greater satisfaction is achieved when the individual performs well in any assigned task. The importance of esprit de corps and its relationship to group success should be stressed. Children can learn to relax by engaging in physical activity as well as learning to enjoy participation in a variety of physical activities. Continued participation in these activities outside of school is an important outcome of the physical education program. The child may also acquire an enjoyment of games and sports as a spectator and learn to appreciate the excellence that is displayed in high-level athletic performance. Children should be made aware of the role of sport throughout history and should understand the important influence that sport has had on our American heritage. They can also develop a knowledge and appreciation of contemporary sport as it influences culture and provides an international language respected and appreciated by all nations.

Sportsmanship. Each child should develop the ability (1) to cooperate and take turns, and (2) to win and lose gracefully, and (3) to follow and lead through a planned program of sportsmanship. Developing allegiance to a team, a knowledge of how to follow rules and regulations, consciousness of safety to others, and respect for the differences in others enhance the development and maturity of the individual. Children can also de-

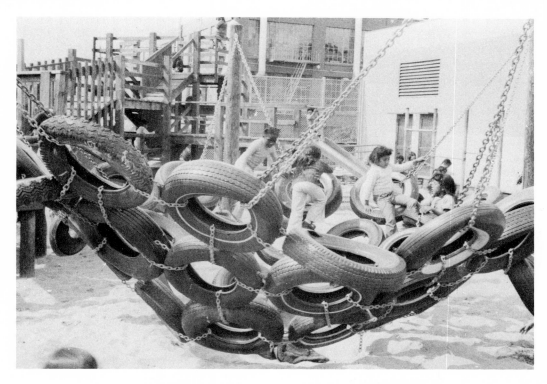

Fig. 1-12. Creative equipment provides variety in movement activities.

velop emotional self-control during periods of physical and mental stress and can develop a sense of honesty and integrity while participating in games as well as being conscious of safety for self and others. However, it must be recognized by teachers that sportsmanship is not inherent in physical education activities but must be planned for and overtly applied by the participant.

RATIONALE FOR THE BALANCED APPROACH TO PHYSICAL EDUCATION

In order to provide interesting, exciting, and meaningful experiences for each child in line with the principles described, we suggest a balanced approach to teaching physical education. *The major purpose of this text is to blend the best* of all physical education philosophies and/or approaches, including the traditional games and sports, perceptual-motor, movement education, and physical fitness concepts of physical education into a well-designed pattern of instruction of developmental movement. Each approach singularly has much to offer toward the achievement of the major objectives of physical education. However, a well-planned combination of all basic methods enhances the ultimate development of the maturing child. The following information is presented to acquaint the teacher with some of the approaches of teaching physical education leading toward the fullfillment of the objectives brought forth in the curriculum model displayed in Fig. 1-8. A more detailed description of each method is given in later chapters. Teachers of elementary school children are afforded an opportunity to develop a personal philosophy of physical education and to construct meaningful programs designed to meet specific indi-

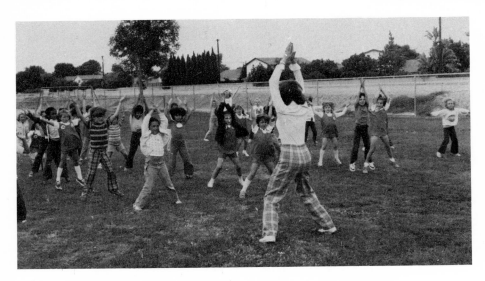

Fig. 1-13. Traditional warm-up formation prior to class activities.

vidual and group needs, using the suggested methods as a guide.

The games and sports approach

The traditional approach in physical education aims to achieve the objectives of physical education through the medium of stunts, dance, games, and sports (Fig. 1-13). The successful accomplishment of these activities contributes to the development of physical efficiency as well as to the development of positive attitudes, appreciation, knowledge, and understanding. Activities should be planned on a progressive developmental basis for each maturational level. At the completion of the elementary school physical education experience, the child should have participated in a variety of lead-up games and sports that emphasize the fulfillment of the objectives proposed. Most traditional activities are presented through a group design rather than on an individual basis, with personal help being given to the children having the greatest difficulty in learning each skill. It is very important in using this approach that the teacher provide adequate equipment and individually modify activities

so that all children have opportunities for full participation in each activity. Games providing activity for a few children at a time should be modified in such a manner that a majority of children have opportunities for physical participation.

Children gain leadership experience by being squad leaders or team captains. In the games and sports approach, the teacher plays a dominant role, becoming involved in the presentation and demonstration of the skill or game to be learned. This phase of the physical education program is teacher directed and planned to meet the needs of the majority of the children in the class.

Movement education

The movement education approach emphasizes individualized programs of motor development (Fig. 1-14). Through this method children become acutely aware of their physical abilities and learn to use them effectively through a problem-solving technique. One of the salient points of this approach is that there are many correct ways to solve movement problems that are proposed by the teacher. Although some movements and

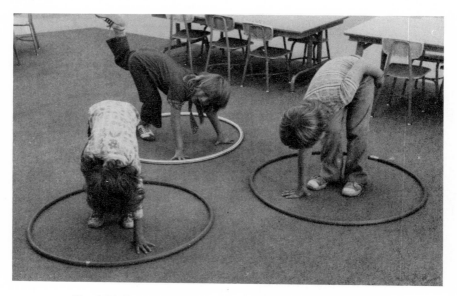

Fig. 1-14. Solving problems through movement experiences.

postures may be more efficient or effective in the solution of the problem, children seldom fail in their attempt.

The technique of discovering how they move enables children to understand their physical capabilities and develop sequential movement patterns from the knowledge acquired. The objectives of physical education are accomplished through a much less structured approach, and failure is kept to a minimum as each child finds a personal solution to the problem at hand. The movement education approach allows children to increase their own motor ability at their own rate. The established goals for the participants are realistic and attainable, since all goals are developed on an individual basis. The informal atmosphere allows for effective social development, so that often one child communicates the solution to the problem to another child. The teacher plays a less dominant role in the movement education approach and acts more as a guide than as a director. Through this method, the teacher finds time for individual instruction, and the child finds time to create new movement patterns.

Although this approach sometimes is viewed falsely as a laissez-faire method, successful programs require much teacher preparation and a thorough knowledge of the participants' needs and abilities.

Physical fitness

The physical fitness approach should include a basic understanding of exercise physiology for all levels. This method of teaching physical education strives to develop muscular, skeletal, and cardiovascular-respiratory systems of the body. Activities are of a vigorous nature and often include intensive competition between teams or groups of children. The program is directive in nature, and children have fewer planned opportunities for social development.

The program should be planned in such a manner that the children experience the conditioning effect of activities designed to develop the heart, lungs, and muscles (Fig. 1-15). Children should discover that when they run, their hearts beat faster. The teacher should take advantage of this phenomenon and take

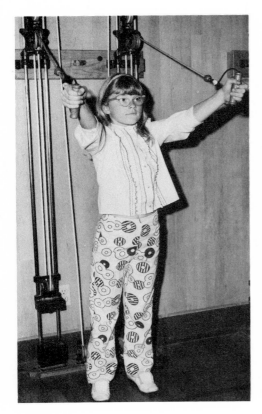

Fig. 1-15. Equipment aids the development of muscular strength.

time to explain the values of physical conditioning in relation to total health. (See Chapter 10.)

Children should become aware of the values of living a physically active life as early as possible and should begin to plan their own programs of physical conditioning. In today's society, modern conveniences have eliminated much of the physical work involved in our daily activity; therefore, it becomes increasingly important to emphasize this aspect of physical education in a well-balanced program.

The perceptual-motor approach

The perceptual-motor approach is a task-oriented method of teaching physical education (Fig. 1-16). Mastery of perceptual-motor tasks prepares children for future learning and understanding of the world in which they live. Perceptual-motor tasks should include both gross and fine motor skills. Locomotor patterns, body awareness and body image, balance tasks, tension recognition, and the ability to relax all play a major role in this method of teaching physical education.

The program is teacher directed, with each child developing motor skills based on individual requirements. The program has a success-oriented approach, each activity beginning at a level at which the child can accomplish the skill. Although this phase of the program has greater emphasis at the lower levels or with children having movement difficulties, it should be a planned part of the total physical education program experience. If movement is combined with sense modalities, a positive body awareness and a favorable self-image are developed. (See Chapter 11.)

Children with learning difficulties often are poorly coordinated and have definite perceptual problems. Although there is a paucity of research indicating that improvement in motor development relates to improvement in classroom skills, there are strong indications that success in motor development activities and the achievement of a favorable body image of oneself have some carry-over to success in the classroom.

No longer can one use only the traditional approaches to material presentation and expect the students to establish acceptable attitudes toward living a physically active life. The day is long past when a teacher can present a stereotyped program from a curriculum guide and expect all students to absorb all material presented at the same rate of learning, much less to develop a sound attitude toward physical education, health, and recreation. The physical education curriculum should be a blend of teaching approaches to satisfy the needs and reach the developmental level of each child.

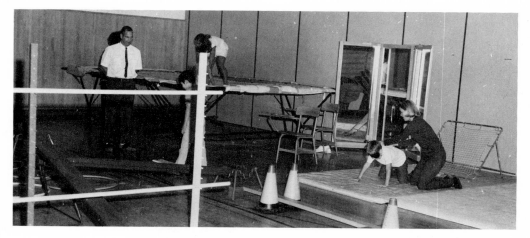

Fig. 1-16. Perceptual-motor activities.

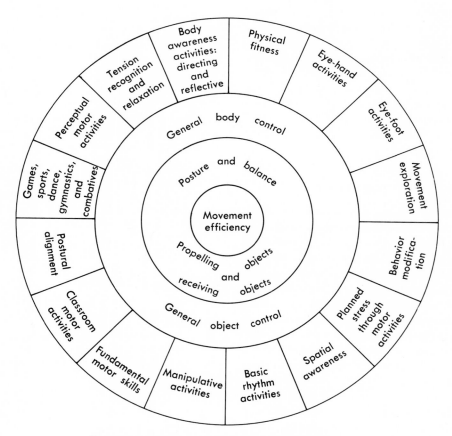

Fig. 1-17. Movement efficiency developmental model.

Each teacher must attempt to find the best way to present program materials in exciting and meaningful ways. There is no reason why all students cannot achieve personal satisfaction in physical education as long as the teacher develops the program within each child's individual potential. This can be accomplished only if the teacher takes time to work individually with each student and to develop programs in line with individual needs presented at different rates of learning.

The teacher blends the science of learning with the art of teaching. And if this is done, not only should learning be enjoyable to the student, but also there should be tremendous satisfaction for the teacher. The smile on a child's face when a skill is accomplished is rewarding to the teacher who knows that personal pride and positive self-control are being developed. There is no better arena than that of physical education to afford children opportunities to develop to their fullest potential. The total developmental model (Fig. 1-17) graphically displays how each physical education approach and developmental task contributes to the achievement of movement efficiency in a balanced manner.

HOW TO USE THE TEXT

The text is designed to follow the child motorically from conception through age 12 years. For effective use of the material it is necessary for the reader to understand our philosophy, which encompasses a balanced approach to elementary physical education—a philosophy that encourages teachers to use a variety of teaching approaches and methods selected on the basis of the age group involved and the lesson being taught. In addition, the reader should become familiar with the differences in learning approaches and understand curriculum development as presented in Part One. From this base,

one is challenged to learn as much as possible about child developmental stages as described in Part Two. Part Three explains in detail specific information required for special program emphasis. When using the activities detailed in Part Four, the reader should refer back to the theory chapters for specific learning approaches, teaching techniques, and class organization.

CLASS ACTIVITIES

1. Develop a justification for physical education that encompasses your personal philosophy.
2. Discuss the need for physical efficiency in our modern society.
3. Develop a short paragraph that describes the aim of elementary physical education.
4. Discuss the strengths of each of the four approaches to teaching physical education as described in this text.

REFERENCES

1. Bookwalter, K. W., and Vanderzswaag, H. J.: Foundations and principles of physical education, Philadelphia, 1969, W. B. Saunders Co.
2. Educational Policies Commission: The central purpose of education, Washington, D.C., 1961, National Education Association Publishing.
3. Hetherington, C. W.: The school program in physical education, New York, 1922, World Book Co.
4. LaPorte, W. R.: The physical education curriculum, ed. 6, Los Angeles, 1955, University of Southern California, College Book Store.
5. Nixon, J. E., Flanagan, L., and Frederickson, F. S.: An introduction to physical education, ed. 6, Philadelphia, 1964, W. B. Saunders Co.
6. United States Bureau of Education Bulletin no. 35, Washington, D.C., 1918, United States Government Printing Office, pp. 5-10.
7. Williams, J. F.: The principles of physical education, Philadelphia, 1964, W. B. Saunders Co.

RECOMMENDED READINGS

Anderson, M., Elliot, M. E., and LaBerge, J.: Play with a purpose, New York, 1972, Harper & Row, Publishers, Inc.
Fait, F. H.: Experiences in movement, Philadelphia, 1976, W. B. Saunders Co.
Kirchner, G.: Physical education for elementary school children. Dubuque, Iowa, 1970, William C. Brown Company, Publishers.
Sweeney, R. T., editor: Selected readings in movement education, Reading, Mass., 1970, Addison-Wesley Publishing Co., Inc.

2

The dynamic teacher

Do you want to be remembered as "my favorite third grade teacher?" Are you able to be patient while working among children who seem to possess an endless supply of energy? Do you think creatively as you seek innovative approaches to make the learning experience enjoyable and meaningful to each child in the class?

If your answer to these questions is yes then your personality is suited to the demands of being a physical education teacher who will promote a strong and healthy self-image in elementary school children. Through creative and enthusiastic planning of a movement skills program, you, the teacher, will serve as the catalyst necessary to achieve the explosion of fun resulting from participation in motor skills and the social development that is savored by each child seeking maximum movement potential. Yes, as a leader and guide, you make the difference between the success or failure of the children with whom you work.

Learning occurs more effectively and efficiently when proper guidance and direction are provided. A well-prepared and well-qualified teacher has a great influence on the amount of learning that will take place. The interest of the teacher in the students combined with knowledge of the field is the foundation for successful experiences in physical education activities. Children are quick to respond to a teacher who sets the ex-

ample by displaying interest and enthusiasm in the subject matter. One must often assume and enjoy playing the role of a child in order to instill the proper mood for youthful participation. Teaching is recognized as both an art and a science and as such allows for the development of meaningful learning experiences. The teacher as a leader guides the child along the correct learning paths, the result being desirable behavioral changes. To provide children with the kinds of changes in behavior that will enhance their positions in society is the role the physical education teacher must play.

Learning to enjoy wholesome physical activity is an identifiable objective of our contemporary society. The teacher who strives for excellence will accomplish this objective through hard work and a desire to be remembered as a good teacher who was successful in his or her instructional endeavors.

PROFESSIONAL PREPARATION

Elementary school physical education teachers should have a thorough understanding of human movement, child growth and development, and contemporary learning theories and techniques combined with a desire to work with children. An adequate program of professional preparation for elementary physical education teachers should include the following aspects:

1. Instruction and practice in the fundamental game skills commonly taught in the elementary schools
2. Instruction and practice in the fundamental rhythm skills commonly taught in the elementary schools
3. Analysis and practice in fundamental skills, gymnastics, combatives, track and field, and perceptual-motor activities for elementary school children
4. Knowledge of the application of principles of anatomy and physiology to the motor performance of children
5. Proficiency in the techniques of movement education as applied to the learning of dance, stunts, and game activities
6. Knowledge of contemporary methods and techniques applied to the presentation of traditional physical education activities in the elementary school
7. Knowledge of the principles of motor learning as applied to elementary age children
8. Proficiency in the perceptual-motor approach to developing motoric sophistication in children
9. Knowledge of the principles, aims, and objectives of elementary school physical education as related to curriculum development

The physical education specialist and the supervisor of physical education should complete additional course work in preparation for effective leadership in public school physical education programs. Since the teacher of physical education in a self-contained classroom will likely have had no more than one course in physical education in preparation for teaching in this area, much can be accomplished through in-service training programs administered by a specialist or supervisor of physical education. When classroom teachers are responsible for teaching physical education, it is imperative that a plan be developed in which

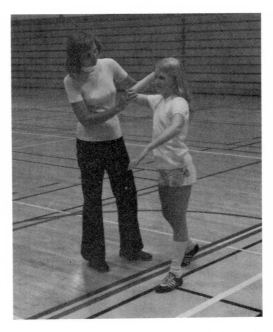

Fig. 2-1. Teacher reviewing correct throwing technique.

regular leadership and guidance are given by qualified resource people who are experienced in elementary school physical education (Fig. 2-1).

PHYSICAL EDUCATION SPECIALIST

The physical education specialist should be a staff member involved in the total elementary school program. It is increasingly important for this individual to be aware of the classroom activities of each group of children involved, since coordination between classroom and playground must take place if integration is to be accomplished. The specialist should work closely with the classroom teacher in developing physical education activities. Although the classroom teacher has a greater opportunity to know the children in a variety of situations, it is the responsibility of the physical education specialist to obtain as much knowledge as possible about the children with whom he or she works. The kinds of behavior

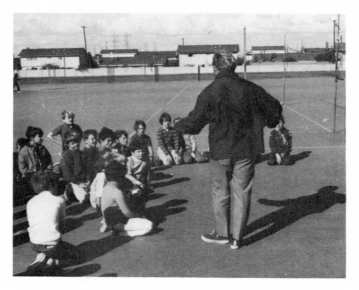

Fig. 2-2. Physical education specialist introducing a lesson.

exhibited by certain children in the class-room should lead to the development of a physical activity program that will enhance the individual needs of those involved. Since the specialist should have more information and ability regarding physical activity programs and their value for the children in the elementary program, it should be his or her responsibility to act as the voice of the school in matters pertaining to physical education. There should be no one better prepared to interpret what is happening in the physical education class to parents and other interested community participants than the specialist in physical education.

The specialist should have a greater wealth of material and have a greater knowledge of the variety of games and approaches to teaching physical activities than the classroom teacher. This knowledge should aid in the development of programs that are best suited for the various age groups involved. Working with the classroom teacher and sharing ideas regarding the total educational experience are major responsibilities of the physical education specialist (Fig. 2-2).

PHYSICAL EDUCATION SUPERVISOR

Although the supervisor of physical education seldom gets directly involved with the teaching of children, it is his or her responsibility to work with the teacher in the self-contained classroom or the physical education specialist to help design successful curricular plans and to act as a resource person in suggesting new and innovative ideas in material presentation. A supervisor of physical education must continue to improve his or her knowledge of physical education by attending state and national conferences, and must carry the material back to his or her colleagues. A supervisor of physical education should continually draw on personal experiences and share knowledge and training with the teachers with whom he or she works. A good supervisor will instill enthusiasm into the teachers and encourage continued development of successful physical education programs. If program and teacher supervision is effective the program will improve and the children will reap the benefits.

CLASSROOM TEACHER AND PHYSICAL EDUCATION

In a self-contained classroom the teacher has the advantage of being responsible for all subject areas taught. It is much easier for the teacher to coordinate learning in the other aspects of the educational program with physical education when he or she is involved in the total program. It is quite easy for the classroom teacher to determine whether it would be beneficial to teach an American folk dance when the children are studying early American history or more advantageous to present dance as a self-contained unit. Coordinating physical education activities with English, mathematics, and social studies can readily be accomplished when one is responsible for designing the total curriculum of the children involved. However, proper guiding of the learning experiences in the most successful manner demands preparation and understanding of physical education activities. It is also easier to allow for continuity of experiences and to provide for proper emphasis in physical education activities in relation to the total school program.

Teacher traits

Although we prefer the use of specialists in physical education, most programs are the responsibility of the classroom teacher. The following traits and factors are important for successful teaching of physical education.

Attitudes. Children are quick to observe the attitude that a teacher has toward presenting a particular subject to them. It is imperative that the teacher of physical education maintain the attitude that physical education is an important phase of the total educational process. The teacher of elementary physical education finds little difficulty in motivating children in movement activities; however, a lack of teacher interest and the inability to provide exciting and in-

teresting activities through a behavioral approach can turn the physical education period into one of boredom and unhappy experiences. Teachers will have difficulty in helping children develop favorable attitudes toward physical education if they are not convinced that the activity has worth in the educational scheme. If all children are able to participate in activities that are fun and are suited to their individual needs and if they understand the value of the activity, favorable attitudes toward physical education should develop.

Humor. The ability to laugh at one's own successes and inadequacies is a trait that each teacher of physical education should possess. At the end of a tiring day when patience has been tried to the breaking point, the teacher with a sense of humor can salvage a potentially damaging situation and turn it into one that is fun for all. In order to make teaching a rewarding and satisfying experience for both the teacher and the student, it is necessary to maintain a good sense of humor. The more trying the experience, the more important it is to laugh. Having fun is one of the greatest motivating factors a teacher can utilize in presenting a successful lesson in physical education.

Enthusiasm. Each teacher should possess a genuine enthusiasm toward physical education activities. The children should observe a behavior that presents physical education as the greatest subject in the school curriculum. A lack of enthusiasm can lead to other faults in developing a successful program, such as failing to prepare adequately for the lesson to be taught and looking at physical education as a "free play" period rather than giving adequate preparation to a subject area that is as important as any other in the curriculum. Enthusiasm is contagious. If the teacher is excited about the day's lesson, the children will experience a beneficial, fun-filled activity period (Fig. 2-3).

Personality. An enthusiastic personal-

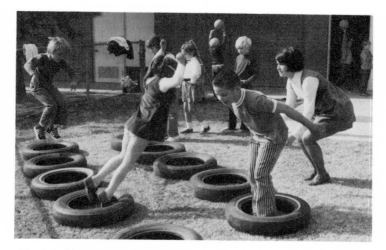

Fig. 2-3. Classroom teacher encourages proper jumping techniques.

ity is one of the prime factors necessary for effective teaching. The impression that a teacher makes on students is a strong motivating factor toward successes or failures in the learning environment. The individual who is always ready with a kindly smile, is friendly to all, and is empathetic toward the problems of developing children has little difficulty in presenting an effective lesson. Students like a teacher who is consistent, fair, cooperative, and dependable in all educational pursuits.

One of the greatest assets a teacher can have is confidence in his or her ability to teach physical education. Confidence in a subject area builds a personality that thrives on success. Making excuses for one's inadequacies is a sign of weakness and results in loss of respect from the students, making teaching difficult.

Appropriate dress, habits of neatness and cleanliness, and a pleasing voice are attractive personality traits.

Each teacher should undertake a program of self-evaluation to determine where improvements can be made in his or her personality. This personality evaluation should be an ongoing process of eliminating the weak points and emphasizing as many of the favorable attributes as possible.

Above all, the teacher should attempt to be himself or herself. Although there is much to be gained by observing a successful teaching performance by another, it must be remembered that there are many excellent ways of presenting an effective lesson. Those who take advantage of their own personalities will be happier and much more successful than those who emulate others.

The following personality traits are suggestive of favorable teaching behaviors. The children are more receptive to physical education when the teacher:

1. Is enthusiastic in lesson presentations
2. Gives individual instruction in teaching skills
3. Is concerned with student enjoyment in class
4. Has a happy, friendly personality that is reflected during instructions
5. Encourages students to achieve their best within their own capabilities
6. Utilizes innovations, ingenuity, and variety in class presentations
7. Speaks in a voice that is pleasing to the ear and easily understood
8. Participates in class activities
9. Is well skilled and demonstrates in class

10. Exhibits patience and understanding with students facing difficulty in learning a skill
11. Praises student achievement regardless of level or degree
12. Develops a class atmosphere in which students are not afraid to make mistakes
13. Is willing to listen and help students with problems
14. Provides for total social contact
15. Is trim and physically fit

Health. Physical education is a demanding subject to teach. A teacher who lacks strength and stamina will often tend to neglect the physical education period. The teacher who does not maintain an adequate fitness level often uses the physical education period as a chance to rest and recuperate rather than to develop a good sequential program of physical activity for the children. Teaching excellence in physical education requires an enthusiastic approach that involves a certain amount of physical effort. The teacher must arrive at school at a fitness level that is conducive to the development of and participation in active physical education games and sports. The children in the class incur the greatest loss when a low health status is maintained by the teacher.

Creativity. Creating new approaches to physical education is one of the most exciting and interesting activities for the teacher. To develop creativity the teacher of physical education must have a strong background in the skills and activities to be taught. The greater the knowledge of the subject matter the more opportunities for creativity will be at hand. In some instances teachers have avoided creative approaches to instruction for fear of receiving criticism from more conservative peers or rigid community groups. However, the teacher too often fails to engage in creative activities because of a lack of knowledge of the subject matter at hand. Creating new activities or new ways of playing games and encouraging the children to do the same can be an exciting phase of physical education.

Creativity cannot be left to chance; it must be planned for and situations must be presented in which children have the opportunity to express themselves in a new and challenging manner. The teacher who listens with an open mind and encourages children to try out their ideas shows a respect for their attempts to do something new and often is able to learn something. New ideas or solutions to problems should not be thrown out until the children have had an opportunity to try them. Children can learn by evaluating their own solutions and often are given too little credit for knowing the difference between success and failure in problem-solving activities. Creativity should be encouraged whenever possible, since it is a way of growth that cannot be duplicated through any other aspect of the school program. Planning situations that encourage creativity should be a part of each program of physical education.

Participation. A question often asked is whether or not a teacher should participate in the physical education activities of the day. Children enjoy having an opportunity to participate in group activities in which the teacher is involved. If a teacher is well skilled, there is an added incentive, since he or she gains a definite personal respect by being able to successfully execute the skill. Through participation in activities with the children, the teacher becomes a co-worker rather than a director. In most cases, children are quite pleased when this occurs and often put the teacher to the test.

If teachers are to participate in the activities, they should be properly dressed for games and sports so as not to be limited to an observational role. A teacher who participates with the children on a regular basis finds that the class response is excellent and that the activity is most enjoyable for teacher and children alike (Fig. 2-4).

Striving for excellence. Teachers of

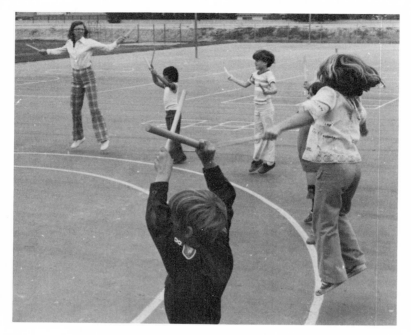

Fig. 2-4. Classroom teacher displays enthusiasm by participating with the class.

physical education should continually strive to improve the teaching-learning situation in their classes. Sharing problems in class organization and successes in the presentation of materials can be a tremendous aid in developing teaching excellence. Teachers should begin with themselves and determine what their greatest needs are in improving the instructional program of physical education. After determining these needs, they should share them with other individuals on the staff or with the supervisor of physical education and should develop a plan to solve the particular problems involved. The important aspect of this procedure is, first, to identify the problem areas and then to seek ways of solving them. Too often a teacher shows little improvement in the instructional program because of a lack of knowledge of how to present the material in an interesting and exciting manner. Individual and small group meetings should be established from time to time to discuss new tech-

niques in material presentation. Teachers should strive to reach their fullest potential in developing excellence in teaching. This can be accomplished only if they recognize the fact that the teaching-learning situation can be improved and that dedication to excellence is necessary for improvement to take place. Successful teaching in physical education is best developed when the teacher:

1. Makes participation in physical education activities an enjoyable experience
2. Is thoroughly convinced of the values of physical education activities in the school program
3. Maintains a good sense of humor and is flexible in the approach to teaching physical education
4. Encourages the children to develop the ability to participate in physical education activities on their own
5. Requires the children to maintain high standards of performance in physical education activities

6. Encourages the children to evaluate the successes or failures of the activities in which they participate
7. Allows the children the opportunity to help in the development of the physical education program
8. Encourages good performances in physical activities by praising the children in successful performances
9. Evaluates the physical education experience and uses the information gained to develop future programs

Class organization. Each teacher of physical education should strive to enhance the instructional program by utilizing sound organizational techniques. Provisions should be made to ensure that children have the fullest opportunities for participation in class activities. The following suggestions are offered as guides to successful class organization:

1. A daily program of physical activities is recommended to best serve the needs of the children in elementary schools.
2. The length of the class period should vary according to the purpose of the lesson and the needs of the children involved.
3. Children should be grouped according to size, ability, and activity interests.
4. Activities should be arranged to provide for individual instruction in learning skills.
5. Adequate equipment should be provided to allow for full participation by all class members.
6. The lesson should provide for the development of leadership experiences.
7. The program offered should be in line with the needs and interests of the children participating in the activity.

If adequate time is given to organizing a class for effective teaching, there will be a twofold return of enjoyment and understanding of physical education. The teacher who plans well will realize the full potential of class participation and successful performance in physical education skills.

Guidance. Physical education teachers should be concerned with the total development of an individual and should not limit their role to one of supplying vocational information. When physical education specialists are responsible for program activities, they enjoy distinct guidance advantages that the teachers of other disciplines usually do not experience. The physical education teacher often has contact with the same children for consecutive years. This continued experience along with the informality of the student-teacher relationship allows for a guidance function not available in any other school subject. Since physical education deals with children in movement activities, individual strengths and weaknesses appear more readily than elsewhere in the school. The play area is an excellent laboratory for studying the individual. A child's personality is usually more observable in action situations than in the confines of the traditional classroom. Although the need for personal guidance increases with the age of the child, there is evidence that problems in health and personal social adjustment formerly associated with older children are now prevalent at the elementary level.

Safety. The desire for new experiences, excitement, and adventure and a need for group recognition are identifiable needs of elementary school children. These needs are satisfied by certain vigorous activities involving close contact with others and the introduction of specialized equipment that results in certain risks to the participants. The element of danger in activity is often the motivating factor needed for full participation and enjoyment by certain individuals. Too often the attempted solution to the risk factor is deletion of the activity from the curriculum. This should not be the case. With proper class organization and a definite

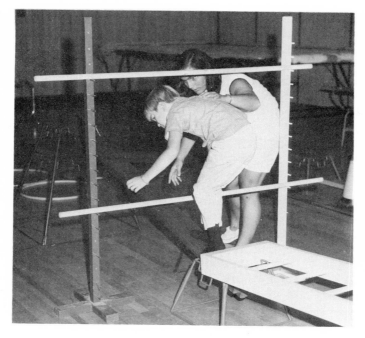

Fig. 2-5. Spotting children provides a safe skill development environment.

safety plan, activities such as touch football, wrestling, tumbling, and swimming can be safe and enjoyable for all. When planning for a safe play environment, the school should apply the following principles:

1. Employ qualified personnel to teach physical education.
2. Provide for adequate protective equipment when needed.
3. Insist on the strict enforcement of rules during play.
4. Provide suitable play areas properly maintained.
5. Ensure that the participants are properly conditioned so that undue fatigue does not occur.
6. Establish a routine safety check of all equipment utilized.
7. Anticipate potential safety hazards and establish local rules when dangerous situations may arise.

If the teacher plans proper safety measures and develops an accident prevention and safety procedure unit, most accidents will be avoided and the child can develop without fear of injury (Fig. 2-5).

PROFESSIONAL SKILLS
Evaluation

Evaluation is a continuous and important part of any physical education program. If program progress toward meeting immediate and long-term goals in physical education is to be verified, it is necessary for the teacher first to determine the level and needs of the children participating in the program. In order to guide the children in the proper direction, the teacher should measure the physical performance level of each child in the class (Fig. 2-6).

Evaluation can be accomplished through a variety of techniques. Teacher observation, developmental scales, knowledge tests, motor ability tests, and physical fitness measurements are used not only to aid in program development and

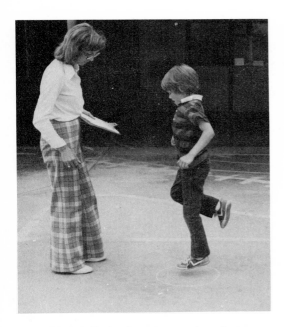

Fig. 2-6. Evaluating movement control.

improvement but also to interpret the program to children, parents, and the community.

Evaluation should be used as a tool to improve the instructional program and to motivate children to achieve individual goals. Because humans seek goals by nature, they learn tasks best in an environment where objectives for learning are clearly presented. Care should be taken to avoid setting group standards too high, which may curtail individual progress. Emphasis should be placed on the advancement of each child toward individual aims. Establishing reasonable behavioral objectives on the basis of maturation and readiness levels provides the teacher with an ongoing method of program evaluation and allows the children to understand their goals.

A sound evaluation program provides for a system of accountability to determine the degree to which program objectives are met. A behavioral objective is a specific course of action that is measurable, observable, and within the reach of the individual child.

Many factors are inherent in the evaluation process. Extreme care must be taken by the teacher when selecting a measurement device. The following questions should be considered by the teacher: Do I understand how to administer the test? To what extent will the test measure motor competencies or reveal deficiencies in movement? Does the test have norms? Is the test reliable? Does the evaluation procedure take into consideration the age and sex of the child?[6]

Determining movement competencies. Screening the child's ability to move efficiently has many purposes, some of which are to detect the child's most obvious movement problems, to stimulate the child to seek self-awareness through self-testing, to motivate the child to want to improve, and to provide a means by which teachers can compare the child's progress with that of other children. In general, teachers can establish whether or not children in their classes are performing appropriately to their particular growth and developmental level. A child who continually performs lower than the average of a class may be indicating the need for special assistance through testing and programming. An assessment procedure in physical education may have as its primary goal self-realization on the part of the child whereby personal insights are gained as to his or her individual strengths and weaknesses. Often testing has as its major goal the motivation of a child to work harder in a particular endeavor. Probably one of the least desirable goals of evaluation is the comparison of one child with another for the sake of giving grades; however, because reports must be made to school officials and parents and teachers are held accountable for a child's progress, testing that makes comparisons may be a necessity.

Although there are many different types of instruments that assess physical competency, they usually provide only superficial indications of a child's true movement proficiency. Geneally speaking, tests that measure motor ability may be divided into two categories: observational surveys or checklists and quantitative measurements. Within each of these two categories, assessment tools may be designed for either large or small group or individual evaluation.

Learning to observe accurately is one of the most important skills of a teacher. Observations can be made through several avenues, namely, through the use of developmental scales, through observing selected motor patterns using a survey or checklist, or through careful analysis of a particular task or problem in technique.

Developmental scales are usually the evaluation instrument of choice for infants and preschool children. Popular developmental scales such as the Bayley,[4] Gesell,[10] and Denver[9] are commonly used for young children up to the age of 4 or 5 years. Most instruments of this type are concerned with observing typical behaviors at a given age. The behavioral categories that commonly are depicted are gross motor control, fine motor control, language and communication, adaptive behavior, and socialization.

Another type of observational approach used is a survey or checklist that indicates how a child moves or the pattern of some particular movement. This observational survey or checklist method may be concerned with relatively general performance areas or with detailed areas as are presented in an instrument such as Godfrey's Movement Pattern Checklist.[11]

Observing skills. An important factor that should be a part of every physical education teacher's repertoire is the recognition of successful or unsuccessful motor performance. Teaching the skill to observe correctly is a critical phase of the teacher education program that must not be overlooked. Teachers often see that there is difficulty in skill performance but are unable to perceive the prob-

lem. If skill performance is to be corrected in a positive direction, it requires that each teacher have a specialized knowledge and understanding of the tempo, balance, coordination, and esthetics of the movement required. Inexperienced teachers usually try to observe too much and often do not see a simple error, such as stepping forward with the wrong foot while executing a throwing skill. On the other hand, many teachers see only errors and fail to reward children who have performed successfully. The development of accurate and efficient observational techniques in the identification of motor skill abilities takes much practice.

The skill of movement observation can be developed and is not limited to the physical education specialist. Classroom teachers in particular need in-service training in proper skill observation techniques. Teachers need help to be able to see accurately what is observable as a child plays. The following suggestions are offered for the teacher who desires to improve this evaluation technique that is so essential for successful learning to take place:

1. Become as knowledgeable as possible about the skill to be taught.
2. Focus on one thing at a time when observing skill development.
3. Progress from individual to small group to total group observation.
4. Develop a checklist for developmental progress in learning skills.
5. Seek help from specialists to check on accuracy of observational techniques.

When using observation techniques, the teacher makes a skill analysis over a period of time, and must plan for it to take place in a specific environment. The value of teacher observation in relation to the learning process must not be underestimated. Although subjective in nature, observation becomes more objective as the teacher becomes more comfortable with it through practice and attains a greater understanding of correct movement patterns.

Motor ability testing. If a teacher needs to have more definitive information than an observation technique can offer, a standardized motor ability test might be the instrument of choice. Note that motor ability tests are usually highly selective in the skills they measure and that no one assessment tool is able to measure all of the elements that comprise motor ability. Some attributes necessary to success in a wide variety of movement skills are strength, flexibility, endurance, power, speed, agility, balance, reaction time, and coordination, as well as the complex interaction of almost countless perceptual factors such as time, direction, speed of movement, angle of movement, and visual figure ground, to mention just a few.[6]

Although group tests may be an effective tool to aid program development, it should be noted that they have some weaknesses. A major fault is their inability to accurately determine specific motor deficits; however, while both observational surveys or checklists and motor ability measurement instruments fail to fully determine why a child may move poorly, they can reveal those children who may require more definitive diagnostic testing. When classroom teachers identify children with severe movement problems, ideally they should refer them to a movement specialist for individualized assessment. The specialist may elect to further observe the children's movement characteristics or choose to use a diagnostic test designed to reveal motor deficiencies, such as the Oseretsky Test of Motor Performance,[8] the Stott General Test of Motor Impairment for Children,[15] or Ayres' Sensory-Integration Test Battery.[3] The teacher should be aware that in most cases an entire test battery need not be given if some preliminary screening has been performed. Once the extent of motor deficit has been determined, a remedial program can then be instituted.

A Basic Motor Ability Test with seven subtests is presented here as an example of a relatively simple and fast screening device that measures a number of discrete movement factors necessary for success in a wide variety of play activities. The specific tests are *bead stringing* as an indicator of dexterity, *target throwing* as an indicator of eye-hand coordination, *back and hamstring stretch* as a measure of flexibility, *standing long jump* as an indicator of the amount of strength and power in the legs, *face down to standing* as a measure of total body agility, *static balance* as a measure of stationary posturing, and, finally, *chair push-up* as a measure of arm strength and endurance. Children who fail to score over the twenty-fifth percentile on three or more of the seven subtests are deemed to require more definitive testing and perhaps remedial programs.

Basic motor abilities test*

Specific administration and scoring procedures. The examiner must follow the administration and scoring procedures precisely. Before each subtest is administered, obvious permanent and temporary physical disabilities that would adversely affect the child's motor performance must be noted. It is also imperative that the child being tested thoroughly understand the directions to each subtest. Therefore the examiner must demonstrate as well as verbally explain each aspect of the test before it is executed. Establishing good rapport with the child and encouraging him or her to put forth the best effort cannot be overemphasized. The testing room should be free from all distractions. It is desirable to follow the order in which the subtests are presented here to maximize performance and attention and keep muscular fatigue to a minimum.

---

*Adapted from Basic Motor Abilities Test in Arnheim, D. D., and Sinclair, W. A.: The Clumsy Child, St. Louis, 1975, The C. V. Mosby Co.

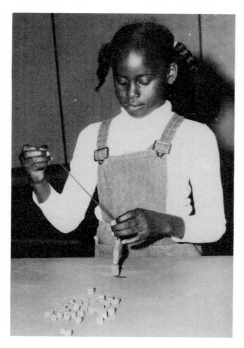

Fig. 2-7. Bead stringing. (From Arnheim, D. D., and Sinclair, W. A.: The clumsy child, St. Louis, 1975, The C. V. Mosby Co.)

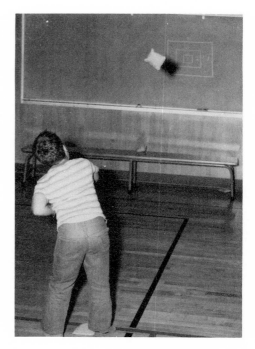

Fig. 2-8. Target throwing. (From Arnheim, D. D., and Sinclair, W. A.: The clumsy child, St. Louis, 1975, The C. V. Mosby Co.)

SUBTEST 1: BEAD STRINGING (Fig. 2-7)

Purpose: To test bilateral eye-hand coordination and dexterity.

Materials: The ½-inch beads supplied with the Stanford-Binet test set, an 18-inch, round shoelace with a ¾-inch plastic tip and a knot tied at the end of the shoelace, a stopwatch.

Procedure: Place the beads and lace before the child. Demonstrate by putting two beads on the lace while explaining that speed is essential. The beads merely have to be on the lace; the child should not waste time stringing the beads all the way down to the knot.

Time limit: 30 seconds.

Scoring: Record the total number of beads strung in the 30-second period.

SUBTEST 2: TARGET THROWING (Fig. 2-8)

Purpose: To test eye-hand coordination.

Materials: A target consisting of three squares measuring 5, 11, and 18 inches on each side attached to a wall with the bottom 4 feet from the floor, fifteen 4 by 5 inch beanbags.

Procedure: Children from 4 to 5 years of age stand behind a restraining line 7 feet from the target and those from 6 to 12 years of age stand behind a restraining line 10 feet from the target. The difference in throwing distances is to minimize the adverse effects of the lack of arm strength in younger children. The tester demonstrates by throwing two bags at the target while explaining that the small square has a value of 3 points, the middle square a value of 2 points, and the large square a value of 1 point. The child is then told to score as many points as possible in 15 throws.

Scoring: The total score is determined by adding the points earned in the 15 throws. If a beanbag lands on the line between two squares, the larger score is awarded.

SUBTEST 3: BACK AND HAMSTRING STRETCH
(Fig. 2-9)

Purpose: To test the flexibility of back and hamstring muscles.

Materials: A 1-meter rule or yardstick.

Procedure: The child sits on the floor with legs fully extended and heels approximately 6

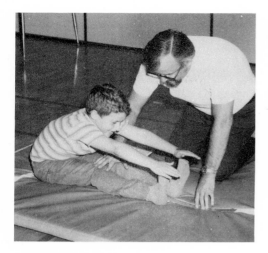

Fig. 2-9. Back and hamstring stretch. (From Arnheim, D. D., and Sinclair, W. A.: The clumsy child, St. Louis, 1975, The C. V. Mosby Co.)

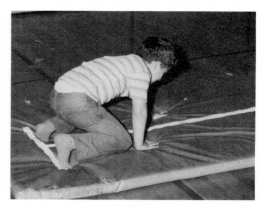

Fig. 2-11. Face down to standing. (From Arnheim, D. D., and Sinclair, W. A.: The clumsy child, St. Louis, 1975, The C. V. Mosby Co.)

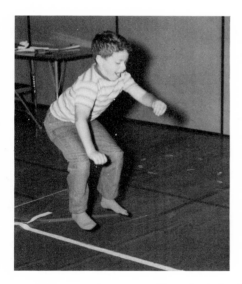

Fig. 2-10. Standing long jump. (From Arnheim, D. D., and Sinclair, W. A.: The clumsy child, St. Louis, 1975, The C. V. Mosby Co.)

inches apart. The 1-meter rule or yardstick is placed between the child's legs with the 10-cm or 10-inch mark even with the heels. Keeping the knees straight, the child bends forward, reaching down the rule as far as possible without bouncing. Three attempts are allowed.

Scoring: Record the farthest point reached by the child's fingertips in the three attempts. Measure to the nearest centimeter

or ⅛ inch. The child receives a score of 0 if his or her fingers reach the heels, a positive score if they go beyond the heels, and a negative score if they do not reach the heels.

SUBTEST 4: STANDING LONG JUMP (Fig. 2-10)

Purpose: To test the strength and power in the thigh and lower leg muscles.

Materials: A 1-meter rule or yardstick, a nonslippery surface for taking off and landing.

Procedure: First the tester demonstrates and explains the proper way to jump. Then the test is executed by swinging the arms back, bending the knees, and swinging the arms forward and extending the legs at the moment of takeoff. A maximum of three trials is allowed.

Scoring: The longest jump of the three trials is recorded in centimeters or inches measured from the point of takeoff to the heel nearest the takeoff point.

SUBTEST 5: FACE DOWN TO STANDING
(Fig. 2-11)

Purpose: To test speed and agility in changing from a prone to a standing position.

Materials: A 4 by 6 foot mat or carpeted surface, a stopwatch.

Procedure: The tester demonstrates twice while explaining that the child is to start on his or her stomach with the forehead touching the mat. On the command "Go," the child rises to an erect standing position with the knees straight. The child repeats this cycle as many times as possible.

Time limit: 20 seconds.

Scoring: Record the number of times the child is able to get to a standing position within the 20-second time limit.

SUBTEST 6: STATIC BALANCE (Fig. 2-12)

Purpose: To test static balance first with eyes open and then with eyes closed.

Materials: Blindfold, stopwatch, two balance boards—one 2 inches wide, the other 4 inches wide.

Procedure: The tester demonstrates on each board, explaining that either foot may be used but the hands must be kept on the hips with the nonsupporting foot behind the other knee. First the child is given one trial on each board with the eyes open and then repeats with the eyes closed or blindfolded. If the child refuses the blindfold or is unable to keep the eyes closed, the test should be considered incomplete.

Time limit: A maximum of 10 seconds per trial.

Scoring: Record the total number of seconds the child can maintain a balanced position. Criteria for discontinuing a trial are touching the foot to the floor, removing either hand from the hips, or opening the

eyes. The total number of seconds the child scored in the four balance tasks is also recorded.

SUBTEST 7: CHAIR PUSH-UPS (Fig. 2-13)

Purpose: To test arm and shoulder girdle strength.

Materials: A stopwatch, a chair or bench measuring 14 to 18 inches above the floor, a wall against which the feet may be braced.

Procedure: The examiner demonstrates twice while explaining to the child that a front-leaning rest position should be assumed with legs together, feet against the wall, arms fully extended, and the body forming a straight line from head to feet. To execute the push-up the arms are bent until the chest touches the chair or bench, then the arms are straightened and the front-leaning rest position is resumed.

Time limit: 20 seconds.

Scoring: The number of correct push-ups counted within 20 seconds.

Text continued on p. 39.

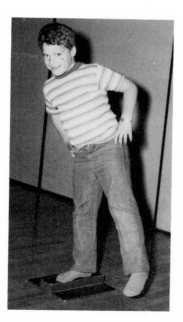

Fig. 2-12. Static balance. (From Arnheim, D. D., and Sinclair, W. A.: The clumsy child, St. Louis, 1975, The C. V. Mosby Co.)

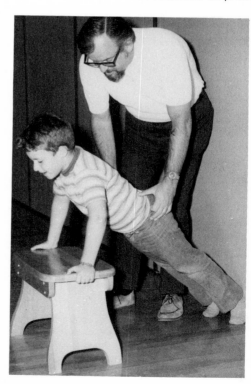

Fig. 2-13. Chair push-ups. (From Arnheim, D. D., and Sinclair, W. A.: The clumsy child, St. Louis, 1975, The C. V. Mosby Co.)

Norms: Basic Motor Ability Tests
Sex: Male   Age: 4 years

Per-centiles	Bead stringing	Target throwing	Back and hamstring stretch		Standing long jump		Face down to standing	Static balance	Chair push-ups
			(cm)	(in)	(cm)	(in)			
90+	10	22	52	28¾	130	51¼	10	18	9
75	7	16	45	25⅞	100	39⅜	8	15	7
50	5	10	36	22⅜	89	35	6	10	5
25	3	3	27	18¾	60	23⅝	4	7	2
1	1	1	18	15¼	30	11¾	2	3	0

Sex: Male   Age: 5 years

Per-centiles	Bead stringing	Target throwing	Back and hamstring stretch		Standing long jump		Face down to standing	Static balance	Chair push-ups
			(cm)	(in)	(cm)	(in)			
90+	12	24	52	28¾	139	54¾	11	22	15
75	9	19	44	25½	110	43¼	10	17	10
50	7	15	33	21¼	97	38¼	7	11	8
25	4	8	25	18	70	27⅝	5	8	7
1	1	5	15	14⅛	40	15¾	3	3	4

Sex: Male   Age: 6 years

Per-centiles	Bead stringing	Target throwing	Back and hamstring stretch		Standing long jump		Face down to standing	Static balance	Chair push-ups
			(cm)	(in)	(cm)	(in)			
90+	14	23	50	27⅞	156	61⅜	15	27	18
75	11	17	42	24¾	133	52⅜	13	20	14
50	8	9	32	20¾	104	40⅞	10	16	9
25	5	1	22	16⅞	75	29½	7	8	4
1	1	0	13	13¼	49	19¼	5	3	1

Sex: Male   Age: 7 years

Per-centiles	Bead stringing	Target throwing	Back and hamstring stretch		Standing long jump		Face down to standing	Static balance	Chair push-ups
			(cm)	(in)	(cm)	(in)			
90+	15	28	47	26¾	171	67¼	16	28	19
75	11	21	39	23½	146	57⅜	14	18	15
50	9	12	29	19⅝	115	45¼	11	16	10
25	6	3	19	15¾	83	32¾	8	9	5
1	3	1	10	12⅛	52	20½	4	4	1

Sex: Male   Age: 8 years

Per-centiles	Bead stringing	Target throwing	Back and hamstring stretch		Standing long jump		Face down to standing	Static balance	Chair push-ups
			(cm)	(in)	(cm)	(in)			
90+	15	36	46	26¼	173	68⅛	15	30	14
75	12	28	38	23⅛	151	59⅜	13	20	15
50	10	18	28	19¼	123	48⅜	11	15	11
25	7	8	18	15¼	96	38¾	8	9	6
1	4	2	8	11¼	69	27¼	5	4	1

Sex: Male   Age: 9 years

Per-centiles	Bead stringing	Target throwing	Back and hamstring stretch		Standing long jump		Face down to standing	Static balance	Chair push-ups
			(cm)	(in)	(cm)	(in)			
90+	15	34	47	26¾	185	72¾	18	30	19
75	13	28	39	23½	163	64¼	16	24	15
50	11	19	27	18¾	132	51	12	17	12
25	9	11	16	14½	102	40¼	8	10	7
1	6	2	5	10¼	72	28¼	5	4	3

Sex: Male   Age: 10 years

Per-centiles	Bead stringing	Target throwing	Back and hamstring stretch		Standing long jump		Face down to standing	Static balance	Chair push-ups
			(cm)	(in)	(cm)	(in)			
90+	17	40	46	26¼	192	75⅝	19	30	21
75	15	32	45	25⅞	172	67¾	16	25	16
50	12	23	31	20⅜	148	58¼	12	18	11
25	8	14	17	14⅞	123	48⅜	8	11	6
1	5	5	4	9¾	99	39	5	5	1

Sex: Male   Age: 11 years

Per-centiles	Bead stringing	Target throwing	Back and hamstring stretch		Standing long jump		Face down to standing	Static balance	Chair push-ups
			(cm)	(in)	(cm)	(in)			
90+	17	42	48	27⅛	207	81½	21	31	25
75	15	34	40	23⅞	181	71¼	17	26	19
50	12	24	29	19⅝	147	57⅞	13	19	12
25	10	14	19	15¾	121	47½	8	12	4

Sex: Male   Age: 12 years

Per-centiles	Bead stringing	Target throwing	Back and hamstring stretch (cm)	(in)	Standing long jump (cm)	(in)	Face down to standing	Static balance	Chair push-ups
90+	16	42	52	28¾	208	81⅞	20	32	21
75	14	35	42	24¾	195	76¾	17	27	17
50	12	26	31	20⅜	166	65⅜	13	19	12
25	10	16	19	15¾	137	53⅞	10	10	7
1	8	7	7	10⅞	108	42½	5	7	3

Sex: Female   Age: 4 years

Per-centiles	Bead stringing	Target throwing	Back and hamstring stretch (cm)	(in)	Standing long jump (cm)	(in)	Face down to standing	Static balance	Chair push-ups
90+	10	22	52	28¾	129	50¾	10	17	8
75	8	17	47	26¾	99	39	8	15	6
50	5	11	36	22⅜	89	35	6	11	5
25	3	3	28	19¼	60	23⅝	4	8	2
1	1	1	19	15¾	30	11¾	2	2	0

Sex: Female   Age: 5 years

Per-centiles	Bead stringing	Target throwing	Back and hamstring stretch (cm)	(in)	Standing long jump (cm)	(in)	Face down to standing	Static balance	Chair push-ups
90+	11	22	50	27⅞	135	53⅛	10	21	15
75	9	18	43	22½	108	42½	9	19	10
50	7	14	32	20¾	95	37⅜	7	13	8
25	4	7	27	18¾	67	26⅜	5	9	7
1	1	4	15	14⅛	35	13¾	2	5	4

Sex: Female   Age: 6 years

Per-centiles	Bead stringing	Target throwing	Back and hamstring stretch (cm)	(in)	Standing long jump (cm)	(in)	Face down to standing	Static balance	Chair push-ups
90+	13	16	54	29⅜	145	57⅛	16	28	16
75	11	11	46	26¼	125	49¼	13	22	14
50	8	6	35	22	100	39⅜	10	17	8
25	5	1	24	17⅝	74	29⅛	7	8	4
1	2	—	13	13	49	19¼	3	3	1

Sex: Female   Age: 7 years

Per-centiles	Bead stringing	Target throwing	Back and hamstring stretch		Standing long jump		Face down to standing	Static balance	Chair push-ups
			(cm)	(in)	(cm)	(in)			
90+	14	15	48	27⅛	166	65⅜	16	31	16
75	12	11	41	24¼	141	55½	13	24	12
50	9	6	32	20¾	111	43¾	10	14	7
25	6	1	23	17¼	80	31½	7	8	3
1	3	—	14	13¾	49	19¼	4	3	—

Sex: Female   Age: 8 years

Per-centiles	Bead stringing	Target throwing	Back and hamstring stretch		Standing long jump		Face down to standing	Static balance	Chair push-ups
			(cm)	(in)	(cm)	(in)			
90+	16	19	52	28¾	180	70⅞	15	25	16
75	13	11	43	25⅛	155	61	13	19	13
50	10	8	31	20⅜	121	47½	11	11	8
25	7	3	19	15¾	93	36½	8	6	4
1	1	—	8	11¼	63	24¾	5	3	—

Sex: Female   Age: 9 years

Per-centiles	Bead stringing	Target throwing	Back and hamstring stretch		Standing long jump		Face down to standing	Static balance	Chair push-ups
			(cm)	(in)	(cm)	(in)			
90+	16	30	50	27⅞	178	70⅛	16	27	17
75	15	20	41	24¼	156	61⅜	14	20	14
50	11	17	30	20	130	51¼	11	13	9
25	8	14	20	16⅛	104	40⅞	8	7	5
1	5	11	9	11¾	78	30¾	4	4	1

Sex: Female   Age: 10 years

Per-centiles	Bead stringing	Target throwing	Back and hamstring stretch		Standing long jump		Face down to standing	Static balance	Chair push-ups
			(cm)	(in)	(cm)	(in)			
90+	17	32	54	29⅜	192	75½	16	30	19
75	14	25	45	25⅞	169	66½	14	27	14
50	12	18	33	21¼	140	55⅛	11	16	9
25	9	15	22	16⅞	112	44⅛	8	10	4
1	6	10	10	12⅛	84	33⅛	4	8	—

Sex: Female   Age: 11 years

Per-centiles	Bead stringing	Target throwing	Back and hamstring stretch (cm)	(in)	Standing long jump (cm)	(in)	Face down to standing	Static balance	Chair push-ups
90+	17	33	53	29⅛	206	81⅛	16	29	18
75	15	27	44	25½	183	72	14	24	14
50	12	19	32	20¾	154	60½	11	15	9
25	10	10	20	16⅛	124	48¾	9	12	3
1	6	2	9	11¾	95	37⅜	6	5	—

Sex: Female   Age: 12 years

Per-centiles	Bead stringing	Target throwing	Back and hamstring stretch (cm)	(in)	Standing long jump (cm)	(in)	Face down to standing	Static balance	Chair push-ups
90+	17	40	53	29⅛	207	81½	18	25	20
75	15	32	44	25½	189	74⅜	16	20	15
50	13	22	32	20¾	161	63⅜	12	14	8
25	10	12	20	16⅛	133	52⅜	9	7	2
1	8	2	9	11¾	104	40⅞	5	3	—

Administering a test—circuit organization. Administering a pretest gives the teacher a base from which to begin program planning. Testing can be a time-consuming and tiring element if drawn out over a long period. One way to complete it quickly and painlessly is to use a circuit testing procedure. This method has a station, with the necessary equipment, set up for each test. Children are given a score sheet (Fig. 2-14) and rotate from station to station until all tests are completed and recorded. The results of the tests can then be placed on a total class score sheet (Fig. 2-15). Careful preplanning is necessary if test results are to be valid.

Preparation for the test. Using the Basic Motor Ability Test as the screening device, the following items are necessary:

1. An area approximately 30 by 40 feet
2. Ten beads and string, stopwatch, table and chair
3. Target, 15 bean bags
4. Mat or blanket, meter stick
5. Meter stick or tape, toe line
6. Mat or blanket, stopwatch
7. One 2 by 4 by 2 inch beam, one 2 by 4 by 4 inch beam, stopwatch
8. Chair, wall, stopwatch
9. Seven pencils

It is necessary to secure the services of 14 dependable helpers, two for each station. While one helper explains and gives the test the other can record the results on the individual score sheet. Before the testing begins, the helpers must be taught how to give the test and how to score and record the results. By using role playing, the teacher can ascertain the accuracy of the training and make any necessary corrections. The results can be hand tabulated or run on a computer, if available, giving the teacher both individual and class profiles of the children's motoric ability. For example, if the class as a whole scores low in the areas of agility and balance, the teacher should develop the program with an emphasis on games

INDIVIDUAL SCORE SHEET

Name_____ Class_____

Date_____

Basic Motor Ability Test

	Pre	Post
Bead stringing	_____	_____
Target throwing	_____	_____
Back and hamstring stretch	_____	_____
Standing long jump	_____	_____
Face down to standing	_____	_____

	open	close	open	close
Static balance 4" beam	_____	_____	_____	_____

	open	close	open	close
Static balance 2" beam	_____	_____	_____	_____
Static balance total	_____		_____	
Chair push-ups	_____		_____	

Fig. 2-14. Individual test score sheet.

BASIC MOTOR ABILITIES

CLASS LIST (names)	AGE	BEAD STRINGING		TARGET THROWING		BACK AND HAMSTRING STRETCH (centimeters)		STANDING LONG JUMP (centimeters)	
		Pre	Post	Pre	Post	Pre	Post	Pre	Post

Continued.

Fig. 2-15. Total class record sheet.

BASIC MOTOR ABILITIES—cont'd

FACE DOWN TO STANDING		STATIC BALANCE 4″ BEAM				STATIC BALANCE 2″ BEAM				CHAIR PUSH-UPS	
		Pre	Post	Pre	Post	Pre	Post	Pre	Post		
Pre	Post	Open	Closed	Open	Closed	Open	Closed	Open	Closed	Pre	Post

Fig. 2-15, cont'd. Total class record sheet.

that will develop these abilities. Activities such as dodge ball, zigzag runs, and balancing stunts can now be offered for a specific reason.

By giving a posttest at the end of each year, individual and class progress can be measured and program effectiveness determined. Teachers who evaluate children for the purpose of program development design activities that fit the needs of the children rather than that require the children to adjust to the program.

THE LESSON

A well-planned and well-designed physical education curriculum is of little value unless the teacher is capable of translating the material into enjoyable program activities that are suited to the needs and abilities of the children in each developmental level. How does the teacher make use of the curriculum plan suggested for a specific grade level? The following procedure is presented to acquaint the teacher with steps that should be followed in utilizing the yearly plan as a guide to the development of the daily lesson.

1. The teacher should refer to the yearly plan to determine what percentages and types of activities are recommended for the level involved. The teacher can then select the broad categories of activities and can project the actual number of days that the children should participate in each classification.

2. After the time factor in each category has been established, the teacher selects the activities that are appropriate for a specific grade level on the basis of the information presented in Chapter 3 in relation to seasonality, feasibility, and other factors.

3. The teacher can then develop activity unit plans within the yearly time block. The units of instruction will vary from single-day plans in level 1 to monthly or 6-week units for level 3. The unit or monthly plan should be more specific than the yearly plan and include the names of the games or skills to be offered.

4. The unit plan is then converted into detailed daily lesson plans that should include the objectives of the lesson, teacher and student procedures, class formations, space requirements, and equipment needed.

Within the unit plan there are two approaches to scheduling weekly activities. The first is the block plan in which the same activity is scheduled 5 days a week for a set period of time. A 4-week unit in soccer offered each day of the week allows for a concentrated effort in a single activity. Skills are learned quite well under this plan; however, it does not allow for variety, and if some students do not like the activity, a lack of interest and unfavorable attitudes toward physical education may be initiated.

The second approach to scheduling involves a *finger-type* plan in which the seasonal activity is offered 3 days a week with alternate programs on the other 2 days. A soccer unit under this plan would be offered on Monday, Wednesday, and Friday, and dance, volleyball, and other activities would be offered on Tuesday and Thursday. This plan allows for a greater variety of physical activities during each week. In the lower levels in which daily self-contained units are complete, the finger program could involve movement exploration activities on Monday and Wednesday, rhythms on Tuesday, sports and games on Thursday, and self-testing activities on Friday.

Although the physical education teacher should determine which plan best meets the needs and interests of the students at the various program levels, the finger-type plan often allows for better utilization of facilities when space is limited.

HOW CHILDREN LEARN SKILLS

Teachers must know how children learn if lesson planning is to be effective.

For the learner, the perceptual-motor process can be enhanced by methods of teaching that employ sound motor learning principles. Although at this time motor learning is for the most part an inexact science, many practical generalizations have been established that may be employed by the instructor. However, the principles discussed in this section must be considered only as suggestions for improving teaching methods and not as ends in themselves.

The learner

There are many factors that may enhance or adversely alter the learning abilities of the child. Maturation and individual developmental status definitely affect learning and motor skill. The very young child is best equipped to acquire motor skills in the same sequence in which myelinization of motor nerves occurs, that is, gross muscle control followed by fine muscle coordination. Upper-body management occurs before lower-limb management. Large-muscle activities such as running and jumping are mastered before the fine movements required in throwing.[13]

Motivation and interest are always factors in learning. Young children find it difficult to sustain the same activity over a long period of time; therefore, it is best to plan for program emphasis to encompass a great variety of activities. Children usually find that large-muscle exercises provide a pleasant satisfaction or a means of draining undirected energies. What is needed, however, is the proper direction for their excitement. Positive rewards found within the activity itself are much preferred to punishment or even rewards external to the activity. Ideally, the child should find the activity so interesting and exciting that he or she will play it for its own sake rather than for prizes, grades, or trophies. Skill objectives are more easily attainable when they are clearly stated by the teacher and, whenever possible, are agreed to or selected by the child in cooperation with the teacher.

Methods of teaching

Teaching has been called both an art and a science. We must concur with this. Teaching must be effective if learning is to take place; effective teaching requires that many interdependent factors occur simultaneously and in sequence with each other. The discrete variables of the teacher's knowledge of the subject, knowledge of the learner, knowledge of personal strengths and weaknesses, and knowledge of many techniques of communication are but a few factors in the storage of information.[15]

Instruction

Instruction is organized in terms of the sense mode that is used, that is, vision, audition, or kinesthesis. *Visual instruction* or guidance refers to teaching by demonstration, films, video tape, and the like. *Verbal teaching* uses primarily the auditory mode of perception for information input. Instruction through hearing is not considered particularly effective when complex motor responses are required. Motor guidance in teaching utilizes the kinesthetic sense wherein the student feels the correct movement pattern or skill. It is generally agreed that not all children learn best through the same sense channels; therefore, the teacher should employ as many sensory modes as possible.[12]

Knowledge of results

Of extreme importance in learning motor skills is the continuous feedback provided by the senses. Children can acquire greater progress in movement skills when they have immediate awareness of the outcome of their performance. The correctness of a motor act can be assisted directly in terms of scores as in basketball or base hits as in baseball or in terms of verbal description by the teacher. Instant playback of video tapes is an excellent method of acquiring immediate knowledge of performance. Children respond best when they are constantly aware of the results of their motor efforts. The astute teacher will provide the child with cues or signals that assist in the feedback process. Through proper cues the child becomes more alert to what can be seen, heard, and felt.

Practice

The way in which a skill is practiced is of the utmost importance for its mastery. Inappropriate practice habits can produce faulty perception and performance. There are many factors that affect the quality of practicing a movement task, for example, how motivated the learners are, whether they are maturationally ready to learn a new task, and whether they have a basic understanding of the objective to be accomplished. The teacher must provide opportunities for various types of practice, depending on the skill to be learned.

Massing of practice. Movement education programs vary considerably in intensity, ranging from a number of hours per day to a few minutes per week. Some motor development systems purport that the functional capacity of the brain can be altered positively by the constant stimulation resulting from the performance of developmental motor patterns.[7] However, movement education programs vary considerably in quality and in amount of external environmental stimulation required. Most programs claiming perceptual-motor learning as an outcome agree that the learner must have many sensory experiences in order to build a backlog for future responses.

The question for many teachers is how much information should be attempted in a single lesson. Should there be a massing of learning until a skill is mastered, or should there be a distribution of practice? Generally, it has been found that distributed practice is better for the learner and that shorter periods in time, intensity, and repetition allow more efficient learning to take place.[14] Authorities in motor learning generally agree that as a person becomes more proficient at a movement skill, increasingly longer periods of time can be spent at its practice. Consequently, younger children require more practices that are spaced closer together than do older children, and skilled performers can effectively engage in longer practice periods than unskilled performers.[7]

Whole-part-whole method. Whole-part-whole method refers to learning skills in their entirety or learning parts that later are combined to form a complete skill. There are different approaches or combinations of the whole-part-whole concept, such as whole only, part only, part-whole, or whole-part-whole. Any or all of these methods may be utilized by a teacher, depending on the task to be learned and the individual characteristics of the learner. Simple motor tasks can generally be taught in their entirety, whereas more complex activities must be broken into their logical parts. A good teacher will identify and present to the child small whole skill patterns that help to make up the greater whole of the activity. For example, a child may be taught to jump rhythmically in place without a rope, which will later lead to the more difficult task of jumping a complete, circling rope. Part learning is concerned with only a segment of a movement pattern or task and is tied to other segments that will eventually form a complete skill. When a part has been learned well, the next part is attempted. If part learning is to be effective, more complex activities must be joined to one another in a logical sequence of events and in a time period in which the relationship of each part can be clearly understood by the learner. Skill parts learned without relationships often become disjointed and splintered. Ideally, the child sees the whole skill correctly executed, either through demonstration by the teacher or by some other audiovisual means, such as video tape or film. The teacher using the whole-part-whole method continually reminds the child what the entire skill should look like and how the parts will eventually emerge as the completed skill.

Speed of movement. Research indicates that skills should be taught in the same manner in which the learner will ultimately perform them. In other words, the elements of the practice of skills should approximate as nearly as possible those of the actual performance. Slow motion practice provides little benefit in training for fast ballistic type movements. If accuracy is required for the successful completion of an activity, it must be considered from the beginning. Skills like shooting a basketball, kicking a ball, or hitting a golf ball include the elements of both speed and accuracy; consequently, each must be practiced as it will eventually be performed.

Specificity and transfer of training

A difficult area of study in motor learning is specificity and transfer of training. A number of researchers in motor learning have concluded that the learning of motor skills is highly specific for a particular task.[7] To illustrate, Fleishman, in an analysis of the factors required in physical fitness, identifies the following specific attributes: (1) speed of change of direction, (2) gross body equilibrium, (3) balance with visual cues, (4) dynamic flexibility, (5) extent of flexibility, and (6) speed of limb movement. Research points out that from all factors studied, specific skills emerge.[7] With this in mind, the teacher must realize that each child brings to the class a multitude of individual skills that he or she can use in learning different motor tasks. However,

excelling in one activity does not mean that the child will have an automatic ability in another.

Transfer of training implies that one learned task can be used to learn another task. However, if motor learning is specific to the task how may one skill enhance or perhaps hinder another?[12] Knapp terms a previously learned act that aids a new skill as positive transfer. Authorities tend to agree that there is specificity in motor ability and that some similarities can be transferred. For example, throwing a ball overhand is similar to the tennis service and the spike in volleyball. Underhand softball pitching can be compared to horseshoe pitching, an underhand serve in volleyball, or a badminton serve. Intrinsic factors such as adjustment of one's center of gravity or application of a specific force in pushing and pulling activities may be transferred from one activity to another. The teacher can improve the process of transfer by pointing out likenesses and dissimilarities between activities. This is particularly true when the child is engaged in tasks designed to assist in cognition.

Learning approaches

Teachers often find themselves in the dilemma of whether to use the direct or indirect method of teaching when presenting a lesson. Many teachers of physical education feel more comfortable using the traditional or direct approach (Fig. 2-16). Selecting the subject and following the parts of a lesson previously described is a neat and clean procedure and one most learning directors have had some experience in using. With this technique, the teacher plays a dominant role, making suggestions for improvement and corrections as necessary. Introducing the lesson, demonstrating the skill, organizing well-designed practice drills, and evaluating the lesson result in a learning module. When this approach is used, the teacher's physical prowess is a

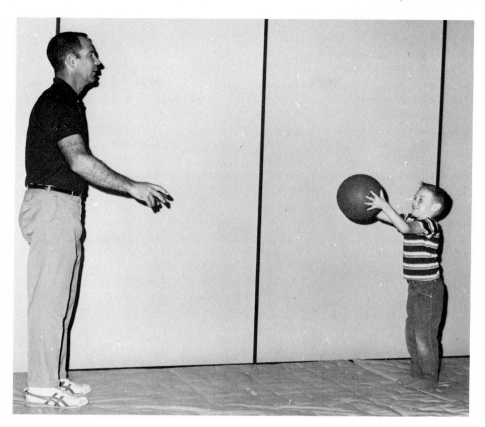

Fig. 2-16. Learning through the direct approach.

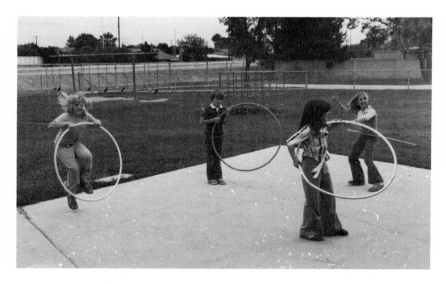

Fig. 2-17. Indirect learning involves individual experimentation.

key to a successful lesson although student demonstrations are acceptable alternatives if individual teacher skills are low. The teacher must be alert at recognizing and correcting errors, often manipulating the child into the correct position for proper execution.

The direct method is most effective in teaching prescribed skills in which the proper form is well established and there is little reason to vary or experiment with a different technique. Such activities as shooting a basketball or punting a football are best taught in this manner.

The indirect approach to presenting a lesson requires as much skill as the direct method but necessitates a definite change in the teacher's role (Fig. 2-17). When using the indirect application, the teacher serves more as a guide to discovery than as a demonstrator. Many teachers initially find it difficult to take a passive role while the class is discovering the technique desired. However, once they understand the role of guide, teachers find joy and satisfaction as they compliment children who have achieved the lesson objective and encourage those who have not to continue to experiment. This avenue of teaching is often associated with problem-solving or movement exploration lessons in which children are seeking the beginning stages of body movement or early object management. (See Chapter 11.)

The indirect method usually is accompanied by a lesson in which many solutions are possible and no single solution is the correct way to achieve a skill. The children are allowed to experiment and discover which way works best for them. This way is often emphasized at the lower age levels but can be used successfully for all ages by increasing or decreasing the complexity of the problem. For example, lessons involving the problem-solving method and relating to body image, preliminary locomotion skills, and creative movement are suited to the indirect approach to teaching.

Teachers of physical education should not rely on one method or approach alone. Teaching excellence results when a blend of the two methods is mastered and the one selected is best suited to the objectives of the lesson presented.

The creative teacher continually seeks to discover new and varied ways of presenting subject matter, challenging the individual to climb the ladder of success with vigor and enthusiasm.

DAILY LESSON PRESENTATIONS

A complete lesson in physical education will include five major parts: introduction, explanation, demonstration, participation, and evaluation. Although all parts of a lesson are important, the emphasis or inclusion of each phase depends on the learning approach selected by the teacher.

Introduction

Introducing the lesson in a positive and interesting manner can make the difference between student enthusiasm and apathy toward the activity. A little research involving the origin of the game or dance will allow the teacher to set the stage for the day's lesson and will serve as a point of reference for the children involved. Visual aids in the form of posters or motion pictures presenting the activity in a stimulating and interesting setting with proficient players can motivate children to pursue the lesson with great enthusiasm. Whenever possible, the introduction should take place in the classroom and should not take time away from the physical education period.

Explanation

The explanation should include the actual specific directions for playing a game or learning a skill. The teacher should know the subject well and use terminology that is easily understood by the children involved. The explanation should be brief and to the point, allowing the children to become involved in the activity as soon as possible. If a complicated game or skill is being taught, the teacher should explain the activity in parts, providing practice periods between directions, until the complete activity is learned. The explanation can be enhanced by using visual aids or combining the explanation with the demonstration. Beginning teachers often spend too much time talking during this phase of the lesson and leave too little time for activity.

Demonstration

Demonstration, like a picture, is worth a thousand words. The teacher who is well skilled and can demonstrate before the class has a definite advantage in the successful presentation of a lesson. Children may interpret the verbal explanation in a variety of ways, but the demonstration presents a visual explanation that is difficult to misunderstand. The teacher can present the demonstration in slow motion, progressing to actual game speed so that all phases of the skill can be easily seen. When the explanation and demonstration are combined, the time for activity is usually increased. Before demonstrating, the teacher must make sure that the skill performed is an accurate reproduction of what is to be learned. If the teacher cannot execute the skill accurately, it is permissible to use one of the better students in the class to demonstrate. This allows the teacher to point out proper positioning and skill techniques to the class without being an actual participant.

The respect the teacher gains by virtue of demonstrating in a professional manner is well worth the time taken to develop personal skills.

Participation

This phase of the lesson should take the majority of time allotted for physical ed-ucation. Children expect to participate during the activity period, and the teacher should prepare the lesson in such a manner that maximum amount of play experience is provided. The quicker children become involved in the activity, the less chance there is for problems to arise, such as lack of attention and interest.

In the lower levels, participation usually involves playing a complete game or activity. In the upper levels, the participation phase may be limited to lead-up skills or drills until such time that the class is ready to play the complete game. In order to alleviate boredom during the drill period, the teacher may substitute a modified game with fewer rules and skills to allow for some game competition during each period. Teachers can have fun creating their own games and often find new and successful approaches to learning an activity through competitive skill drills.

Evaluation

The evaluation period is the last phase of the daily lesson. This phase should take no more than 2 to 3 minutes out of the total period, but it can be one of the most valuable experiences of the day. During this time, the teacher is able to discuss with the class the successes or failures of the day's lesson and offer suggestions for the next day. A note of favorable recognition for a child's excellent play or a brief reprimand to a class that could improve its behavior is more meaningful when done immediately after the experience. Grouping the class briefly before returning to the classroom provides a cooling-off period and allows the teacher to check on injuries and make sure all equipment is returned.

DISCIPLINE

An important factor related to the success of any learning environment is discipline. Teachers of physical education must develop and maintain consistency in class discipline regardless of the learning approach utilized. It makes little difference whether one is involved in a teacher-directed lesson or a pupil-oriented creative movement experience; discipline must be evidenced if learning is to be effective.

Inexperienced teachers often make the mistake of being "too easy" for fear of being disliked by their pupils. However, they soon learn that if firm discipline is employed, students have a respect for the teacher that cannot be achieved through other, substitute means. Since discipline is the key to learning without disruption, each teacher must develop class control skills that are effective and suited to his or her personality and beliefs.

There are many approaches that will work; however, we support a *positive teacher-directed, assertive approach.* This approach is founded on the belief that the teacher must set firm behavioral limits and display consistency in response to both correct and incorrect actions. Each learning director must make students aware of the class behavior desired and be assertive enough to enforce predetermined penalties for not complying. It is also important to reward good behavior, which is often taken for granted by most teachers, since positive reinforcement is a necessary phase of the disciplinary process.[5]

Although the days of the drill sergeant have hopefully disappeared from the education field, individual teachers must set their standards early and be firm enough to ensure that they are adhered to for adequate class control. A well-disciplined class can be an enjoyable experience for both teacher and pupil.

The method used should be developed in a positive manner and should be clearly understood by the students if they are to reach the maximum learning potential of an activity lesson. Some teachers tend to relax during a creative movement lesson; however, freedom of movement during motor skill acquisition does not negate the need for strong teacher control. This control, often not visible to the layman, is critical if disciplinary consistency is to be achieved. For fair and consistent class control, the teacher must

1. Establish the limits of pupil-class behavior
2. Make students aware of the consequences for non-compliance
3. Be consistent in response to student behavior
4. Reward compliance with established class rules
5. Make the students aware that their choice of noncompliance or compliance will result either in a penalty or in a reward

Firm and friendly discipline must be a part of each teacher's repertoire. Without strong teacher direction leading toward student self-direction, the achievement of established educational goals is made increasingly difficult.

PUBLIC RELATIONS

The importance of every teacher being well schooled in the elements of public relations cannot be underestimated. It is particularly important for teachers of physical education to become involved in the development and maintenance of a favorable public relations program. Many parents and community residents view physical education as a frill and have not been oriented to the benefits accrued through a well-designed program conducted under the auspices of the "new physical education."

The public must be informed of the positive values received through participation in a program of this type and bury forever the myth that free play and recess with no direction prevail. Parents must understand (1) how success in motor activities can develop a strong self-concept, (2) the relationship of achievement in motor skills to all learning, and (3) the mental and physical benefits received through participation in vigorous activity.

It is the responsibility of each teacher to take advantage of every possible means available to promote the values of a modern physical education program.

Promotional activities must be developed to sell the program to school administrations, school boards, parents, and the community in general. To help keep abreast of new ideas, one should not overlook the support that can be received from local, state, and national professional organizations. The American Alliance for Health, Physical Education, and Recreation has excellent materials for public information programs.

The following are examples of approaches that have been successful and can serve as guides to help develop political tactics in supporting a discipline that is a key to the well-being of our total society.

Demonstrations

Teachers should be cognizant of the fact that the public tends to support programs it sees and believes in. The active teacher will seek every opportunity to display programs that will enhance the image and understanding of physical education. Service clubs, PTAs, shopping centers, and athletic contest halftimes are excellent places for activity demonstrations to take place (Fig. 2-18). These programs provide the average student an opportunity to perform in front of an audience, a privilege usually reserved for the gifted athlete. When planning a demonstration, the teacher should follow these steps:

1. Determine a theme for the demonstration, such as "Fitness is Fun."
2. Select the participants.
3. Select activities and the order of events.
4. Arrange for rehearsals.

The arrangement of activities on a program is of prime importance. The program should consist of a wide variety of activities, beginning with a fast-moving skill and alternating tempo until the finale, which should have a flair for the spectacular. Demonstrations are most effective when they are designed for a purpose and kept short and on schedule.

As an example, a well-planned mass fitness activity of 1000 or more elementary age children can be accomplished in 6 minutes during a football game halftime. What could be more fun for the children and what better exposure can be obtained than promoting the program in front of thousands of people?

Audiovisual presentations

A slide or movie presentation displaying the physical education program and using local students and faculty as the cast is an extremely effective approach and relatively easy and inexpensive to produce. The narration describing the highlights of the film can be recorded on tape, simplifying teacher responsibilities during the program. Creating a promotional package allows for numerous presentations with but one preparation. Pictures assist in giving a more effective and exciting presentation to the audience. This is especially true when the participants are recognized as "my son!" or "my daughter!"

One of the joys of teaching is creating new and exciting activity programs. This same satisfaction can be achieved through a well-organized public relations program depicting what one is thoroughly convinced is a valuable educational experience.

Displays

A simple yet effective way to promote physical activity is to design special displays. This can be done through the use of photographs, posters, or specialized play equipment. By placing these displays in school showcases or store windows, the teacher can promote the programs to students, parents, and the

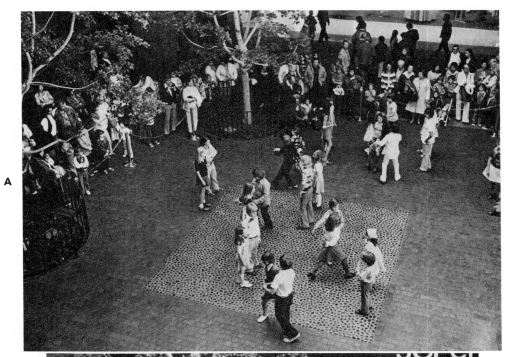

A

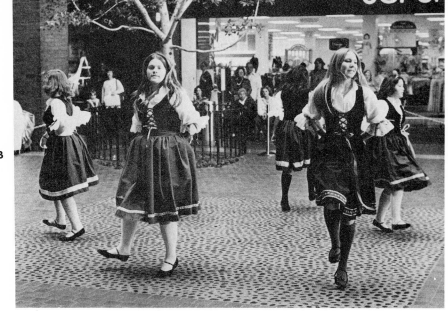

B

Fig. 2-18. Shopping center demonstrations and displays. (Courtesy Los Angeles City Schools.)

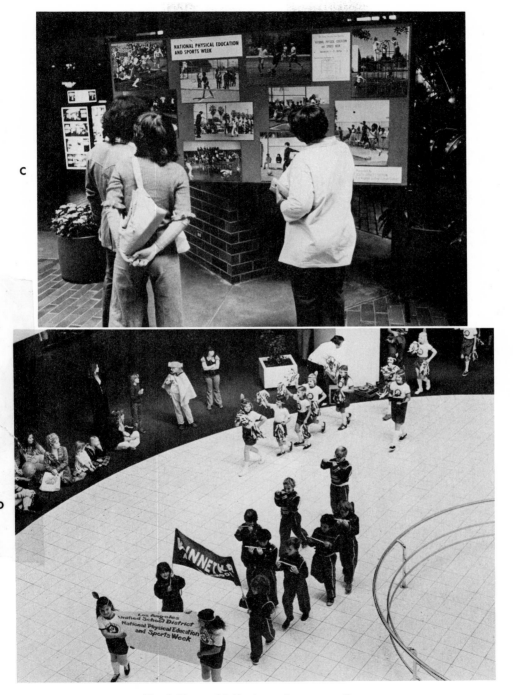

Fig. 2-18, cont'd. For legend see opposite page.

community. This approach to public relations can be an exciting student project and can be easily integrated with other subjects, such as art, history, and geography.

• • •

To summarize, teachers of physical education are important persons faced with a great number of responsibilities. When they accept these responsibilities with pride and enthusiasm, the experiences for all concerned are well worth the effort.

CLASS ACTIVITIES

1. Plan a demonstration of physical education activities for a parent meeting.
2. Observe children participating in a ball game. Select one child who is having difficulty and make recommendations for improvement based on your observation.
3. Discuss ways in which the classroom teacher can work toward excellence in increasing his or her knowledge of physical education teaching.
4. Make a collage of children participating in a variety of play activities.
5. Administer at least two of the Basic Motor Ability Test items to the class.

REFERENCES

1. Arnheim, D. D.: Area I physical activity, general stretch-ing. In Larson, L. A., editor: Encyclopedia of sport sciences and medicine, New York, 1971, The Macmillan Co.
2. Arnheim, D. D., and Sinclair, W. A.: The clumsy child, 1975, St. Louis, The C. V. Mosby Co.
3. Ayres, A. J.: Southern California sensory integrations tests, Los Angeles, 1972, Western Psychological Services.
4. Bayley, N.: Bayley scales of infant development, New York, 1969, The Psychological Corporation.
5. Canter, L.: Assertive discipline, Seal Beach, Calif., 1976, Canter and Associates.
6. Clarke, H. H.: Application of measurement to health and physical education, Englewood Cliffs, N.J., 1976, Prentice-Hall, Inc.
7. Cratty, B. J.: Movement behavior and motor learning, ed. 3, Philadelphia, 1973, Lea & Febiger.
8. Doll, E. A.: The Oseretsky test of motor performance, Minneapolis, 1946, Minnesota Educational Trust Bureau.
9. Frankenburg, W. K., and Dodds, J. B.: The Denver developmental screening test, J. Pediatr. **71:**181-191, 1967.
10. Gesell, A. L.: The first five years of a child's life, New York, 1940, Harper & Row, Publishers, Inc.
11. Godfrey, B. B., and Kephart, N. C.: Movement patterns and motor education, New York, 1969, Appleton-Century-Crofts.
12. Knapp, B.: Skill in sports, London, 1963, Routledge & Kegan Paul Ltd.
13. O'Donnell, P. A.: Motor and haptic learning, San Rafael, California, 1969, Dimensions Publishing Co.
14. Oxendine, J. B.: Psychology of motor learning, New York, 1968, Appleton-Century-Crofts.
15. Singer, R. N.: Motor learning and human performance, New York, 1968, The Macmillan Co.
16. Stott, D. H.: A general test of motor impairment for children, Dev. Med. Child Neurol. **8:**523-531, 1966.

RECOMMENDED READINGS

Canter, L.: Assertive discipline, Seal Beach, California, 1976, Canter and Associates.
Cratty, B. J.: Remedial motor activity for children, Philadelphia, 1975, Lea & Febiger.
Dauer, V. P., and Pangrazi, R.: Dynamic physical education for elementary school children, ed. 5, Minneapolis, 1975, Burgess Publishing Co.
Koontz, C. W.: Koontz child developmental program, Los Angeles, 1974, Western Psychological Services.
Siedentop, D.: Developing teaching skills in physical education, Boston, 1976, Houghton Mifflin Co.

3

Effective program management

Children benefit most from a well-planned and well-organized program of physical activities designed to meet the individual needs of each maturational level. Effective learning in physical education depends on the careful selection of the child's experiences in each grade. Organizing these experiences to provide for a safe, healthy, and interesting developmental program of physical education will do much to ensure that the outcomes of physical education are in line with established objectives. Currently, there is a trend to employ full-time physical education teachers in the elementary schools; however, this trend is progressing at a slow pace because of limited finances in school districts throughout the country. Educational systems moving in this direction have recognized the value of a sound physical education program presented by trained specialists (Fig. 3-1). Another plan is to utilize a supervisor of physical education who serves many schools and is charged with the responsibility of providing classroom teachers with current materials, methods, and techniques for conducting physical education.

Although the need for specialists in physical education is recognized by both teachers and administrators, most elementary schools are still organized on a self-contained classroom basis. Under this plan, the classroom teacher has the full responsibility of organizing the physical education program as well as the many other subject areas offered in the curriculum. Regardless of who has the responsibility for teaching physical education, the fact remains that all activities must be well planned and organized in order to meet the needs and interests of the elementary school child.

In order to achieve the stated objectives of elementary physical education as determined by the individual school or school district, a great deal of effort and deliberation must go into planning the program. Activities must be based on the needs of the children at each grade

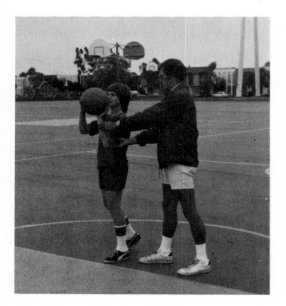

Fig. 3-1. Physical education specialist individualizes instruction.

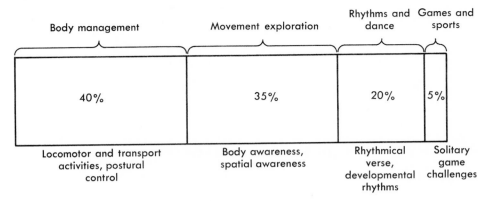

Fig. 3-2. Level 1 activity percentage chart, ages 0 to 2 years.

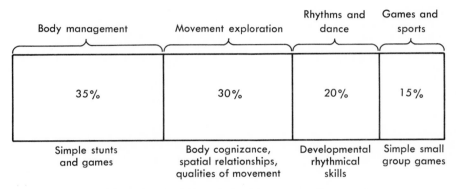

Fig. 3-3. Level 2 activity percentage chart, ages 3 to 5 years.

level. In order to determine the starting point for a physical education program, it is imperative that the teacher evaluate the current status of each child. Teachers can use the motor tests described in Chapter 2 to determine general class competencies and individual student needs.

SELECTING PHYSICAL ACTIVITIES

Before discussing specific factors involved in the selection of physical activities, we will present a classification system to provide for the proper emphasis in selecting activities. There is no unanimity among members of the physical education profession regarding such a sys-

tem. For the most part, the selection of a classification system appears to be the writer's prerogative, depending on the particular approach to teaching physical education. In this text, physical education activities are listed under four categories: body management, movement exploration, rhythms and dance, and games and sports. The accompanying charts list examples of activities provided under each category and suggest percentages for each instructional level (Figs. 3-2 to 3-5).

PLANNING THE PROGRAM

Teachers should begin planning for physical education by developing a yearly plan based on the suggested per-

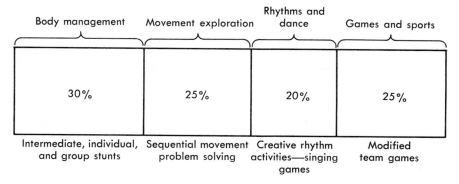

Fig. 3-4. Level 3 activity percentage chart, ages 6 to 8 years.

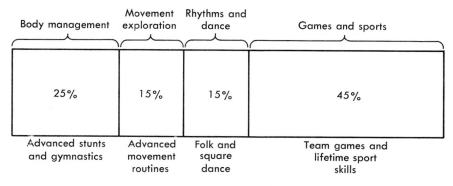

Fig. 3-5. Level 4 activity percentage chart, ages 9 to 12 years.

centages provided for specific developmental levels. This gives the teacher a point of reference from which to develop actual program activities. From this plan, the teacher should then develop monthly, weekly, and daily lessons based on the needs of a particular class. The factors of class size, activity variation, and seasonality should be considered during the selection and planning of the physical education program for each developmental level.

We have designed this text so that activities are presented by developmental levels rather than by grade levels because the abilities of children in each grade vary greatly with growth, maturation, and learning. A fifth grade teacher may find third grade activities quite appropriate

for some in the class, and, conversely, sixth or seventh grade activities may be quite appropriate for a selected few.

Class size

The size of the class determines to a large degree the amount of individual attention that can be given to the children involved. As a general rule, the class size should be commensurate with the developmental abilities and interests of the children. A regular class in physical education should have a maximum of 35 pupils, whereas a class of children with motor deficiencies should be limited to 20 or less. The adequacy of facilities, achievement level of the pupils, and special motor problems are factors to be con-

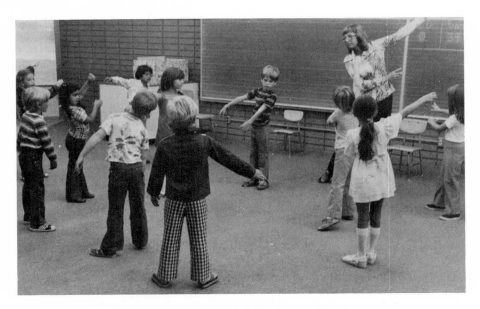

Fig. 3-6. Proper class size improves instruction.

sidered in determining class size (Fig. 3-6).

Activity variation

Physical education provides for a broad choice of activities. Teachers should be careful to include a wide variety of activities when planning the program because the games played over and over each day, month, or year may not meet the needs and interests of all the students in the class. Creating new games or modifying traditional activities adds to the joy of teaching. New activities should be presented, the proper amount of time being devoted to movement education, body management, rhythms and dance, and games and sports. Adequate time allowed for each of the categories requires careful planning to assure a program balance.

The following questions serve as guides to the selection of activities:

1. Is the activity appropriate for the needs of the children based on the preliminary evaluation?
2. Is the activity appropriate to the ability level of the children involved?
3. Are the rules simple enough to eliminate confusion during participation?
4. Have the students played a part in selecting the activity to be learned?
5. Have the students achieved the foundation skills necessary for successful performance in the activity being presented?
6. Are there opportunities for children to develop creativity in movement activities?

Seasonality

Proper attention given to fall, winter, spring, and even summer activities will aid in presenting a program that is conducive to development of an interest in physical education. In areas where seasonal climatic conditions affect participation in certain activities, the physical education program should be planned so that outdoor activities are offered during the best weather conditions. Teachers should also plan their program in line with national sport seasons; attempting to teach children softball skills during the fall does little to develop interest and enthusiasm when football and soccer are in season. Custom and feasibility should

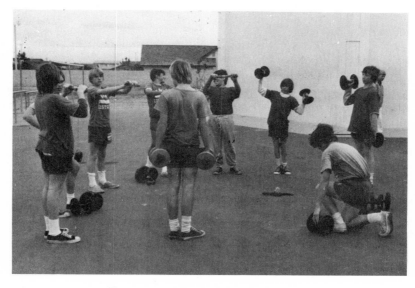

Fig. 3-7. Meeting the physical objective.

play a major part in the selection of activities based on seasonality.

MEETING THE OBJECTIVES OF PHYSICAL EDUCATION

Program activities should be selected in line with their contributions toward the general objectives of physical development, knowledge and understanding, and attitude and appreciation. Each activity considered should be reviewed in respect to its contribution to the developmental outcomes described in Chapter 1. Neglect of a review of this nature often allows only a limited approach to child development through physical activity. A review of the contributions of each activity toward the objectives of physical education will aid the teacher in providing a balanced program at all levels (Fig. 3-7).

Skills for leisure

Activities offered in the instructional program should be utilized in extra class hours and other leisure-time hours. Many activities are acceptable because of their immediate developmental value. How- .

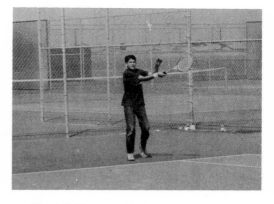

Fig. 3-8. Developing lifetime sport skills.

ever, there should be concern for teaching skills that can be used for maintaining good health and personal satisfaction in adult life. A strong foundation in movement patterns and elementary game skills can set the stage for learning and enjoyment in the more sophisticated sport activities during the adult years (Fig. 3-8). The ability to successfully take part in lifetime sports leads to continued enjoyment and participation in physical activity. Learning skills well enough to play actively encourages individuals to reach the fitness goals so much needed in our sedentary life. (See Chapter 10.)

Feasibility

In selecting activities for the physical education program, the teacher should also consider the feasibility of the activity considered. Such things as adequate time allowances, the availability of proper facilities, and the confidence and ability of the instructor should all be considered before an activity is selected. Attempting to present activities when these three factors have not been properly provided for will usually result in a poor teaching-learning situation that can transform a normally safe and exciting activity into one that is hazardous and uninteresting to the children.

Identifiable needs

Teachers must identify the needs of the children at each developmental level if they are to plan effectively. This can be accomplished through personal observation by the teacher and through a sound program of evaluation. After testing the students, teachers have the opportunity to take students from the point at which they find them to as far as they can go within their own individual and group capabilities. This manner of teaching allows children to achieve levels of skill in physical education that are within their own individual potentials. With the needs of the individuals and group so determined, the teacher will then be able to prescribe a developmental program that will have meaning and be within the capacities of the children (Fig. 3-9).

Program integration and transfer

There are many physically active games that can aid pupils in the classroom subjects of reading, spelling, and mathematics. The blending of body movement

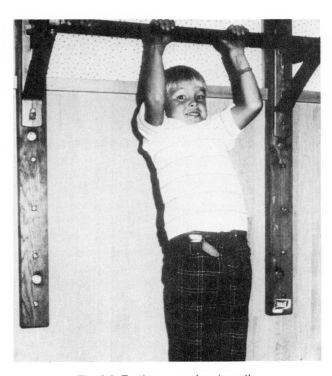

Fig. 3-9. Testing muscular strength.

with academic learning provides great motivational assistance and encourages children to learn cognitive skills without the realization that this type of learning is taking place. Teachers of special education find that motor activities coupled with cognitive activities are of particular value in teaching those children who have learning difficulties. The repetition often found in game situations extends the learning period and enables many children to achieve a specific goal through repeated practice in a fun situation. (See Chapter 12.)

The integration of physical education with other subjects in the school can do much to enhance the total education of the child. Social studies, language arts, music, art, mathematics, science, and in-

dustrial arts afford many opportunities for integration with physical education in the education of the child. A geography lesson can come alive as children participate in a native dance of the country being studied. Encouraging children to write about or describe their favorites sports in an English class might well be the motivating factor necessary to achieve success. A project in a woodshop class can increase the physical education equipment inexpensively; balance boards, stilts, and jumping standards are practical items that can be constructed and used directly in the physical education program. There is no better subject area than that of physical education to discover how the human body functions. Children in a science class can better understand the

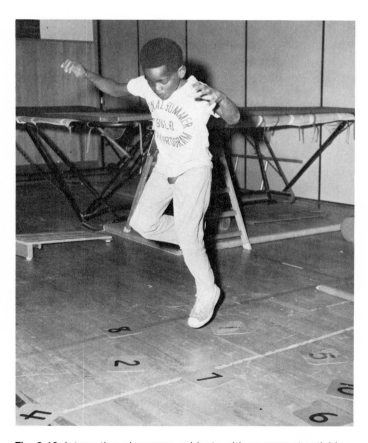

Fig. 3-10. Integrating classroom subjects with movement activities.

values of exercise as they develop charts and graphs on which are recorded their own heart and respiration rates. Projects can develop into interesting discussions regarding growth and development and the maintenance of good health. Sports and games are ideal topics for the art lesson. Posters made by children in an art class make wonderful displays on bulletin boards and often tell a story in a more meaningful way that children understand.

Teachers responsible for physical education should make every effort to integrate physical education with other school subjects whenever possible. Greater participation, interest, and enthusiasm can be generated when the child becomes physically and mentally involved in learning (Fig. 3-10).

Activity progression

In order for children to learn effectively, skills must be developed step by step, one forming a basis for the next. Children must have a good foundation before more advanced skills can be taught. Lessons should have continuity, showing a gradual progression from simple to more complex skills. Children must first be taught fundamental locomotor skills before they can succeed in a game utilizing these skills. Lead-up games comprising individual basic skills, such as around the world, in which the shooting skill required for basketball is developed, should be learned prior to participation in sophisticated official sports and games, such as basketball (Fig. 3-11). Part Four offers progression in a variety of activities and skills so that teachers can present them in a logical order in relation to degree of difficulty.

PROGRAMMING FOR EFFECTIVE TEACHING

In order to provide the most efficient learning situation, teachers of physical education should be familiar with various types of grouping techniques. Grouping pupils is essential in developing a good program of physical education; it provides for a sequential progression of experiences, permits students of equal ability to be together, allows for individual instruction, and provides leadership experience for many children.

For certain activities, the teacher might wish to work with the class as a whole, or in other situations, it might be more desirable to divide the class into smaller groups. The teacher might accomplish this by numbering the children from one to four, or whatever number of groups is desired and then combining the same numbers into groups. The class can also be divided by allowing the children to select their own team members, which is one method of equalizing competition.

The squad system is a very desirable type of organization for the physical education period because it is a controlled yet free program that offers opportunities for child planning, child leadership, and child appraisal. Although the squad system is often looked on as a traditional approach to class organization, the creative teacher can use this system for purposes of individualizing instruction. Since the class is already grouped, this organization allows for greater freedom than might result from presenting the same activities to the total class.

Because of the social immaturity of many children, it is necessary to develop a progressive system of squad selection to eliminate the placing of a heavy burden of responsibility on some children too early in their development. Some classes will be ready to achieve squad organization and will be able to bypass the first or the first and second progressions. It is the teacher's responsibility to determine the starting point on the basis of the maturity, readiness, and ability of the class.

The following system of squad organization has proved to be a successful method of class organization (Fig. 3-12).[2]

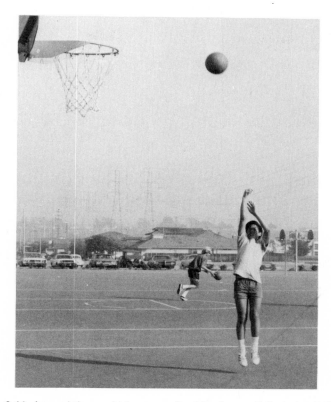

Fig. 3-11. Around the world is an excellent lead-up activity to basketball.

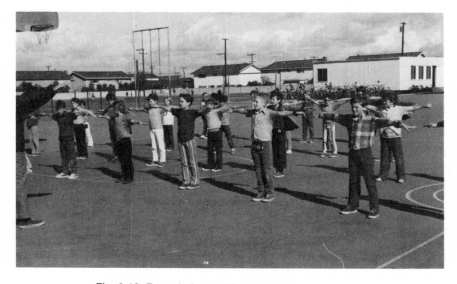

Fig. 3-12. Extended squad formation for warm-ups.

PROGRESSION 1

1. The teacher appoints squad leaders and selects squad members at 3- to 4-week intervals.
2. Squads are assigned to a leader; the leader and the group remain together during the physical education period.
3. During the activity period, the teacher may assign a familiar game on a daily basis; each squad leader is responsible for selecting the equipment.
4. The teacher assigns an activity space to each squad leader; the game and the equipment remain in the assigned location during the time devoted to play.
5. When all squads are ready to play, the teacher gives the signal to begin.
6. After adequate playing time has been allowed, the teacher gives the signal to stop. The children form a line in front of their squad leaders, with the leaders facing the squads, after which a signal to move to the next playing area is given by the teacher. The squad leaders lead their groups, in line, to the next activity, rotating in one direction only. Changes should continue every 5 to 10 minutes, depending on the difficulty of the game, until each squad has participated in all activities planned. First grade children are often not capable of any further squad progression.

PROGRESSION 2

1. The children elect squad leaders.
2. Each squad leader chooses his or her own squad members.
3. The teacher assigns the game and the play space as indicated in progression 1.
4. Each squad begins to play when ready.
5. At the teacher's signal, all squads rotate as indicated in progression 1.

PROGRESSION 3

1. The children elect squad leaders.
2. Each squad leader chooses his or her squad members.
3. Each squad leader selects the game for the day, the choice of the activity being made in the classroom.
4. At the teacher's signal, the squads prepare to rotate as before. This time the squad leaders do not move with their groups but act as leaders of the same games for each succeeding squad. Each squad moves informally rather than in a line to the next activity. The teacher may wish to appoint an assistant squad leader to aid in controlling the group, thereby affording additional opportunities for leadership.

PROGRESSION 4

1. Each child chooses which game to play by standing in front of the squad leader of that particular game and in the place where the game is to take place. If the squad is filled with the maximum number possible, the leader sends the extra children to another squad.
2. Each squad starts to play when the size limit has been reached.
3. At the teacher's signal to stop, each squad lines up in front of the squad leader.
4. At the signal for rotation, the children may go to any game they have not played that day and follow the same procedure as before.

PROGRESSION 5

All steps are similar to those in progression 4 except that a class leader is chosen at the time the other squad leaders are selected, and it is this person's responsibility to give the signal to stop playing, to change squads, or to aid in any way the class agrees on. In the primary grades, class leaders should be rotated on a daily basis to provide a greater number of opportunities for leadership and to eliminate the possibility of one child's being deprived of the opportunity to participate in the games.

• • •

The teacher may wish to experiment to determine the progression of squad organization for which the class is ready. Since the degree of maturity is generally observable, the teacher should be able to select the point at which the class is prepared to begin. It is possible that a class may be ready for one phase of a progression but may not be mature enough to use it in its entirety. In the upper grade levels, squads may be maintained for a longer period of time. Periods of 4 to 6 weeks are suggested as team games are introduced and longer units of instruction are necessary. In order to prevent the problem of having one child always selected last and to alleviate favoritism, the teacher and the squad leaders should meet away from the class so that the children will not know in which order they have been chosen. In coeducational situations, the selection should be made by alternating a boy and then a girl. In order to be more fair, the direction of the choices by the squad leaders should be reversed after each round; for example, with four squads, number four would make the fifth choice and number one squad would make the eighth and ninth choices. Squad leaders can help by maintaining control of their own team members and also can assist the teacher in a variety of routine procedures during the period, such as checking out equipment, taking roll, and helping to plan the daily lesson. Sound squad organization should allow for maximum time utilization and child participation during the physical education period.

It is the teacher who makes the squad system work in ways that will promote creative, interesting, and exciting lessons. If viewed in this manner, it is a method of class organization that can be appropriate for a variety of approaches to teaching physical education.

EQUALIZING COMPETITION THROUGH A HANDICAP SYSTEM

As an alternative to ability grouping, handicapping allows children to achieve success regardless of skill level. Adults have successfully used the handicap system in golf and bowling for many years. the system allows individuals of different skill levels to compete against each other on an equal basis. Physical educators can adapt this method to program planning and ensure fun, fitness, and individual challenges for all elementary students through well-designed activity organization.

While a creative teacher can adapt a variation of this idea in many ways, the following examples of equalizing competition among students of varying skill levels are offered:

Level 1 equals the well-skilled child
Level 2 equals the average-skilled child
Level 3 equals the poorly skilled child

Basketball: Level 1 players must shoot from a farther distance than lower level players for the score to count.

50-yard dash: Level 2 players start 5 yards closer to the finish line. Level 3 players start 10 yards closer.

Dodge ball: Level 1 players are allowed one hit before leaving the circle. Level 2 players are allowed two hits while level 3 players get three hits before having to leave. If level 2 or 3 players are in the winning group twice, these children move up one classification. Colored ribbon or numbers can be used to denote handicap levels and to aid in the identification of the participants.

Although this system is designed for the normal child, it also follows the mainstreaming philosophy of a program for the atypical.

SELECTING STUDENT LEADERS

It is the role of the teachers to provide maximum opportunities for children to experience leadership; however, child leadership is not automatic but must be planned for and taught. Bookwalter aptly states that in developing pupil leadership, the following principles should be applied:

1. Duties must be mutually understood by teacher, leader, and pupils.
2. Full performance of duties must be expected.
3. Authority must accompany the responsibility of leadership.
4. The leader must be acceptable to the group.
5. The leader must be democratic, not autocratic.
6. The leader must guide by example rather than precept.
7. The leader must be positive (implementing) rather than negative (inhibiting) in approach.
8. Satisfactions rather than annoyances must ensue.
9. Creativity potential must be developed.
10. Slower individuals must be encouraged and developed.
11. Superior individuals must be encouraged to attain their capacities.
12. Alternate leadership and followership experiences should be provided.
13. Self-direction and self-expression of all must be promoted.
14. Socially sound standards of behavior must be inculcated.
15. Help in meeting individual needs more fully must be provided.[1]

Leadership experiences should be progressive in nature; teachers should assign small responsibilities that the child is capable of completing successfully prior to an assignment as an assistant or squad leader. Opportunities to report attendance, act as an assistant in group games or stunts, help the teacher record test scores, and perform other assigned duties can help the child develop the ability to serve others and achieve self-realization compatible with the goals of physical education (Fig. 3-13).

Peer teaching

The use of more talented children in a class to lead and teach skills to their peer group can be an effective way of teaching physical education. Children are often motivated by the abilities of the better skilled boys and girls in the class, and their attention and interest are often increased through this approach to learning. The use of physically gifted students to aid the teacher in presenting a physical education lesson can allow for more indi-

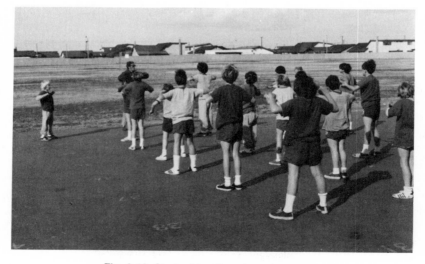

Fig. 3-13. Student leading class exercises.

vidualized instruction and can provide greater opportunities for small-group participation. Peer teaching can be effectively utilized at all levels but should be supervised carefully to ensure that proper techniqu s in both skill and safety are provided (Fig. 3-14).

Don't be afraid to give children responsibility in leading activity lessons. The teacher is often surprized by the ability of young children to lead class activities in a very efficient manner. In many cases, some discipline problems can be eliminated by having children experience leadership responsibilities in the different position of peer teacher. By selecting children who can successfully serve in this capacity, the teacher is able to devise numerous organizational designs that will give greater flexibility and interest in a variety of physical education activities.

Cross-age teaching

Another method that has been successful in the elementary physical education program is that of utilizing the talents of students in the upper grades during the activity period. In this approach, students from a nearby high school or junior high school work under the supervision of an individual responsible for the physical education program. Many of these stu-

dents indicate an interest in the teaching profession and welcome the opportunity to work with younger children. Such a cooperative venture between the schools involved provides an in-service approach to planning and presenting physical education activities. The supervisor of physical education first develops the master program and then assigns each student to a group of elementary school children. The students work with their assigned groups in developing a particular skill or game activity. The utilization of a large number of older students in the teaching-learning situation allows for much individual attention to the group involved and provides a close relationship between teacher and child (Fig. 3-15).

Some schools using this plan have devised a schedule whereby one period of physical education is offered in the morning and one in the afternoon. Half of the class attends during the morning session and the remaining half of the children participate during the afternoon. One of

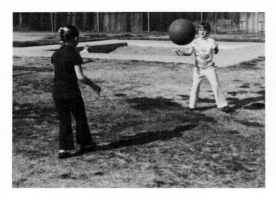

Fig. 3-14. Peer teaching.

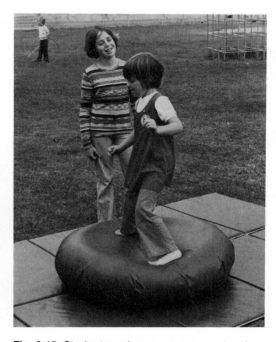

Fig. 3-15. Student serving as a cross-age teacher.

the concomitant values of this approach is that the regular teacher has two periods during the day in which work can be accomplished with a class that is half the size of the normal enrollment. This allows the teacher to give more small-group and individual instruction in the classroom in areas of reading and other subjects than would be possible under the regular program.

The response to this approach to teaching physical education has been quite favorable on the part of both the children and the student aides who act as teachers. Each student aide has the opportunity to evaluate, plan, and participate with the children in his or her group. The possi-

bilities for teaching physical education under this plan are unlimited, but the use of this technique depends heavily on the availability of high school or upper grade students. It should be mentioned that children from the upper elementary grades also have participated in this program with some degree of success.

USING VOLUNTEER PARENT GROUPS

Utilization of parents as aides during the physical education period also has been a successful approach, particularly in the primary grades. Many school districts have parents serve as aides in the

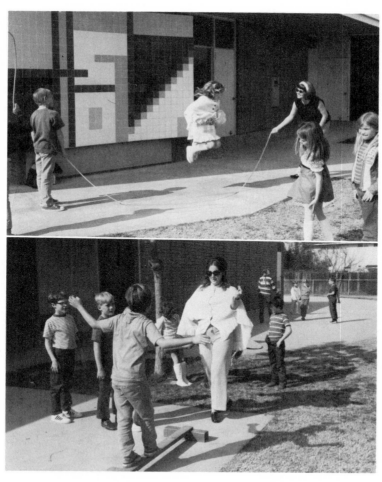

Fig. 3-16. Parents help children develop skills through small group instruction.

cafeteria, attendance office, and classroom. There is no reason why these same parents cannot help to lower the student-teacher ratio in a physical education activity lesson. In many instances, parents can be found who have a physical education background, are highly skilled, and thoroughly enjoy the challenge of teaching skills to children in elementary school. Small-group instruction in selected games or perceptual-motor activities involving balance, coordination, and object manipulation can easily be presented by community lay personnel with minimal orientation. Interested parents can help the teacher develop basic motor skill and self-testing activities after a brief in-service training program (Fig. 3-16). The following suggestions should aid in the development of a successful program:

1. Heterogeneous groups are usually more successful, since the less skilled students often mimic or model the skill patterns of the better students.
2. The children should have readable name tags, and each group should have a color code to aid in class organization and control.
3. A list of sequential directions should be provided for the parents, stating specific skills to stress.
4. A ratio of no more than six children to each parent should be maintained.
5. A teacher should be in charge but be free to circulate between stations to assist children and parents and offer positive reinforcement.

Some ideas for skill stations in which parents can help are as follows:

1. Obstacle course (old tires, cones, and boxes that may be worked in with permanent playground equipment)
2. Ball-handling skills (catching, throwing, bouncing, dribbling, and kicking)
3. Beanbags
4. Balance board
5. Walking beam
6. Jump rope
7. Stilts
8. Hula-Hoop
9. Small group games

HOW TO INDIVIDUALIZE

In order to individualize instruction it is necessary to organize the class in a manner that lowers the student-teacher ratio. In some cases this results in a one-to-one teaching-learning situation. Many teachers are able to accomplish this through the squad system and use of group leaders. Others rely on parent volunteers, cross-age tutors, peer teaching, team teaching, or teacher aides. Whichever the case, the value of individualized instruction rests with the added specific practice received for a definite purpose. Individualized instruction promotes the affective as well a the psychomotor domain through successful accomplishments of specific skills. Effective individualized instruction requires a thorough knowledge of the skill to be learned, the identification of children who are either limited or gifted in the skill, and the organization and presentation of challenges necessary to meet specific needs.

ESTABLISHING CLASS ROUTINES

In order for the teacher to maintain control and the children to feel secure, effective organization of the physical education period requires the establishment of certain class routines. Such things as distribution of equipment, movement from the classroom to the play area, and certain class formations should all be consistent. Once these procedures have been learned, they should be unvarying from day to day so that as much time as possible can be devoted to the activity. The formation selected might be a line, a circle, squads, or an informal sitting position. If the routines are taught properly, the children will be able to go to the play area and return with little or no supervision. It is advantageous at the end of the activity period to meet the children in a group in order to give them opportunities to evaluate the day's lesson. Often this brief culminating activity is filled with teachable moments. It is also an excellent time for the teacher to make sure that no one is injured and to check on all equipment prior to returning to the classroom. Each teacher should develop procedures for collecting equipment, getting drinks, using the lavatory, and changing clothes, keeping the best interests of the children in mind for each individual situation.

The following is a list of suggestions to be considered in organizing for physical education:

1. Establish a designated activity area and class formation in which each physical education class begins.
2. Involve children in motor activity as soon as possible.
3. Make sure that all children have an opportunity to participate in the activity selected.
4. Provide enough equipment so that no child will have to wait for a turn to participate.
5. Include a physical fitness component in each lesson presented.
6. Allow creativity to occur regardless of the lesson presented.
7. Provide leadership opportunities for each child in the class through a rotation system.
8. Explain rules and diagrams in the classroom prior to going to the play area.
9. Develop a system in which equipment is taken to and from the play area in an efficient manner.
10. Establish a consistent method of moving the group to the play area and returning with minimal disruption to other classes.

Lesson planning

Adequate planning is necessary if the teacher is to present a sound physical education program in line with the goals and objectives discussed in Chapter 1. Teachers of physical education should have a yearly, monthly, weekly, and daily plan for activity. In developing the lesson plan, teachers must be aware of the objectives that the children are to achieve and what kinds of experiences will meet these objectives. The physical education program should be planned from kindergarten through the twelfth grade so that there are a variety of experiences that are not duplicated from year to year. Unless teachers understand what has been

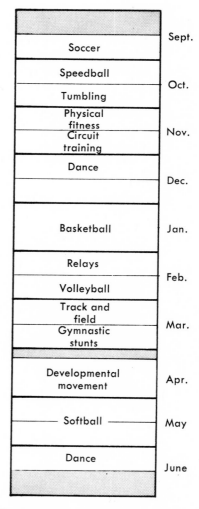

Fig. 3-17. Yearly activity plan for level 4.

learned prior to the grade level currently being taught and what is to come afterward, they will find effective planning increasingly difficult. From the yearly, monthly, or other time block plan, the teacher should be able to develop complete activity units within specific areas of instruction. We have included a sample yearly plan to demonstrate how broad planning relates to the areas of physical education (Fig. 3-17). The weekly plan sets the guidelines for what is to be offered to the students during this period of time (Fig. 3-18). This gives the teacher an opportunity to specifically view the program activities designed for the week. The daily plan is the most specific and provides the teacher with a guide for time allotment, teaching procedures, and suggested formations (Fig. 3-19). After each day's lesson, the teacher should evaluate the successes and failures of the class in order to determine the pace and direction for the following day. It is not always possible to determine that the activities suggested in the plan will be successful when put into practice; therefore, teachers should be flexible and be prepared to make changes in the daily plan of activities that might be more appropriate for

A

	Week No. 1	Week No. 2	Week No. 3	Week No. 4
Monday	Testing	Hokey Pokey Singing games Head, shoulders, knees, and toes	Testing Throwing and striking skills	Basic ball skills (exploration method)
Tuesday	Angels in the snow Shadow pictures Locomotor skills	Simple stunts Crab walk Alphabet Greet the toe	Locomotor challenges Beanbag target throw	Relaxation Wigwag game
Wednesday	Forty ways to get there (mimicry) Reflective activities	Leap frog Over and under Relay with beanbag Chicken Fat record	Lummi sticks Hammer Rhythm challenges Finger play	Singing games Looby Loo London Bridge
Thursday	Hula-Hoop activities Hoop on ground Personal space	Follow me (imagery) Movement exploration activities	Balloon play Volley and hit Working in pairs	Jump rope rhymes and challenges Tin can stilts
Friday	Simple relays using basic locomotor skills	Obstacle course and fitness challenges	Ladder toss Picking daisies Circle pass	Wall dodge Basic ball skills Throwing

B

	Week No. 1	Week No. 2	Week No. 3	Week No. 4
Monday	Review kicking and catching skills	Practice underhand and overhand throw Play overtake ball	Practice fielding fly balls Play work-up	Softball tournament
Tuesday	Review rules Play base kickball	Practice base running Play beatball	Play work-up	Softball tournament
Wednesday	Review force-out rule Play base kickball	Practice batting skills Introduce work-up	Play work-up	Softball tournament
Thursday	Review double-play Play base kickball	Practice pitching skills Play work-up	Introduce softball Play softball	Softball tournament
Friday	Play base kickball	Practice fielding ground balls Play work-up	Play softball	Softball tournament

Fig. 3-18. A, Weekly activity plan for level 2. **B,** Weekly activity plan for level 4.

Name of game: *Nation Ball*   Date: *Nov. 17th*
Behavorial objective: *To dodge, catch, a throw a ball accurately.*
Developmental goal: *Endurance, strategy, agility*
Space and equipment: *Rectangular court with center line*
Time allotment: *25 minutes*

Activities	Teacher procedure	Formations	Comments
2 minutes warm-up	*Have class leader give regular warm-up activities*	*Extended squad formation*	
5 minutes Practice throwing skills	*See that children throw ball properly in preparation for game; give individual help where needed.*	*Corner formation*	*Keep eye on target and follow through*
3 minutes Explain Nation Ball rules	*Keep explanation simple; place class in game situation as soon as possible.*	*Informal*	
12 minutes Play Nation Ball	*officiate game*		
3 minutes Review the lesson and cool down.	*Evaluate the play of the class and check equipment*	*Informal*	

Fig. 3-19. Daily lesson plan for level 4.

successful learning within the abilities of the children.

Planning with children

Children should have every opportunity to help the teacher plan the physical education period. When children help develop routines, suggest needed practice for certain skills, and determine the best way to check out equipment, the program takes on a deeper meaning. Planning can be fun and children will have greater interest when involved in curriculum development. By selecting games and dances, building much

needed equipment, and being involved in general overall planning, students can play a greater part in the educational process. Often the teacher finds children suggesting activities that integrate with other subject areas or have greater appeal than what was originally designed.

Formations

A modern physical education playground will have a variety of circles, straight lines, rectangles, and other figures painted on the activity surface. These permanent lines are helpful to the teacher in organizing the class and are of benefit to any physical education facility. In addition to this, specific formations are needed to provide adequate learning experiences. The following formations are suggested for use in teaching a variety of physical education activities.

Circle. One of the best ways to form a circle is to have the children take positions on a circular marking on the playground or gymnasium floor. If no markings are available, the teacher may take the hand of the first child in a straight line and walk around until he or she joins hands with the person at the end of the line, or the children may join hands by themselves to form the circle. This formation is required in a variety of games of low organization, elementary dances, and warm-up exercises (Fig. 3-20).

Shuttle formation. The shuttle formation (Fig. 3-21) is excellent for practicing handoffs or passing-type skills. It can also be used for certain types of relays, since it allows children to execute a skill and return to their original positions after all have had a turn.

Corner formation. The corner formation (Fig. 3-22) is designed for throwing and catching skills. It also allows the teacher to rotate and instruct the different groups participating in the activity while maintaining a good supervisory position.

Zigzag formation. The zigzag formation (Fig. 3-23) can be used for throwing and

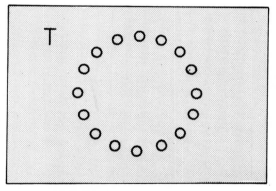

Fig. 3-20. Circle formation.

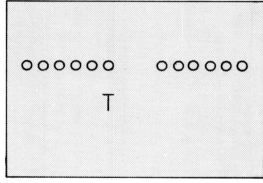

Fig. 3-21. Shuttle formation.

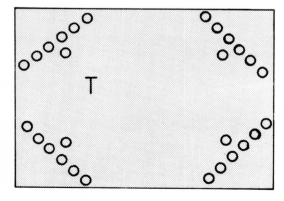

Fig. 3-22. Corner formation.

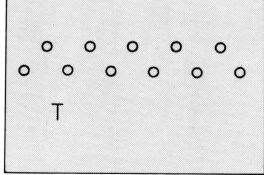

Fig. 3-23. Zigzag formation.

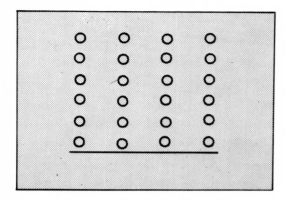

Fig. 3-24. Relay formation.

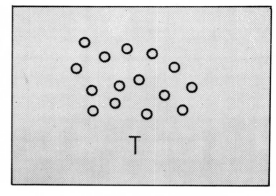

Fig. 3-25. Informal scatter formation.

kicking skills. It works best for small groups.

Opposing lines. This formation is used in many lead-up games and allows the class to be divided into two teams.

Relay formation. If the class is organized into squads, they are already in the relay formation (Fig. 3-24). Little or no movement should be necessary to begin a relay activity.

Informal formation. For creative activities or when no formal positioning is necessary, children are asked only to arrange themselves in a manner in which they cannot reach out and touch their neighbor (Fig. 3-25).

TEACHER'S SIGNALS

A physical education lesson may vary from creative movement to formalized skill development.

Regardless of the type of lesson presented, it is necessary that each teacher develop some type of starting and stopping signal. This signal is used in getting the attention of the children so they can listen for directions. It also helps the teacher establish the control necessary for any lesson to be successful and safe.

When teaching a movement education lesson in which childen are freely moving about an area, if the instructor wishes to give further directions, a signal that can be easily heard and has a specific meaning, such as "freeze," can be used. Children learn to enjoy signals and react quickly to the command presented. In other situations in which activity is of a quiet nature, the teacher may snap the fingers or clap hands to start or stop an activity. A combination of a finger snap to begin and the word "freeze" to stop gives the children an understanding of what is expected of them at each command.

A whistle has long been the symbol of the physical education teacher. It is an excellent piece of equipment for use in the physical education class; however, it should be used sparingly and must convey a specific meaning to the children. When the teacher blows the whistle, it should be done with authority, and it should indicate that all activities must stop, play equipment must be held, and all children must look in the direction of the teacher for further instructions. In the upper elementary grades, the whistle is used for officiating game activities. It should be noted that if whistles are provided by the school, there should be adequate means of sterilizing the mouthpieces.

MOTIVATIONAL AIDS

Each school should be well supplied with illustrated *booklets* of various sports and game activities. A reading table with these kinds of materials can be set up in the classroom in addition to the volumes in the library.

Bulletin boards can provide the children with an opportunity to collect pictures and drawings of in-season athletic performances. Photographs and articles from magazines and sports pages of newspapers can be used for this purpose. In addition to being used for displaying these materials, bulletin boards can be used for posting activity schedules, individual skill records, and self-testing charts. Materials can be arranged in an attractive, interesting, and colorful manner. Displays should be changed weekly so that children will be encouraged to look at the bulletin board.

Motion pictures and *slides* are excellent for introducing new activities to the class. Many companies provide a variety of filmstrips and cartridge movies for use in the instructional program (see Appendix); however, some teachers prefer to make their own slides or movies of performances that often are more appropriate for specific situations. Video tape recordings can also be used for this purpose.

Learning resource center

Each teacher of physical education should encourage the principal or building leader to provide audiovisual materials that can be viewed in a learning resource center. Film loops depicting correct skill movements and slide presentations and audio tapes of historical sports events or outstanding amateur and professional competitors should be available for children to view and hear. Material of this nature, as well as collages and pictures of athletic events and special competitions, may be available in the classroom or library setting. By using audiovisual presentations the teacher can often motivate children to greater performance levels and encourage the slower learner to seek higher degrees of

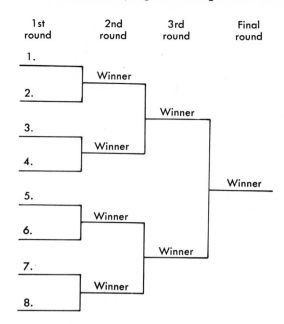

Fig. 3-26. Elimination tournament.

skill. There is no reason why sports and game activities should not be presented in the resource center with material on other learning areas.

Tournaments

Tournaments are excellent motivational aids and stimulate the interest and enthusiasm of children in the upper elementary grades. They are more often thought of as being in the extraclass program; however, they can be a valuable part of the instructional program, particularly during the team sports units. The type of tournament selected depends on the amount of time available, the type of activity, and the number of teams or individuals involved. Teachers should select the tournament that best complements the class activity.

Elimination tournament. A single-elimination tournament is the easiest and quickest way to arrive at a winner (Fig. 3-26). It is best used when there are a large number of teams, limited facilities,

Round 1	Round 2	Round 3	Round 4	Round 5
1-6	1-5	1-4	1-3	1-2
2-5	6-4	5-3	4-2	3-6
3-4	2-3	6-2	5-6	4-5

Fig. 3-27. Round robin tournament.

and a short period of time to complete the tournament. If the number of teams of individuals entered equals a power of two, such as 2, 4, 8, 16, or 32, it is not necessary to have any byes, but if the number of teams or individuals does not equal a power of 2, then the next higher power of 2 must be selected to complete the first round. The number of byes is determined by taking the next higher power of 2 and subtracting the number of teams involved; for example, if 9 teams are competing, there will be 7 byes in the first round: the next higher power of 2 after 9 is 16, and subtracting 9 from 16 leaves 7. Teams drawing byes are automatically placed in the second round.

Round robin tournament. This tournament has the advantage of offering maximum participation when time and facilities permit; it is the most satisfactory method of organization. The winner is the team that has the greatest number of wins after playing all the other teams. Numbers should be substituted for the names of teams or players to simplify the rotation in a robin tournament. There will always be one less round than there are teams entered in the tournament; for example, six teams would yield five rounds. The numbers of the teams should be written in sequence in a counterclockwise direction as indicated in Fig. 3-27. Team number one should be held stationary while the rest of the teams are rotated one position in a counterclockwise direction for each round. At the end of five rounds, all teams will have had the opportunity to compete against one another. If the number of teams is uneven, add a bye and follow the same procedure as outlined

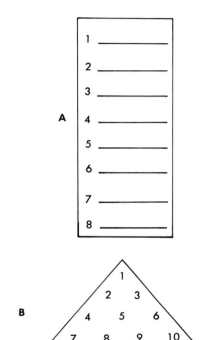

Fig. 3-28. A, Ladder tournament. **B,** Pyramid tournament.

previously. After the schedule is completed, team names may be substituted for the numbers.

Ladder or pyramid tournaments. Ladder tournaments provide continuous competition and are best used for individual or dual activities. The object is to climb to the top of the ladder or pyramid and remain in that position until the tournament is completed. The names of players or teams are listed separately on cards or tags and arranged on the rungs of the ladder by chance. One advantage the ladder or pyramid tournament is that it

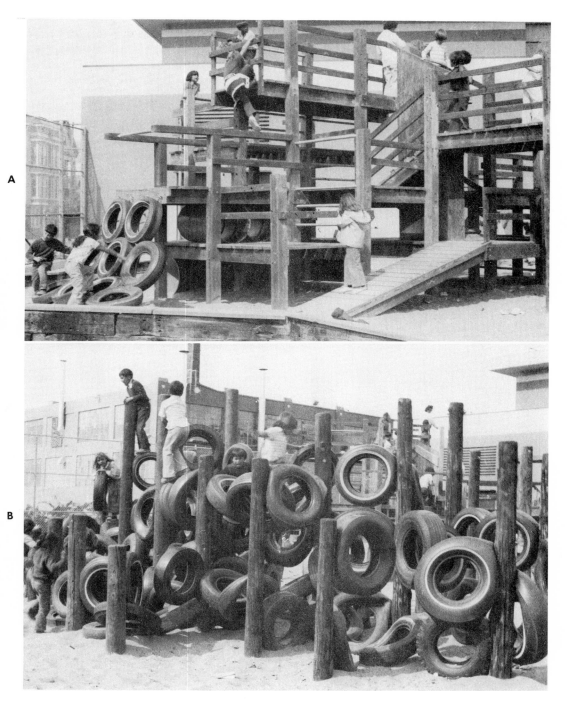

Fig. 3-29. Imaginative play areas encourage participation.

takes little supervision, since the students usually arrange their own matches and report the results. In a ladder tournament a player may challenge only the first or second player immediately above his or her own name. If the higher player wins, they remain in their original positions, but if the challenger wins, they exchange positions on the ladder. Pyramid tournament players may challenge any team or individual on the row directly above them or in the same row directly to their left (Fig. 3-28).

Although there are many other types of tournaments, the ones just described are most commonly used in elementary schools.

FACILITIES

Modern construction technology augmented by creative design has made it possible to develop physical education facilities that are esthetically pleasing,

functional for a variety of activities, and economically sound. For the most part, indoor physical education facilities are specific in nature; however, they often serve more than one purpose, ranging from an auditorium to a gymnasium. Today, most experts agree that multipurpose use of activity space is a realistic concept and one that aids in the justification of financial expenditures.

When planning physical education buildings, individuals must be willing to consider new designs and materials such as the cable-tent structure or the air bubble concept. Using these new construction techniques, costs can be kept relatively low compared to the traditional physical education structure.

Physical education facilities should be well planned and provide attractive play areas (Figs. 3-29). Adequate space is important to the success of the program and should be designed to place few limitations on the type of activities that can be

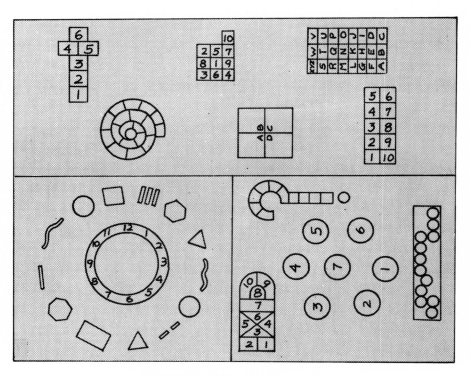

Fig. 3-30. Multipurpose play area.

offered. It is a sound policy to seek professional advice when planning a new structure. Combining this help with the physical education teacher's description of the functional use of the area should result in a team approach to building that will meet economic standards without sacrificing activity space. Creative design encourages innovative program development in both indoor and outdoor activities.

Outdoor facilities

The American Association for Health, Physical Education, and Recreation recommends that there be a minimum of 5 acres of land plus 1 additional acre for each 100 children in an elementary school. Part of the play area near the school buildings should be blacktop and be large enough to accommodate basketball and volleyball courts with enough open space for games of low organization (Fig. 3-30). The remaining area should be of natural or artificial turf with fields marked for football, soccer, and softball activities. Lines burned in natural turf by an asphalt-base liquid will usually last the length of a sport season, eliminating continual marking.

Primary play area

A separate small playing area should be set aside for the younger children. Climbing apparatus, slides, sandboxes, and other selected equipment are placed in this area. Fencing off the area provides a safe play space and helps to prevent injury from activities participated in by older children. Fig. 3-31 is an example of an outdoor primary physical education facility.

Indoor facilities

Indoor facilities may range from the grade-level classroom or multipurpose room to the professionally designed gymnasium. The indoor facility should be free from protruding objects and should have permanent floor markings painted in bright colors. Separate locker rooms with complete facilities for boys and girls should be located adjacent to the gymnasium. Adequate storage is necessary for proper maintenance of equipment and supplies. Specific designs of physical education facilities may be found in the following publications:

1. Planning areas and facilities for health, physical education, and recreation: Athletic Institute, Merchandise Mart, Chicago, Ill. 60654 and American Association for Health, Physical Education, and Recreation, 1201 Sixteenth St., N.W., Washington, D.C. 20036.
2. Equipment and supplies for athletics, physical education, and recreation: Athletic Institute, Merchandise Mart, Chicago, Ill. 60654 and American Association for Health, Physical Education, and Recreation, 1201 Sixteenth St., N.W., Washington, D.C. 20036.
3. School sight analysis and development: California State Department of Education, 721 Capitol Mall, Sacramento, Calif. 95814.
4. Facilities and space allocations for physical education: Outdoor teaching stations for elementary and intermediate public schools, Bulletin 40, 1967, Bureau of Health, Education, Physical Education, and Recreation and Bureau of School Planning, 721 Capitol Mall, Sacramento, Calif. 95814.

Equipment

The following equipment is recommended for indoor and outdoor facilities. Indoor equipment includes two three-speed record players, dance drum, climbing rope, jumping boxes, trampoline, basketball standards, volleyball stan-

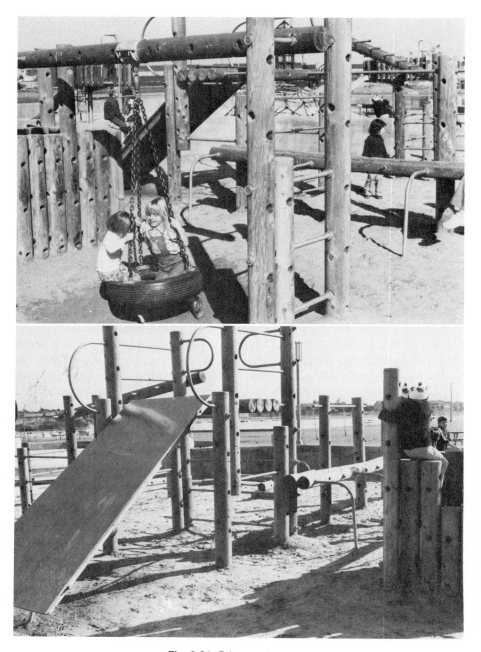

Fig. 3-31. Primary play area.

dards and net, gym scooters, Stegel or similar piece of climbing apparatus, and gymnastic mats.

Outdoor equipment includes creative climbing and play apparatus, horizontal bars, horizonal ladders, balance beam, tetherball standard, basketball standards, volleyball standards, softball backboards, soccer goals, swings, free-form sandbox, track and field equipment, long-jump pit, high-jump pit, and standards, and perceptual-motor obstacle course.

Creativity in design

Although certain requirements and standards are necessary to ensure adequate play space and equipment, the creative physical education teacher should promote new designs in facilities and play equipment. There is a trend to move from the flat asphalt jungle to creative play areas arranged with slopes, paths, and natural equipment that encourages developmental play. Innovative planning and promotion will often result

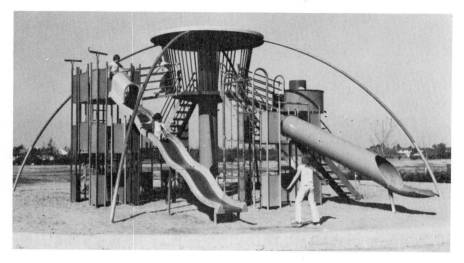

Fig. 3-32. Creative equipment design.

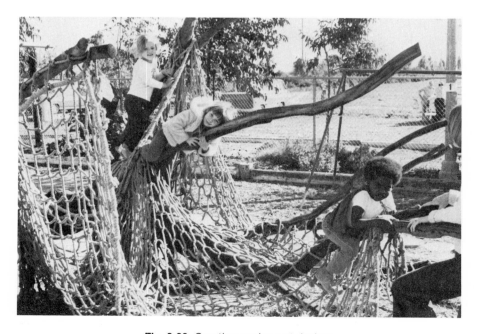

Fig. 3-33. Creative equipment design.

in the achievement of play equipment far beyond normal expectations. One often discovers that children are not concerned with highly sophisticated equipment but seek the thrill or challenge of maintaining balance or demonstrating their physical prowess by swimming, jumping, balancing, and traveling for fun on the craziest of inventions.

Parent volunteers may be of use in

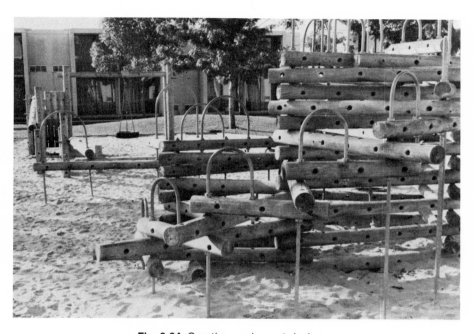

Fig. 3-34. Creative equipment design.

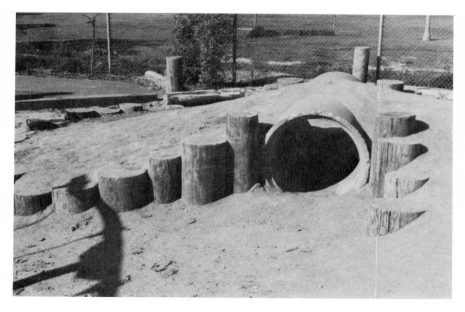

Fig. 3-35. Creative equipment design.

playground construction. Many parents are construction engineers, heavy equipment operators, and carpenters and would be willing to assist in a school playground project if asked. Building your own playground can be fun and rewarding for those participating in a group project for the benefit of the children. Many items, such as tires, telephone poles, and cable spools, can be obtained free of charge in most areas. Through creative planning, exciting equipment can be constructed with minimal cost to the school or community (Figs. 3-32 to 3-35). When entering into a project of this type, it is advisable to seek professional help for a structually safe design.[3]

Equipment children can make
(Fig. 3-36)

Ball scoop: cut a portion of a plastic bottle straight off at the bottom or off at a slant. Scoops are excellent in developing hand-eye coordination and encouraging success by enlarging the catching receptacle.

Panty hose rackets: holding a wire hanger by the hook, pull the center of the longest side until it forms a diamond. Curl up the hook end to form a handle. Cut one leg off the panty hose and slip it over the top of the racket so the toe fits snugly over the corner

opposite the handle. Pull the stocking firmly over the diamond shape and wrap excess stocking around the handle. Tape around the handle to form a grip. The racket works best with a Ping-Pong ball or golf Whiffle Ball.

Stocking balls: crush two double sheets of newspaper into a ball. Place paper ball into toe of a stocking and twist it to close in ball. Pull stocking back over ball again and twist. Continue until all stocking is used, then tuck remaining ends together and seal with masking tape.

Tin can stilts: punch two holes on opposite sides of the bottom of a juice can. Run a rope through the holes and tie ends together. The length of the string depends on the child's height.

Bowling pins: place ¾ inch of sand in the bottom of a round plastic bottle and replace the cap. Paint on numerals or letters for game adaptations.

Supplies

Enough supplies should be provided so that each child can participate without extensive waiting periods for a turn at the skill. If possible, each child should have a piece of equipment when a skill is being taught. Available supplies should include utility balls of all sizes, soccer balls, volleyballs, softballs, footballs, bats, basket-

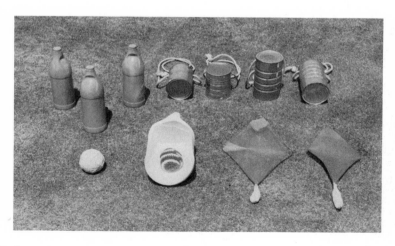

Fig. 3-36. Equipment children can make. Ball scoop, panty hose racket, stocking ball, tin can stilts, and bowling pins.

balls, beanbags, measuring tapes, dance and rhythm records, long jump ropes, individual jump ropes, colored pinnies, whistles, stopwatches, Hula-Hoops, selected geometric shapes, stilts, and parachutes.

INVOLVING THE COMMUNITY

Obtaining community input in relation to program organization and conduct is one way to ensure that parents have a better understanding of what the school is attempting to accomplish. A contemporary approach is to initiate a needs assessment program involving students, community, teachers, and administrators. For a needs assessment program to be successful it should:

1. Have a broad-based selection process for participants
2. Be conducted at the local school level
3. Provide community awareness through publicity and interaction of interested persons
4. Have regular progress reports
5. Provide for accomplishment of goals through action-oriented implementation
6. Disseminate findings in layman's language

The needs assessment process first involves the establishment of a school-community planning committee comprised of the principal or his or her representative; curriculum coordinator; teachers of physical education; students; representatives from city government, business, and industry; and senior citizens. The purpose of the planning group would be to first, recommend types of community representatives, determine people-selection procedures, and establish a calendar of meetings. Second, the planning group would organize a conference for all interested groups.

The following is a sample needs assessment conference program that can be used as a guide:

8:30	Refreshments
9:00	Welcome those attending and define purpose of the meeting
9:15	Divide into groups of six to eight people
9:30	Evaluate "what is," identifying program problems
10:00	Determine "what should be," brainstorming ideas
11:00	Report to the total group and record recommendations
11:30	Develop plans for action
12:00	Adjourn

Brainstorming

The prime vehicle to be used during the conference is brainstorming. This is a technique that often begins with a dream and ends in action. Brainstorming is free-wheeling, no-holds-barred, off-the-top-of-the-head talk, about a specific subject or subjects, hopefully to come up with some ideas that have not been brought forth before. During brainstorming it is important to accept all thoughts without evaluating their worth. This keeps the channels open and the creative flow of ideas coming. No matter how "far out" ideas may seem, they often open up leads to other avenues of thought that ultimately offer a solution or a new look at the problem.

Brainstorming is usually at its best in a small group of from six to eight people in which there is much opportunity to interact and develop each other's ideas. Attacking a problem in this manner, through unlimited ideas from group members, usually results in a plan that will remove the obstacle blocking the goal or provide an alternate plan for bypassing the block and reaching the goal. Individuals participating in the brainstorming approach usually find it is an interesting and informative way of building group unity and working toward problem solutions.

Programs of this nature are comparatively easy to organize, and through community involvement, plans can be made to develop curricula, facilities, and equipment. Much can be accomplished through this group process since common interests serve as a base for action-oriented improvements. This team approach to educational improvement provides an excellent opportunity to enhance the relationship between the comunity and the education system.

CLASS ACTIVITIES

1. Develop a yearly plan of physical activities for children in level 3 using the suggested time percentages in the activity chart in the text.
2. Plan an in-service program for parent volunteers showing major topics to be discussed.
3. Create a new game for level 4 children, using nontraditional equipment.
4. Design a physical education resource center, listing materials that should be included for use.
5. Visit an elementary school and design a remodeling plan to modernize facilities and equipment.
6. Select a lifetime sport activity and develop a sequential program of instruction for all levels.
7. Establish a handicap system for any one of the following activities: four square, wall ball, tetherball, and volleyball.

REFERENCES

1. Bookwalter, K. W.: Physical education in the secondary schools, New York, 1964, The Center for Applied Research in Education, Inc.
2. La Salle, D.: Guidance of children through physical education, New York, 1946, A. S. Barnes & Co., Inc.
3. Lehrer, R., and Sparks, N.: Play power, San Francisco, 1976, Volunteers to Beautify Our Schools.
4. Pestolesi, R. A., and Sinclair, W. A.: Creative administration, Englewood Cliffs, N.J., 1978, Prentice-Hall, Inc.

RECOMMENDED READINGS

Aitken, M. H.: Play environment for children: play space, improved equipment and facilities, Bellingham, Washington, 1972, Educational Designs and Consultants.

American Association for Health, Physical Education, and Recreation: Essentials of a quality elementary school physical education program, Washington, D.C., 1970, The Association.

American Association for Health, Physical Education, and Recreation: Organizational patterns for instruction in physical education, Washington, D.C., 1971, The Association.

American Association for Health, Physical Education, and Recreation: Planning facilities for athletics, physical education and recreation, Washington, D.C., 1974, The Association.

Bucher, C. A.: Foundations of physical education, ed. 7, St. Louis, 1975, The C. V. Mosby Co.

Ezersky, E., and Theibert, P.: Facilities in sports and physical education, St. Louis, 1976, The C. V. Mosby Co.

Hewes, J. J.: Build your own playground, Boston, 1975, Houghton Mifflin Co.

Mosston, M.: Teaching physical education, Columbus, Ohio, 1966, Charles E. Merrill Publishing Co.

Pestolesi, R. A. and Sinclair, W. A.: Creative administration in physical education and athletics, Englewood Cliffs, N.J., 1978, Prentice-Hall, Inc.

THE DEVELOPING CHILD

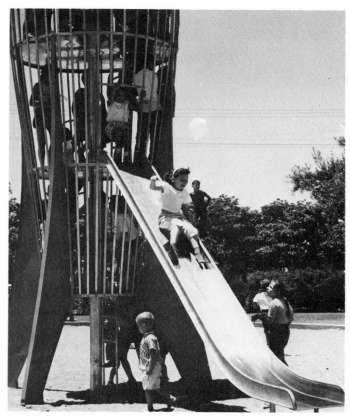

Photo by Linda Brundage

Part Two describes the child's physical, emotional, and mental characteristics in the periods of development from conception through late childhood. Special consideration is given to the importance of motor development and physical education during these periods.

4

Beginning: from conception through toddling

There is no more important time in human existence than the period from conception through toddling. One must marvel that from a single egg no larger than the period at the end of a sentence grows the miracle of new life, free to move about the terrain on two relatively small feet. This chapter discusses selected developmental events in the life of the new person and their relationship to behavior.

PRENATAL DEVELOPMENT

Because many of the events that occur between the time of birth and the first unassisted step are continuations of the prenatal period, it is important to briefly discuss this 9-month span in the light of maximizing future development. Life in utero is characterized by four basic features: orderly cell division, differentiation, unification, and integration. Following the union of the male sperm with the female ovum, the new life rapidly develops through a predetermined genetic plan, progressing through the germinal, embryonic, and fetal stages.

Germinal period

The germinal period is the first stage of prenatal development following conception; it is during this time that the fertilized egg attaches itself to the uterus. This period lasts about 2 weeks and is characterized by rapid cell division and the beginning of a new life.

Embryonic period

The embryonic period is from the implantation of the fertilized egg until the embryo is recognizable as a human fetus. This period covers an estimated time span of 6 weeks, or from the second to the eighth week after conception. During this period the embryo develops the necessary equipment for survival in the womb. The embryonic stage can best be described as the period in which cells begin their differentiation into the specialized tissues of organs and organ systems. The outer layer of cells is the first to differentiate and will later form the skin and nervous system. The next cells to take on unique qualities are in the middle layer, and they eventually will develop into such tissues as muscles, bone, lymph glands, heart, and blood vessels. The inner, cellular layer forms the organs of digestion and breathing. Although only about $\frac{1}{5}$ inch in length after 28 days of growth, the embryo has a primitive heart, simple kidneys, a liver, and a digestive tract, as well as rudimentary eyes, ears, and a nose.[13] Because the nervous system is necessary to the functioning of the body as a whole, the brain and spinal cord demonstrate the most rapid growth when compared to other body structures.

During the first 8 weeks after conception the number, size, and specialization of cells increase. Any situation, external or internal, affecting the mother can adversely affect the growth of the embryo. The embryo is particularly susceptible to viral diseases, such as rubella, or German measles, or to certain drugs that might affect cellular growth.

Fetal period

Around the end of the second month after conception the embryo measures about 1 inch in length and weighs ⅔ ounce.[13] It now has all the features essential for recognition as a human and, therefore, is considered a fetus. The fetal period extends from about the eighth week after conception until the time of birth (Fig. 4-1). Rapid, uniform, progressive growth characterizes the cellular and tissue development during this period. The new human being gradually has changed from a mass of diffused and undifferentiated cells to a highly organized and interrelated group of organic systems. The early fetus is distinguished from the embryo by the presence of rudimentary arms, legs, and organs essential for independent life after birth. The hard skeletal system begins to replace the

soft, cartilaginous skeleton by accumulation of bony minerals (Fig. 4-2).

Motor behavior before birth

Probably the first movements of the embryo are of the mouth because the muscles of this area are the first to develop. At 6 weeks after conception a reflex response can be elicited if the mouth is stimulated. During the third month after conception the fetus displays increased spontaneous movement and can turn the head, push the legs, bend the elbows, make a fist, bend and fan the toes, move the thumb, bend the wrist, squint and wrinkle the forehead, open the mouth, and press the lips together, all without the mother feeling the movement of the now 3-inch fetus. Activity is increased during the fourth month, with the fetus getting stronger and increasing in length by two or three times and in weight by as much as six times. At about 4½ months after conception the once light movements of the fetus now have become sharp kicks and pushes as strength increases. The movement behavior of the fetus during the fifth month is one of great activity with movements that are from side to side, up and down, and even completely around as in a somersault. Fetal movements continue to get stronger up to the end of the eighth month after conception with progressive development of the nervous and muscle systems. Because the eighth and ninth months are the time when the fetus gains considerable weight, the space for movement becomes more confined. The fetus, for the most part, completely stops moving at about 2 weeks before birth because of settling into the mother's pelvic floor.

Developmental direction and integration

As previously discussed, the developmental and maturational direction from the earliest period of life is generally from the head downward to the feet and from

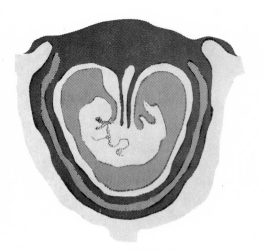

Fig. 4-1. Human fetus.

the center of the body or midline outward to the fingertips.[20] This pattern of development is continued when the fetus gains motor control first of the head, then of the trunk, then of the arms, and finally, of the legs, after which the baby begins to kick within the mother.

During development in utero, the fetus' motor behavior follows closely the progressive cellular development established at the time of conception. For example, the early fetus expresses movement that is arrhythmical and asynchronous. Gradually, the fetus acquires the ability to perform less random and diffuse movement. This tendency toward motor behavior that is more rhythmical and synchronous is the result of maturation and an integrating process within the expanding nervous system. An important aspect of neurological maturation is myelinization of some nerves within the nervous system, which refers to the development of a fatty substance that coats the

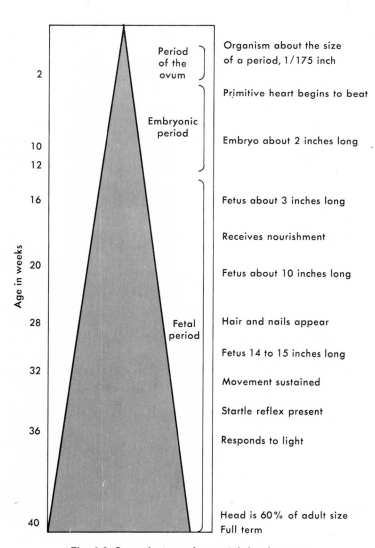

Fig. 4-2. Some factors of prenatal development.

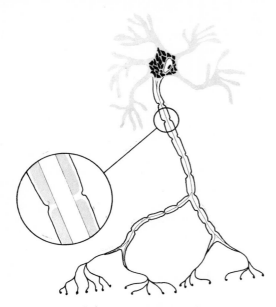

Fig. 4-3. Myelinated nerve.

nerve, serving as insulation against misdirected nerve impulses.[14] Myelinization of the nerves allows for an increased speed of muscle action and more precise movement, as well as an increase in muscle strength (Fig. 4-3).

Prenatal movement education

Movement education, broadly speaking, starts before birth during the fetal period. If one considers movement as an integral part of an individual's total behavior, then movement education must be considered as beginning in the prenatal environment. The mother-to-be who is physically and emotionally healthy and who engages in daily activity establishes an in utero environment that is conducive to proper development both before and after birth.

Increasingly, we are gaining the knowledge that prenatal development can be adversely affected by the unhealthy living habits of the mother, such as ingesting nicotine into the system through smoking, consuming large quantities of alcohol, or taking various legal or illegal drugs.[2] Excessive stress can also be damaging to the fetus. Although a mother-to-be should be physically active, developmental disturbances, such as those described by Ausubel[3], can be caused by excessive activity resulting in exhaustion by the mother, which may lead to an increase in lactic acid and carbon dioxide in the fetal bloodstream, producing a faster heart rate and increased physical activity. Also, fear, rage, and emotional distress in the mother may lead to functional problems of the fetal intestinal tract that affect nutritional absorption and may create a decrease in the general motor reaction threshold and hyperactivity, which could continue after the birth of the baby.

In general, the fetus is subject to both internal and external stimuli and can react positively or negatively to them. Between the first and third months in utero the fetus' movements are distinct. At this time it can react to sound, light, and even the mother's position changes. It is well known that 7 months after gestation sounds can be heard by the fetus even through the amniotic fluid in which it resides. While still in the mother, the fetus can be stimulated to increase its heart rate and general activity through musical sounds directed to the mother's abdomen.[12] Therefore, one must agree that from conception to birth, life unfolds in a predetermined manner and that neither is the mother an incubator nor the unborn baby a parasite, but the two, together, are an interacting dynamic duo.

FIRST DAYS AND WEEKS AFTER BIRTH

Giving birth to a new person is one of the most beautiful events that nature has to offer. Through a tortuous route the newborn twists, turns, and struggles as it is pushed to the outside world. To make the birth process less traumatic for both mother and newborn, doctors are increasingly using less medication and encouraging mothers to learn relaxation and muscle control. A mother who is aware of her own body movements during the last hours prior to birth, who is relaxed and unafraid, and who is able to run, wander, swim, or mount stairs without effort will more easily accomplish the movement performance of giving birth.[9] To ease the physical and psychological shock to the newborn, some doctors are changing their obstetrical methods to take into account that the neonate is truly aware of a variety of sensations. The birth is not hurried, sounds are kept to a minimum, and lights are subdued. The newborn is eased from the mother and placed on her bare abdomen. When the pulse ceases in the umbilical cord, it is cut and tied, and then the newborn is placed gently in warm water that approximates the temperature of the womb that was the newborn's home.[16] Infants born with a minimum of trauma are helped to start life without the usual pain, confusion, and fear.

The neonatal period is one of adaptation to a different environment and lasts for about 2 weeks. The newborn emerges with a large, unstable head that is one-quarter the size of the body. In the first 3 or 4 days the newborn most commonly sleeps as much as four fifths of the day. Following the fourth day, the newborn's sleep time drops to about three quarters of the day. At this time any discomfort the newborn experiences causes random activity of the entire body. Contrary to the idea that newborns do not move a great deal, they have been observed to make as many as 50 movements per minute.[13] Movement is essential in newborns for muscle exercise and strength. Following the developmental direction, movements of the head and arms are common, leading to the emergence of upright posture, manipulation, and perception. The newborn makes throaty sounds as well as grunts, mews, and sighs; sneezes to clear the nose; and yawns to gain extra oxygen.

Full-term newborns come into the world with many sensory abilities; for example, they can distinguish light from dark and can focus on an object when they are 3 or 4 weeks old.[21] Newborns can discriminate between loud and soft sounds; however, the senses of touch, taste, and smell are far better developed than the senses of hearing and sight.

Reflex and motor behavior

As mentioned earlier, movement begins in the second month of prenatal life. During the third month in utero, spontaneous movements of the arms, legs, shoulders, and fingers are possible, and 3½ months after conception, almost all the reflexes the newborn will have are present.[13] A reflex is defined simply as an involuntary response to a stimulus (Fig. 4-4). Reflexes are specific, purposeful, and adaptive and occur below the conscious level of the individual. Essentially the newborn is a reflex organism. Responses come from stimulation by the newborn's own body or by the environment.

At birth, reflex behaviors fall into two broad categories: survival and posturing. Newborns survive because they can root, that is, turn automatically toward their mothers' breasts when the sides of their mouths are touched, such as when the nipple touches the lips; because they can swallow the milk in their mouth; and because they can cry when uncomfortable, sneeze when there is something in the nose, cough to clear the throat, breathe, hiccough, vomit, and eliminate waste spontaneously.

Full-term newborns can move their heads weakly up and down and from side to side but are unable to hold their heads in a steady midline position. They can flex, straighten, and randomly move their arms about. The baby can grasp a rod when pressure is applied to the palm and hold on tight enough to be pulled up off the mattress (grasp reflex). The trunk, on the other hand, has relatively few available movements. The most apparent are

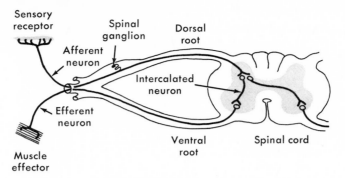

Fig. 4-4. Simple reflex arc.

bending the trunk and straightening the back slightly. The legs, at this time, bend, straighten, kick, jerk, rotate, and tremble. When the bottom of the newborn's feet are stroked, the toes extend upward and fan out. If a loud noise is made or support is taken away from the newborn, the Moro or startle reflex occurs. In normal newborns, the Moro reaction is a symmetrical response with both arms moving out to the sides and upward and the legs extending downward. Failure of a Moro reflex to appear at birth or a reflex that is still prevalent after 4 months of age can mean a neurological dysfunction or delay in maturation.

Of particular importance to the newborn's resting postures are the tonic reflexes, which direct the newborn's early motor and cognitive development.[5] They are the labyrinthine reflex and the symmetric and asymmetric tonic reflexes. The labyrinthine reflex is stimulated by putting the newborn either on the back or the abdomen. If the newborn is placed on the abdomen, flexor tonus is increased, and if he or she is placed on the back, extensor tonus is increased. The symmetric tonic neck reflex is stimulated by moving the newborn's head when he or she is in either the front- or back-lying position. If the head is gently pushed downward when the newborn is in the front-lying position, the knees will automatically flex, the buttocks will elevate, the elbows will bend, and the hands will clench.

Conversely, if the newborn is placed in the back-lying position and the head is pushed gently backward, the arms will straighten, the hands will open, and the legs will be elevated. In contrast, the asymmetric tonic reflex creates tonus that causes the newborn to assume a fencing-like position. When the newborn is laid on the back, if his or her head is turned, the leg and arm on the same side straighten and those on the opposite side become flexed or drawn up. If the head is gently turned to the opposite side, the opposite reflex pattern will occur. These early postural reflexes provide the newborn with the beginnings of body awareness and understanding that there are two sides to the body.[5] The asymmetric tonic reflex gradually becomes less obvious in the first 6 months of life, but obvious remnants may be present as late as the second or third year of life.

Another reflex that is obvious at birth is the stepping, or placing, reflex, which some authorities believe to be the basis for bipedal locomotion. This reflex appears by the tenth day after birth and is usually suppressed by the sixth week. To stimulate the stepping reflex the newborn is supported around the trunk in an upright position, pressure is then applied to the soles of the feet and the newborn performs a step. The newborn is in the reflex stage of learning until the primitive reflexes are suppressed and voluntary movements begin to predominate.

Table 4-1. Early normal developmental characteristics: gross motor behavior

Age*	Major events
4 weeks	Turns head to side. Holds hands in fist. Has sagging head. Shows tonic neck reflex. Displays crawling movment of legs.
8 weeks	Lifts head. Turns from side to back. Sits with support. Pushes self with arms and lifts chest.
12 weeks	Crawls prone. Holds head steady for 5 seconds. Raises chest off mattress. Holds hands mostly open.
16 weeks	Keeps head steady when sitting. Attempts to right self when tilted. Bears some weight on feet. Likes to sit.
20 weeks	Sits unsupported. Pulls self to sitting position. Supports weight on forearm and lifts head.
24 weeks	Lifts chest off floor. Bears some weight on feet. Controls head. Crawls backward. Reaches out with each hand. Stands by holding on. Rolls over from back to stomach.
28 weeks	Bounces self. Rocks on hands and knees. Supports weight on feet. Begins to crawl forward. Steps when supported under arms.
36 weeks	Crawls by moving hands and knees. Shows hand preference. Sits unsupported. Pulls self to standing position. Pulls self to sitting position.
40 weeks	Pulls self to feet. Stands by holding on. Creeps on hands and knees over obstacle 2 inches high. Stands unsupported for 1 minute.
48 weeks	Pulls self up to side of crib. Walks alone. Creeps by using hands and feet.
56 weeks	Walks short distances. Starts and stops. Walks backward. Throws objects. Stands up from lying on back.
62 weeks	Walks smoothly. Creeps upstairs. Stoops and stands up. Ascends stairs by walking.
18 months	Ascends stairs by marking time. Jumps in place. Walks sideways. Walks without falling. Runs awkwardly. Pulls toy.
24 months	Walks backward. Runs in preference to walking. Squats on floor. Descends ladder carefully by marking time. Jumps from 18-inch height with help. Throws object overhead.

From Arnheim, D. D., Auxter, D., and Crowe, W.: Principles and methods in adapted physical education, St. Louis, 1977, The C. V. Mosby Co.
*The ages at which the major events noted here occur are approximate.

INFANCY

An infant has been described as a child who is not over 2 years of age or who is not walking independently. Infancy is the period in which the individual must learn to eat solid food, walk and use many small muscles, gain some control over the elimination processes, acquire the basis for speech and begin to communicate, coordinate the eyes, develop a predictable cycle in sleeping and eating, and progress from a completely helpless state to one of relative independence.[13]

Posture control and mobility

During infancy the infant gains control of posture, acquires locomotor skills, and uses the hands in a purposeful way (Table 4-1). The events leading to mobility in the upright position are numerous, but those that stand out most are: sitting with some support, sitting alone, crawl-

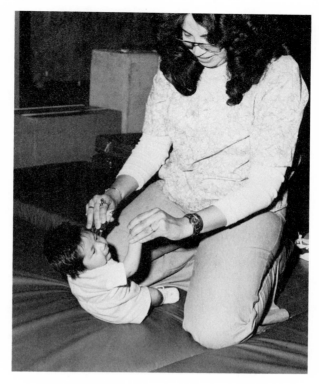

Fig. 4-5. Infant showing immature head and trunk control.

ing, creeping, walking with some support, and walking alone. Starting as a completely grounded, helpless organism dominated by the force of gravity, the infant suppresses primitive reflexes and gains in matruation, strength, and confidence in order to move freely and explore the environment.

In general, posture and movement of the infant follow maturation of the central nervous system; the spinal cord predominates in the first 2 months of life, the brain stem from 4 to 6 months and the midbrain from 6 to 10 or 12 months; finally the highest center, the cerebral cortex, takes primary control.[10]

In the beginning, the infant's body parts move independently with movements that are swimminglike and random. Gradually, movements become synchronized with the larger muscles gaining control before the smaller ones

(Fig. 4-5). Between 1 and 3 months of age, the infant can lift the head while lying on the abdomen. At this time the infant can also squirm and twist and sometimes even unintentionally roll to the side; however, not until about 3 months of age does the infant turn over from back to front. Nervous system maturity and muscle strength come slowly. At about 3 months of age, the infant can sit without support and push its chest off the floor with the arms. One of the most important events in mobility is crawling, in which the infant, keeping the abdomen in contact with a surface, attempts to move forward by first pushing or pulling with the arms and then pushing with the legs. Sitting without support with the head held steady appears at about 4 to 5 months of age, and creeping or moving about on hands and knees takes place around the eighth or ninth month after birth.

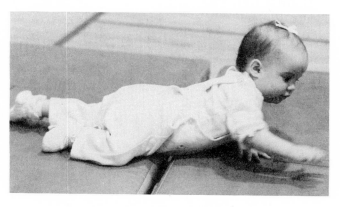

Fig. 4-6. Nine-month-old infant creeping.

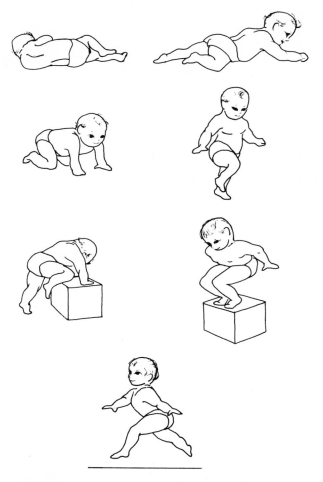

Fig. 4-7. Sequential development of posture and locomotion.

The ability to move about the environment in an upright posture on the two small surfaces of the feet must be considered one of the human being's greatest attainments (Fig. 4-6). The infant has been preparing for independent walking for many months; however, it is not until countless physiological and anatomical factors have been acquired that the infant can move with relative safety from the four-point, quadrupedal position to the very unstable, fully upright, bipedal position.

Bipedal locomotion progresses from the time the infant first tries to pull himself or herself up on the side of the crib, to moving around the room holding onto furniture, to walking free of support, to toddling about with feet spread and arms raised at about 15 months, to finally walking in a mature manner at around 4 years of age.[14]

A child is considered a toddler when he or she can move independently, although unsteadily, in the upright posture. At 18 months, the toddler can walk very fast but labors at getting started and, once going, finds it very hard to stop. At 2 years, the young child is still refining the walking pattern, but just a few more months growth and maturation allow the child to walk sideways; the child may even try to walk backward and displays a semblance of reciprocal or cross-lateral use of the arms (Fig. 4-7).[6]

Arm and hand control

To see, reach, grasp, and manipulate objects is, like walking, one of a human being's greatest assets (Table 4-2). Through this process the environment can be thoroughly explored and things created. As the eyes become coordinated, so do the arms and hands. There are three very important aspects to using the arms and hands in a coordinated manner: the use of the arms in reaching, the use of the hand in grasping or seizing an object, and the function of the hand in letting go of an object.

In the newborn the arms are, for the most part, kept out to the side of the body. When one arm moves, often the other arm mirrors the same movement. The act of reaching does not appear in the normal infant until about 4 months of age, at which time performance is asynchronous and poorly coordinated. When the infant reaches the entire body becomes involved with the action. At this time the infant finds it very difficult to overcome the stronger muscles that want to keep the arms bent rather than allow them to straighten. As maturation of the nervous system occurs, better motor differentiation together with increased control of the eyes allows the arms to be better directed, particularly at around 5 months of age when both the infant's arms have moved more to the midline of the body. At about 6 months of age, the infant can coordinate the process of seeing an object, reaching for that object, and grasping the object with some adroitness. However, not until the age of 6½ or 7 months will the infant reach with one arm, mainly the right arm, in preference to the other. The reason why the majority of people are right-handed is unknown; however, it is known that speech, language and right-handedness are controlled by the left side of the brain.[14] Hand preference should take place in the first 18 months of life.

Prehension, the act of grasping or seizing an object, is present at birth in the form of the grasping reflex. Because the newborn's hands are closed in a fist, the act of grasping must wait until they are opened at about 3 months of age. The thumb, at birth, is held either free or encased by the fisted fingers. Grasping, at 6 months, is initiated by the entire hand with a gradual shift, through maturity, toward the thumb, or radial, side of the hand, becoming radial palmar grasp at 6½ months of age. At 9 months the infant grasps with the fingers rather than the palm of the hand. As the use of the fingers becomes the rule rather than the exception, the infant is able to deal with increasingly smaller objects. At 8 months

Table 4-2. Early normal developmental characteristics: small muscle

Age*	Major events
4 weeks	Holds hands fisted. Attends to objects. Holds onto ring.
8 weeks	Swipes at objects. Begins to coordinate head and eyes.
12 weeks	Shows one- and two-arm control. Looks at interesting object and waves arms. Looks alternately at object and hands. Brings hands to front of body.
16 weeks	Holds hands mainly open. Brings hands to object. Reaches for objects. Picks up objects with palm.
24 weeks	Examines objects. Searches for hidden objects. Reaches for objects. Transfers objects from one hand to other. Visually tracks to midline. Lifts cup. Begins to rotate wrists horizontally.
28 weeks	Grabs objects with palms. Scoops raisins. Shows some hand preference.
32 weeks	Bangs objects on table. Tracks moving objects. Demonstrates rudimentary thumb opposition.
36 weeks	Rings a bell. Demonstrates pincer grasp. Takes objects out of container. Bangs objects together.
40 weeks	Releases objects awkwardly. Plays with fingers. Puts object into container. Holds own bottle. Attempts to hold three 1-inch cubes in one hand. Bangs two cubes together at midline of body.
48 weeks	Releases object easily. Chews and swallows. Makes marks with pencil.
64 weeks	Builds tower of two cubes. Puts raisins in box. Scribbles. Dumps raisins from container.
18 months	Picks up cereal with pincer grasp. Builds tower of four 1-inch cubes. Makes circular scribbles. Turns pages.
24 months	Builds tower of five 1-inch cubes. Turns pages of magazine one at a time. Unwraps paper covering from box.

From Arnheim, D. D., Auxter, D., and Crowe, W.: Principles and methods in adapted physical education, St. Louis, 1977, The C. V. Mosby Co.
*The ages at which the major events noted here occur are approximate.

the infant uses the thumb with the first finger in a pincerlike manner and at 9 months begins to use the thumb in a very rudimentary way. Not until around 16 months of age is thumb opposition apparent, and not until 2 years can the infant perform a mature thumb opposition bilaterally and simultaneously.

Because the flexor muscles of the fingers overpower the extensors, releasing an object requires more maturity than grasping it. An essential event occurs at about age 2½ months that may be called the *vital release*, which is the combination of grasping and letting go of an object in sequence. However, it is not until about 9 months of age that the infant can release or drop an object by volition. At 15 months the infant has integrated the use of the eyes with the hands and has accomplished the grasp and release functions necessary to successfully place one block on another, and by 18 months of age the infant can build a tower of four blocks.[14] Also at 18 months the infant can throw a ball from a standing position.[14] Coordination of the arms and hands is essential if the child is to adequately explore the surroundings and perform one of the most difficult of motor skills—writing.

Vocalization

Communication through purposeful vocalization can be considered an important outcome of the long period of dependency that the human being must

Table 4-3. Early normal developmental characteristics: language and communication

Age*	Major events
0	Exhibits undifferentiated birth cry.
4 weeks	Watches person moving. Makes demand cry. Makes throaty cry.
8 weeks	Attends to person's voice. Shows discomfort. Gurgles. Coos.
12 weeks	Makes different sounds when touched or played with. Tenses when lifted. Shows vital or differentiated crying when cold, uncomfortable, or hungry.
16 weeks	Turns head to sound of voice. Recognizes mother. Laughs. Experiments with voice.
20 weeks	Turns to sounds. Shows displeasure. Responds to voices.
24 weeks	Responds to anger. Displays nonrhythmical crying. Babbles.
28 weeks	Squeals. Makes "M-m" sound. Smiles at mirror. Demands attention. Tries to imitate speech.
32 weeks	Combines babbling and gestures. Combines two syllables. Displays rhythmical babbling.
36 weeks	Cries to gain attention.
40 weeks	Understands "no." Waves bye-bye. Looks for hidden object. Imitates sounds. Says "da-da" and "ma-ma."
44 weeks	Shakes head "no." Says one word. Imitates new sounds. Listens to words. Anticipates playing pat-a-cake.
48 weeks	Knows own name. Indicates personal desires. Commands through gestures.
52 weeks	Knows names of objects. Shows likes and dislikes. Imitates words. Possesses three-word vocabulary. Anticipates being scolded. Responds to "Give it to me."
64 weeks	Points to things wanted. Shows variety of emotions. Possesses five-word vocabulary.
18 months	Knows three body parts. Imitates talking. Possesses 10 word vocabulary. Hums and sings to self. Uses words to indicate wants.
21 months	Tries to follow directions. Knows five body parts. Leads adult to object. Exhibits great curiosity. Connects three or four words. Possesses 20 word vocabulary.
24 months	Follows simple commands. Refers to self by name. Knows how some objects work. Names most objects played with. Imitates parents speech. Expresses two- or three-word sentences.

From Arnheim, D. D., Auxter, D., and Crowe, W.: Principles and methods in adapted physical education, St. Louis, 1977, The C. V. Mosby Co.
*The ages at which the major events noted here occur are approximate.

undergo (Table 4-3). Simply stated, communication is the transferring of information by some symbolic form from one person to another. Language, in the usual sense, refers to communication by means of the voice; however, there are nonlinguistic means of human communication using postures, attitudes, gestures, and facial expressions. Vocalization occurs mainly through the control of expired air passing through the vocal cords, or larynx. Although the acquiring of motor skills necessary for speech is very important, it is, to some people, less dramatic than the acquisition of mobility in the upright posture.

As in the development of all motor responses, there is a hierarchy of events leading to mature speech. Vocal sounds at birth are represented by undifferentiated sounds, such as crying, yawning, sneezing, and coughing. Undifferentiated crying is replaced, at about 3 months of age, by differentiated crying, also known as *vital crying*, indicating the infant's response to discomfort, such as pain, cold, or hunger. Meaningful sounds, such as phonemes, or babbling and lallation, occur at about 6 months of age.[17] The ability to echo speech sounds appears at about 7 months and is maintained throughout life. Other speech milestones are considered by some observers to occur at about 20 months, when the child can name an object, and at about 4 years of age, when simple sentences are produced.

Sensory awareness and perception

Although the sensory functions of the full-term infant are at a relatively primitive level, all the brain cells are present. Through variation in experiences and environmental stimulation, the various senses are enhanced. The sensory organ receptors are designed to respond to specific stimuli: light, heat and cold, stretching of muscle fibers, pressure on joints, vibrations, and chemical stimulants that differentiate tastes and smells. The perceptual process is what gives meaning to the stimuli coming to the brain by way of the sense organs.[7]

Sensory awareness is composed of four basic factors: reception, perception, conceptualization, and expression. The sense organs are the means by which stimulation is brought to the organism. When the stimulation has reached the brain, it must be perceived or decoded in order to be interpreted. Once it is interpreted, the stimulus must be associated to past events that have been stored in the brain, a concept or idea must be made, and then some expression or overt behavior must occur. Many learning theoreticians consider the gaining of posture and locomotor control to be basic to the perceptual-conceptual process.[12]

Visualization. The newborn responds immediately to light by moving or twitching the eyelids. This light reflex may also elicit the Moro or startle reflex. There are indications that some colors can be perceived, particularly blue and green.[14] The infant will follow a movement or object with the eyes when only 2 weeks old. At approximately 3 months of age, infants can visually perceive an outline, and at 8 months, they can identify the detail of a configuration from a varied background, which is the beginning of figure-ground perception. However, it is not until almost 1½ years of age that coordinated focusing of the eyes occurs. At this time three visual functions can take place simultaneously: the oculomotor system can coordinate six pairs of eye muscles in the process of convergence or the simultaneous turning in of the eyes in order to focus on near objects, the thickness of the eye lenses can be muscularly altered, and the eyes can accommodate incoming light by dilating and constricting the pupils.

One may equate the maturing of the child's visual accommodation and convergence with taking the first step, speaking the first word, and opposing the thumb to the index finger.[17] At approximately 2 years of age the child can visually differentiate unlike objects, such as the brother and the cat or the house and the car. The 4-year-old child is often mature enough to differentiate among shapes, sizes, and varied visual symbols.

Vision may be defined as the comprehension of information that is gathered in the brain through the eyes and reconstruction of this information into conceptual images that have meaning. It involves sight, perception, integration, and conception. Vision, therefore, must be considered in terms not only of sight but also of the entire, developing individual.

Audition. Auditory development is apparent late in the fetal stage. At birth the newborn will respond to noise with the Moro reflex pattern. At 3 months of age, the infant responds more specifically to threatening sounds and appears to be able to focus attention on particular voices and sounds. At 4 and 5 months, the infant becomes able to localize a sound by turning the head in the direction of the stimulus. Auditory maturity parallels the development of language.

Tactility. For the maturing human organism to move efficiently, it must have tactile competence. Tactility may be defined as "a system for gaining information from the cutaneous surfaces of the body by means of active or passive contact."[4] Touching and feeling involve the excitation of not only skin receptors but also the entire motor system. Tactility is, in essence, dependent on the ability to touch, move, and manipulate the environment. Through their tactile abilities, children can discriminate and discern familiar objects held in their hands. This is an ability necessary to the eventual accomplishment of high-level motor tasks. The combination of feeling and movement is known as the *haptic sense.*

Stroking the newborn's skin at birth will elicit various skin reflexes, such as the grasping reflex. An infant, at approximately 5 months of age, is able to differentiate and react to sensations that can affect its survival, such as pain, wetness, and temperature irregularities. At 13 months the infant can discriminate nonpain stimuli, such as roughness or smoothness. At 16 months the infant becomes aware of the third dimension and realizes that all objects are not flat but may have depth. At 2 years the child can feel and determine the difference in shapes of objects, such as blocks or balls. However, it is not until approximately 4 years of age that the child is able to accurately identify the unique features of objects by touch alone.

Socialization and play

Two very important aspects of the development of the infant and toddler are socialization and play (Table 4-4). The human being's gregariousness and need to be with people is a response learned from the first interactions with the mother.[18] There is a direct relationship between emotional and psychological development and development of socialization.

At birth the newborn is completely dependent upon someone else for survival, and this is the time when the newborn learns to trust the environment and most particularly those who are in charge of its needs. Trust or mistrust of the world may begin even before birth, depending on the type of emotional climate that the mother has established for herself and for her infant.

During early development, sociality and play are closely associated. At birth the newborn expresses few outward signs of being interested in people; however, it does respond to the soothing sounds of the parent, rhythmical rocking, and gentle stroking of the skin. At 1 month of age the infant can distinguish between an inanimate object and a person, stares at faces, and babbles and coos at things that move. By the second month after birth, the infant becomes aware of adults, responding to them with a smile. By the third month the infant begins to talk when talked to and engages in spontaneous play by pulling on the blanket and looking at his or her hands when they are brought in front of the face. In the fourth month the infant instigates socialization by smiling first when an adult comes near. At this time the infant initiates play by playing with the hands and pulling blankets over the head. At 5 months the infant smiles at itself in a mirror and smiles at a smile. The 6-month-old infant is quick to recognize family members but a bit standoffish when strangers come into view. Play at this time is a matter of playing with the feet and smiling and talking to a mirror. Seven months of age is a time for playing peek-a-boo games and becoming more suspicious of strangers.

Table 4-4. Early normal developmental characteristics: social and adaptive behavior

Age*	Major events
0	Responds to sounds. Responds to persons. Responds to brightly colored objects.
4 weeks	Shows awareness of persons. Searches for nipple. Regards persons' faces.
8 weeks	Smiles when talked to. Shows excitement when being approached by adult. Looks for source of sounds.
12 weeks	Likes to be around persons. Anticipates being fed. Plays with own fingers.
16 weeks	Shows pleasure with certain toys. Laughs with persons. Plays with hands. Recognizes bottle. Brings objects to mouth. Is aware of self in mirror.
20 weeks	Plays peek-a-boo. Smiles at familiar person. Shows displeasure when toy is taken away. Inspects own hands.
24 weeks	Smiles at image in mirror. Wants to be talked to. May fear strange persons. Holds own bottle.
28 weeks	Makes noise to gain attention. explores objects. Sucks food from spoon. Chews bananas and bread. Pats own image in mirror.
32 weeks	Plays pat-a-cake with help. Watches persons. Says "da-da" and "ma-ma." Uncovers toy.
36 weeks	Brings arms in front of face. Uses fingers to feed self from dish. Defends own possessions. Drinks from cup with some spill. Responds to questions.
40 weeks	Plays pat-a-cake. Likes to play. Looks at pictures in book. Responds to "no-no."
52 weeks	Puts everything into mouth. Uses fingers to feed self crackers. Chews in circular manner. Jabbers with expression. Imitates words. Plays nursery games.
64 weeks	Exhibits solitary play. Pulls socks off. Brings spoon to mouth. Drops things from crib and high chair to gain attention. Cooperates in dressing. Plays ball. Speaks two words.
16 months	Carries personal things. Dips spoon in dish. Indicates when diapers are wet. Unzips large zipper. Identifies common clothes.
18 months	Demonstrates side-by-side play. Is very possessive of own things. Helps feed self. Imitates scribbling. Follows simple directions.
21 months	Helps in washing self. Drinks from cup. Helps remove own clothes. Makes two-word sentences. Makes basic wants known. Identifies objects in picture.
24 months	Takes shoes off if laces are loosened. Feeds self with fingers. Holds and hugs doll. Pulls off own clothes.

Adapted from Arnheim, D. D., Auxter, D., and Crowe, W.: Principles and methods in adapted physical education, St. Louis, 1977, The C. V. Mosby Co.
*The ages at which the major events noted here occur are approximate.

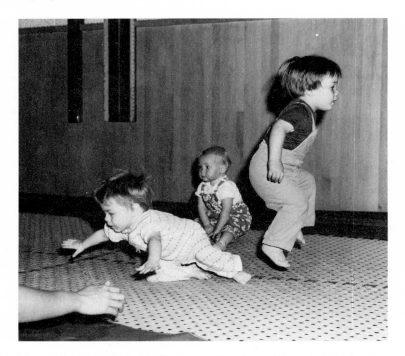

Fig. 4-8. A child 18 months old will play next to other children but seldom interacts.

During the eighth month, the infant seems to put everything in the mouth, biting on toys, clothing, and blankets. The 10-month-old infant can now play pat-a-cake and wave bye-bye and play for long periods alone.

The 1-year-old infant's world expands to include other people, particularly those who like to play chase and make faces that can be imitated. At 1 year of age the infant is very able to show such complex social behaviors as fear, anger, affection, jealousy, and even sympathy.[14] By 15 months of age the infant is a whirlwind of activity, getting into everything, exploring, and being very concerned with the newfound freedom of locomotion. The hands are now free to pull, lift, and feel the environment. While at 15 months the infant is engrossed with a newfound freedom and desires solitary play, the 18-month-old infant seeks out social approval from family, becomes increasingly aware of other people, and will even play next to another child without pushing or

shoving (Fig. 4-8). The 18-month-old must still be considered an infant, but at 2 years of age, the child almost suddenly has become a preschooler and is no longer highly dependent but able to toddle about and be more tolerant of other children, play side by side with them, acknowledge that they are there, and even occasionally play with them.

EARLY DEVELOPMENTAL STIMULATION

There can be no doubt that the human organism requires a variety of stimulation, both externally and internally, in order for growth and development to take place.[8,15] The presence or absence of stimulation can be a key factor in whether or not children reach their full maturational potential (Fig. 4-9). The drive to be stimulated is commonly called seeking behavior; much as flowers seek sunlight, people search out sensory stimulation when it is lacking.

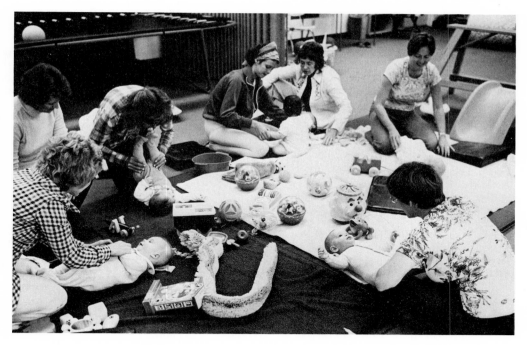

Fig. 4-9. Early stimulation is necessary for children to reach their full potential.

The period from birth, and perhaps even before birth, to 18 months of age is crucial for the child's physical, mental, and emotional development. When there is insufficient sensory stimulation, deprivation often occurs, leading to retardation.[11] For example, children who do not receive adequate maternal care may become intellectually, socially, or physically impaired or may even die. Children, especially very young children, should be given a rich environment of movement, touching, hearing, and seeing experiences.[19]

Concerns for physical education

One must consider physical education an inseparable part of all education that must be included in the full spectrum of life from birth to old age. As discussed previously, motor behavior probably begins in utero when the mother's own physical and emotional well-being is in some way transmitted to her unborn child. Although the physical educator, in the usual sense, is not trained to work at the nursery school level, many of the children he or she works with at the preschool and primary levels may have many residual characteristics of very young children, therefore requiring programming at that level of development. Activities that are specifically designed for the physically very young individual are presented in Chapter 13. These activities are classified as level 1 and are concerned mainly with basic body management.

CLASS ACTIVITIES

1. Observe two babies of different ages and record the number of movements each executes in a 1-minute period.
2. Visit a toy store and identify toys that are designed for infants and toddlers. Are the toys appropriate for the indicated age? If not, why?
3. Demonstrate, in order of their occurrence, the events leading up to mature use of the hands.
4. Demonstrate, in order of the occurrence, the events leading up to walking.
5. Plan a perceptual-motor stimulation program for an infant who is developmentally 8 months of age.

REFERENCES

1. Arnheim, D. D., Auxter, D., and Crowe, W.: Principles and methods in adapted physical education, St. Louis, 1977, The C. V. Mosby Co.
2. Arnheim, D. D., and Sinclair, W. A.: The clumsy child, St. Louis, 1975, The C. V. Mosby Co.
3. Ausubel, D. A., and Sullivan, E. V.: Das kindersalter, Munich, Germany, 1974.
4. Barsch, R. H.: Enriching perception and cognition, vol. 2, Seattle, 1968, Special Child Publications, Inc.
5. Bender, M. L.: The Bender-Purdue reflex test, San Rafael, Calif., 1976, Academic Therapy Publications.
6. Corbin, C. B.: A textbook of motor development, Dubuque, Iowa, 1973, William C. Brown Co., Publishers.
7. Cratty, B. J.: Perceptual and motor development in infants and children, New York, 1970, The Macmillan Co.
8. Diem, L.: Die menschliche bewegung, Schorndorf/Stuttgart, West Germany, 1976, Hofmann-Verlag.
9. Diem, L.: Selected session materials from summer workshop: motor development and the young child, San Diego, 1976, San Diego University Press.
10. Fiorentino, M. R.: Reflex testing methods for evaluating C. N. S. development, Springfield, Ill., 1963, Charles C Thomas, Publisher.
11. Hebb, D.: Organization of behavior, New York, 1949, John Wiley & Sons, Inc.
12. Kaluger, G., and Heil, C. L.: Basic symmetry and balance: their relationship to perceptual motor development, Prog. Phys. Ther. 1:132-137, 1970.
13. Kaluger, G., and Kaluger, M. F.: Human development, St. Louis, 1974, The C. V. Mosby Co.
14. Knobloch, H., and Pasamanick, B., editors: Gesell and Armatruda's developmental diagnosis, New York, 1974, Harper & Row, Publishers, Inc.
15. Koch, J.: Total baby development, New York, 1977, Wyden Books.
16. Leboyer, F.: Birth without violence, New York, 1975, Alfred A. Knopf, Inc.
17. LeWinn, E. B.: Human neurological organization, Springfield, Ill., 1969, Charles C Thomas, Publisher.
18. Rarick, G. L., editor: Physical activity: human growth and development, New York, 1973, Academic Press, Inc.
19. Ribble, M.: The rights of infants, New York, 1967, Columbia University Press.
20. Stott, L. H.: Child development, an individual longitudinal approach, New York, 1967, Holt, Rinehart & Winston.
21. Young, P.: Babies can communicate at birth, The National Observer, July 24, 1976, pp. 20-21.

RECOMMENDED READINGS

Frank, L. K.: On the importance of infants. New York, 1966, Random House, Inc.

Helmuth, J., editor: Exceptional infant. The national infant, vol. 1, New York, 1967, Brunner/Mazel, Inc.

Koontz, C. W.: Koontz child developmental program: training activities for the first 48 months, Los Angeles, 1974, Western Psychological Services.

Prudden, S.: Creative fitness for baby and child, New York, 1972, William Morrow & Co., Inc.

Stoddard, M.: For a more perfect baby, Twin Falls, Idaho, 1972, Standard Printing Co.

Stone, J. J., and others, editors: The competent infant, New York, 1973, Basic Books, Inc., Publishers.

5

Building: from 2 to 5 years of age

The period from 2 to 5 years of age represents one of the most dramatic periods, if not the most dramatic period, that the human being goes through. It is a time of great transformation, almost as startling as a butterfly emerging from its coccoon; the infant has changed into a unique person who has all of the fundamental behavior traits of humankind. The early childhood period is the time for integration of movement with perception; for toilet training; for learning to communicate effectively both in verbal and nonverbal ways; for acquiring skills in self-care and independence, such as, eating, dressing, bathing, relating to other people, and learning how to distinguish right actions from wrong actions.[9] The early childhood period is a crucial time for gaining awareness of self, and a very important time for developing self-esteem and a feeling of personal worth (Fig. 5-1).

GROWTH AND PHYSICAL DEVELOPMENT

From conception on, physical growth and development proceed in an orderly manner. In the period covering 2 to 5 years of age, directional growth and body control continue to take place from the head to the foot and from the center of the body outward. Although the progression of maturational events is predictable for each individual, they occur at differing rates of speed, making each child a unique person.

During early childhood the toddler's body shape changes from round to more linear.[6] Probably the single most outstanding growth attribute of early childhood is the increase in height. The lengthening process that takes place during the early childhood period is ascribable to the rapid growth of the long bones and trunk, with leg length increasing significantly as compared to trunk length. For example, the head of the 2-year-old child, like that of the infant, is approximately one-fourth the size of the entire body and is one-fifth the size of the body by age 5 years.

The very rapid tissue growth that occurs during the first 2 years of life gradually decelerates by age 5 years and levels off until the time of rapid pubertal growth. Weight gain follows the same pattern as height, with the very young child gaining from 3 to 5 pounds per year. In general, muscle growth during infancy and early childhood is proportional to the child's growth as a whole; however, this changes as the child reaches approximately 5 years of age, when major weight gain is related mainly to the increase in the amount of muscle tissue.[6]

DEVELOPING BODY CONTROL

Gaining control of body movements follows the same pattern as physical

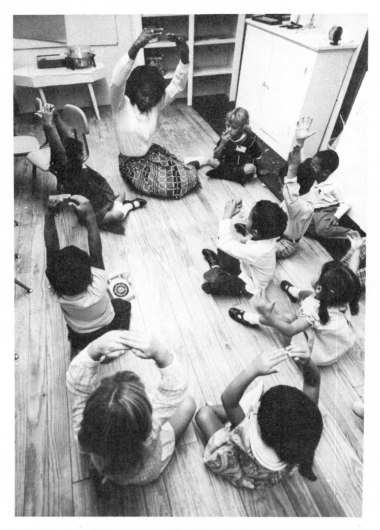

Fig. 5-1. The early childhood period is a major time for gaining self-awareness and self-esteem. (Courtesy Michael D. Sullivan.)

growth and maturation. Following the directional sequence of cephalocaudal and proximodistal development, body control proceeds from the head downward to the feet; from the trunk outward to the arms, hands, and fingers; and from the hips to the legs and, finally, the toes.[8] Gross motor control precedes fine motor control; in other words, activities that require the predominance of large muscles for their execution usually can be accomplished by the child before those activities that mainly use small muscles.[1]

Basic locomotor skills

By the time children reach their second birthdays they can, for the most part, transport themselves in the upright position, besides having a mastery of those preliminary skills that have led up to walking. As the toddler's typical stance with bent knees and legs wide apart gradually changes to one with straight legs and a narrower base of support, other more complicated patterns of moving the body occur. For example, the preschooler learns to run, climb, jump, hop, and gal-

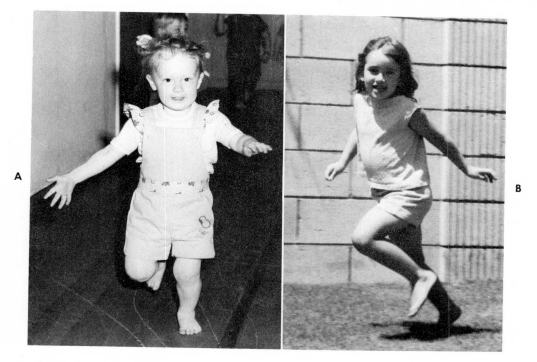

Fig. 5-2. A, A typical 2-year-old child running with arms out to the side for balance. **B,** A 4-year-old running, beginning to show a more efficient use of the arms.

lop and may even develop a rudimentary manner of skipping as well as other special skills for propelling the body, such as ice or roller skating, tricycling, or perhaps even bicycling or swimming.

Running. As discussed in Chapter 4, a fully independent walk does not occur until about 15 months of age, when the child is able to rise from the floor in a completed upright posture and begin to toddle. At 18 months the toddler can usually walk quickly in a straight line and at 2 years the young child seldom falls and can demonstrate a somewhat uncontrolled and inefficient running ability with obvious difficulty in starting, stopping, and turning (Fig. 5-2).

Running must be considered a direct outgrowth or extension of the walking pattern. In walking, one foot moves ahead of the other with the heel of the forward foot touching the ground before the toe of the opposite foot pushes off and the arms

and legs moving in synchronous opposition.[15] Basically, there are three phases in the running pattern: the pushoff, the flight, and the landing.[1] The major difference between running and walking is that in the middle phase of the running pattern the body is not supported. As speed in running is increased, the body must be inclined forward with its weight placed increasingly on the balls of the feet.

Before the young child is able to run, as with all body control events, sufficient strength, balance, and coordination must be developed. Muscle strength must be present to such a degree that the child's body can be pushed forward and upward into the flight phase. Dynamic balance and postural control are also prerequisites, allowing maintenance of the body segments in their proper alignment throughout the entire running pattern. There must also be a smooth interaction between the muscles of the arms and legs to allow their opposition to one another.

Generally, the beginning runner displays an exaggerated movement around the long axis of the body with stiff arms that swing from side to side, knees that rotate outward, and feet that are wide apart with toes outward. Gradually, as maturation and learning occur, there is less body rotation, arms begin to swing easily and bend at the elbows, knees and feet begin moving in a straighter line with the base of support as it becomes narrower.[15] Between 2 and 3 years of age the preschooler acquires a smoother running pattern but still has difficulty in executing quick changes of movement. The 4- to 5-year-old child, on the other hand, can stop and turn quickly, and by the time the child reaches 5 or 6 years of age, the adult style of running has usually been acquired.[6]

Climbing. Climbing is one of the many fundamental skills that emerge directly from the locomotor patterns of crawling, creeping, and walking (Fig. 5-3). As with all other body transport skills, a certain level of strength, balance, and coordination must be present before climbing can take place. Often, the infant who has just learned to creep will attempt to ascend stairs using a similar creeping pattern. The 15-month-old child can normally go up a flight of four or five stairs in a creeping fashion with ease but will have great difficulty in coming back down those same stairs. In the early period of learning to descend stairs, the child may attempt a head first approach; however, this will soon be forsaken for a safer, backward method.

At 18 months of age, the toddler can usually walk up stairs in the upright posture by holding onto a hand for security; 3 months later the young child can ascend independently by holding onto a bannister and by 2 years is able to go up and down stairs without assistance.[8,10] In general, even though climbing stairs in the upright posture has been achieved, de-

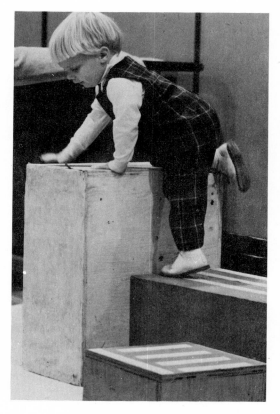

Fig. 5-3. At 2 years of age many children are challenged to climb.

scending will be accomplished by creeping backward. In its initial stages, walking up and down stairs is performed by the marking time, unilateral method, or in other words the child steps up on the riser with the same foot each time and brings the trailing foot up on the same riser, meeting the leading foot. It is not usually until about 3 years of age that the child can demonstrate the alternate foot ascent of the stairs and not until 4 or 5 years that the alternating foot descent is demonstrated.

It should be noted that ladder-climbing skill development follows a sequence similar to that of stair climbing but may appear a little later, depending on the availability of equipment and the distance between the rungs to be traversed. In both stair and ladder climbing, the young child can accomplish the climbing sooner if the rungs are closer together and the slant is not too severe.

Opportunities to climb are major requirements for a chld's total motor development. Skill in climbing a variety of obstacles increases significantly between the ages of 3 and 6 years. There is a great need during the preschool years for available climbing equipment, such as trees, jungle gyms, boxes, and nets, to satisfy children's natural desires to test themselves and their environment.[6]

Jumping and hopping. As was noted in the section on running, in order to propel the body in such a way that it becomes suspended in space requires a complex integration of many neurophysiological attributes. The basic skills of jumping and hopping stem directly from the locomotor patterns of walking and running. To project himself or herself into the air without tumbling out of control requires the child to have a great deal of courage and self-confidence, along with the appropriate level of maturation. One should also note that as children attempt new and challenging movements it is very common for them to revert to motor behaviors that are typical of more primitive and seemingly safer methods until such time as learning and confidence emerge.

Jumping. In general, a child first learns to jump a distance and from a height and then learns to jump an obstacle. There is a very close relationship between learning to climb stairs and learning to jump from a height. The first indication that children are ready to experience jumping is when they can run. The first jump occurs when the 2½-year-old child performs a large step from the lowest stair riser while holding onto the hand of an adult for security. At about this same age the child is beginning to jump up and down on the floor with both feet.[2]

In general, jumping from a height progresses through many preliminary events but mainly stems from the initial pattern of an exaggerated step downward, land-

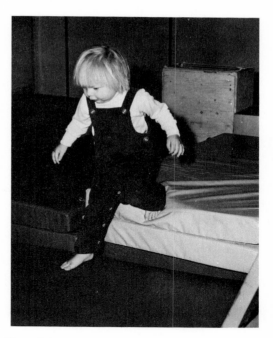

Fig. 5-4. Learning to jump from a height starts with an exaggerated step down.

ing on the lead foot (Fig. 5-4). From this beginning pattern, the child progresses to stepping off with one foot and landing on the opposite foot, to jumping from a height with both feet and landing on both feet (at about the age of 32 months), and to finally jumping down by taking off with one foot and landing on two feet (at about 3 years of age). In most cases, the child of 3 years has mastered fairly well jumping from varying heights that measure up to 18 inches.[15]

Distance jumping, on the other hand, occurs from the time children jump in place with both feet, at about 28 months; to when they can run and leap from one foot to the other, which is about the time they can make an exaggerated step from a height; to about 3 years of age, when they can make a standing jump forward with two feet, landing on both feet. The next and most difficult sequence after the distance jump occurs at about 3 years of age. It is running and jumping forward from one foot and landing on both feet and is like the long jump in track and field. Between the ages of 3½ and 4 years, a large percentage of children can demonstrate an effective standing broad jump, and at 5 years, may even be able to jump a distance of 5 feet.[8] Note that jumping over an obstacle is considered to be more difficult than jumping from a height or distance and does not normally appear in the child's jumping repertoire until after 3 years of age. At this time a two-foot jump can be performed over an obstacle about 8 inches high, ending with a two-foot landing. In general, one may expect children to be effective jumpers by approximately 4½ years of age.[7]

Another jumping skill that gradually emerges out of the two-foot, in place jump is the ability to perform a vertical jump for height. By the age of 4 years, the child should be able to spring into the air, reaching as high as possible, when asked to touch a specific object positioned overhead.[15] In all jumping tasks that require the child to go forward or as high as possible, the arms and legs must be coordinated for maximum thrust. The beginning jumper jumps stiffly, with little bending of the knees and little forward and upward swing of the arms. As development occurs, arms and legs become a coordinated unit to maximize jumping distance or height. Rope jumping commonly begins at about 5 years of age.

Hopping. One-foot hopping, although more difficult than jumping, is a basic locomotor skill stemming from the pattern of walking and running. The action of hopping may be described as lifting the body into the air by jumping off one foot and landing on the same foot. One-foot hopping is considered to evolve out of the two-foot, jumping in place pattern. Before children are able to properly coordinate a hop on one foot, they must be able to perform a one-foot static or stationary balance, which is commonly possible at 2½ years of age, and have enough strength to propel their bodies off the ground. A child of 3½ years usually can initiate from one to three hops on one foot; a child of 4

years, six hops; and a child of 5 years, ten hops. It is not until 6 years of age, however, that the typical child can perform as a fully proficient hopper.[4,8]

Galloping and skipping. Galloping and skipping are advanced extensions of the walking and hopping patterns. Galloping, which is performed by a walk and leap, usually does not appear before the fourth year of life and does not become well established before 6½ years of age.[3] The skipping pattern commonly is acquired somewhat after galloping is learned. Skipping must be considered one of the most, if not the most, difficult skills in basic locomotion. Its proper execution requires the performer to step-hop alternately on each foot in a smooth rhythmical transition from one foot to the other. At age 4 years, a child might attempt a rudimentary type of skipping step-hopping with one foot only and walking on the other foot.[4] About 14% of all children can demonstrate a true skip using each foot in an alternate manner at 4 years of age, 22% at 5 years of age, and 90% at 6 years of age (Table 5-1).[7]

Developing other forms of transportation. The preschool period is a time for developing a vast array of transport methods. Swimming, bicycle riding, and skating are but a few skills that can be learned during this time, depending on the available opportunities. The newborn, at 11 days of age, makes swimming movements when placed in water. This reaction is commonly known as the swimming reflex and normally becomes disorganized or no longer present at about 5 months of age; however, if training continues, the infant can develop the ability to move independently in the water.[11] Toddlers have been taught to swim as far as fifteen feet in a pool and have become very proficient swimmers by 5 years of age.[6,8,11] A 2-year-old child can pedal a tricycle once the walking pattern has been well established, although the coordination of the eyes with the hands for the purpose of steering is not well developed. If locomotor skills and

Table 5-1. Normal developmental characteristics: gross motor behavior

Age*	Major events
27 months	Jumps off floor with both feet. Balances on one foot for 1 second. Ascends ladder carefully by marking time.
30 months	Walks straight line. Throws ball 4 feet or farther. Jumps from 18-inch height with one foot forward. Rides tricycle. Broad jumps 4 inches. Ascends ladder by marking time. Can walk on tiptoe.
36 months	Descends stairs by marking time. Jumps from 24-inch height with help. Jumps from 8-inch height with feet together. Hops on foot one or more times. Balances on one foot for 2 seconds. Kicks stationary ball. Climbs freely over furniture.
42 months	Hops ten or more steps with both feet. Hops four or more steps on one foot. Throws 3-inch ball 6 feet. Walks heel to toe on a line for 10 feet. Balances on one foot for 5 seconds.
48 months	Ascends ladder by leading with alternate feet. Broad jumps 24 inches. Balances on one foot for 8 seconds. Hops on one foot. Catches object that has been thrown. Jumps in place with two feet. Jumps from 24-inch box with two feet.
52 months	Displays highly synchronous walking. Descends stairs by leading with alternate feet.
56 months	Descends ladder by leading with alternate feet. Hops seven or more steps on one foot. Throws 3-inch ball 10 feet.
5 years	Skips. Walks backward heel to toe. Walks like adult. Gallops. Throws 9-inch ball 10 feet. Hops ten or more steps on one foot.

Adapted from Arnheim, D. D., Auxter, D., and Crowe, W.: Principles and methods of adapted physical education and recreation, ed. 3, St. Louis, 1977, The C. V. Mosby Co.
*The ages at which the major events noted here occur are approximate.

postural balance patterns are well established, a 4-year-old child may even be able to ride a two-wheel bicycle; however, this skill is not normally possible until 5 or 6 years of age.[8] It may also be of some interest to elementary school teachers that children unable to coordinate the use of a two-wheel bicycle with training wheels by 5½ years of age, in actuality, may not have adequately inhibited the primitive tonic neck reflexes, which prohibit them from moving their heads independently in relation to the rest of their bodies.[13]

Balance

The maintenance of equilibrium while engaging in a variety of locomotor and nonlocomotor activities is called balance.

As children gain in posture control, they also gain in their ability to perform static (stationary) and dynamic (moving) balance activities (Fig. 5-5). (See Chapter 8.) Balance "generally reflects the efficiency and the integration of the muscular system (particularly the reflexes that enable children to unconsciously adjust their postures to the upright), of ocular control, and of the vestibular apparatus (inner ear)."[4] One may assume that from the time the fetus moves within the mother or adjusts to the mother's changes of posture, the ability to balance is being developed; however, it does not stand out as a major ability until the infant becomes a toddler. The 2-year-old child will attempt to stand on a walking board that is 4 inches high by 3½ inches wide by 8 feet long and when just a little older, will walk

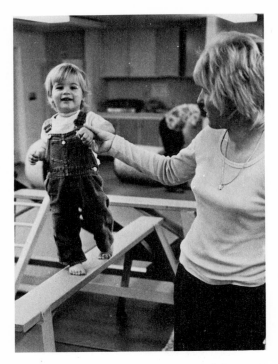

Fig. 5-5. Learning to balance is one of the most important human achievements.

the same board by a one-foot-on–one-foot-off method.[2] At 3 years of age 50% of the children should be able to walk along a 1-inch line for a distance of 10 feet. Three-year-old children can usually balance on one foot for 3 to 4 seconds, but it is not until they reach 4 years of age that they can statically balance on one foot for 10 seconds and walk a circular line. At 4½ years of age children can alternately walk a 2½-inch wide balance beam.[2] By the time children have reached their fifth birthdays, they have acquired the degree of maturation in both static and dynamic balance necessary to allow them to learn such varied skills as roller and ice skating, skiing, and two-wheel bicycle riding.[6]

Controlling projectiles in play

The early childhood and preschool years are a time for building basic skills in play, particularly those concerned with the management of objects in space. The four skills that are essential to effective play in the young child, as well as for preparing the child for advanced sports activities in later years, are throwing, catching, kicking, and striking. Their development closely parallels the child's maturation in the large muscle control necessary for posture, locomotion, and balance and in the small muscle control of the hand, foot, and eye required for fine movement activities.

Throwing. One might speculate that throwing begins when an infant voluntarily lets go of an object; however, most authorities describe it as occurring when the sitting infant rejects some unpleasant or unwanted object by either pushing or tossing it away.[5] At 1 year of age, paralleling ocular-motor and manipulative development, throwing is begun crudely but with some accuracy. However, it is not until about 2 years of age that the young child is able to impart both distance and accuracy to the throw.[6] At age 2 years, the child performs throwing only by raising the arm above the level of the shoulder. The movement is immature and jerky with little or no use of either the body or legs. Between the ages of 3 and 5 years, preschool children begin to rotate their bodies and lower their throwing arms so that they are approximately in line with their shoulders; however, their feet still remain planted. A major accomplishment occurs between the ages of 5 and 6 years when the child learns to step forward with the same foot as the throwing arm. A mature throwing pattern, with the opposite foot stepping forward, should not be expected until the child has reached 6½ years of age.[15]

Catching. Effectively perceiving a moving object in space requires many sophisticated perceptual abilities. The child must be able to adjust to the different sizes of objects, to the distance the object must travel, to how the object is projected, to its direction, and to the speed of its flight.[15] The age at which these perceptual abilities occur is highly variable, depending, of course, on maturation and on the child's opportunities to gain experience with a variety of objects in different situations. Catching, although in many ways more complicated than throwing, is highly dependent on the development of the coordinated use of both hands in grasping and the teaming or coordination of both eyes.

In catching, large ball control comes before effective small ball handling. A child usually learns to manage a rolling ball first by trapping it when it has been rolled between his or her spread legs and develops the skill to the point that the rolling ball can be stopped by running directly to it. Catching an object in the air after it has been thrown is one of the most difficult body control skills. At about the age of 2 years, children can begin to deal effectively with the rolling ball and at 3 years, can begin to manage the airborne ball. At 3 years, when instructed, the preschooler will stand in one place with the arms stiffly outstretched and receive a gently tossed object. With the continued experience of having a large 14½-inch ball, a beanbag, or other manageable object thrown, the child progresses from the rigid arms to a more shovellike appearance, with elbows relaxed and hands wider apart. At the age of 4 years, the child's elbows are bent but are still held in front of the body; however, the child now begins to anticipate the throw by leaning slightly forward and will make a grasp at the ball as it comes within range. The 4-year-old child is also beginning to use more of the hands and arms instead of trapping the object against the body.[15] Gradually, as skill at catching progresses, the child's arms are brought to the sides of the body and, by age 5 or 5½ years, the arms reach out to receive the ball and give way to it as it approaches.

A fear factor may creep into the child's catching behavior, as demonstrated by closing the eyes and turning the head, especially if there is a history of being hit in the face by some projected object, usually a ball. Unless confidence is restored to the child immediately, this fear reaction may undermine future efforts at ball catching. Children who are fearful can learn to catch softer and more manageable objects such as fleece balls, balloons, ropes, or beanbags.

Kicking. The ability to kick a stationary ball on the ground appears when a child is able to run and balance momentarily on one foot. Eighteen-month-old toddlers can normally perform rudimentary kicking by walking into a large ball and pushing it forward with their legs or bodies.[10] Gradually, young children begin to learn to push the ball with just one foot,[6] then with experience, they learn to swing their legs into the ball. As with most beginning skills, there is little use of the body or arms. When the child has attained the degree of balance and strength necessary to stand on one foot for a longer period of time, the swing of the kicking leg increases; however, the leg is still relatively stiff. With time, the child increases the backswing, leans the body forward on contact, and follows through with the kicking leg. The 4-year-old child who has had opportunities to practice the kick gradually acquires an effective stationary kick in which the knee and hip bend before contact; however, not until 5 years of age will the child be able to kick effectively for distance and accuracy, and not until 5 or 6 years of age will the punt be introduced into the kicking repertoire.

Punting is a very difficult skill and can be accomplished only when the child is able to balance extremely well on one foot and to lean the body forward while at the same time dropping the ball and kicking it before it hits the ground. Learning to punt usually occurs after the child has mastered the stationary ground kick.[15]

Striking. The skill of striking objects that have been projected into space is not as predictable as throwing, catching, or kicking. Although striking appears to start from the overarm hitting action (much like throwing), as a skill it does not have

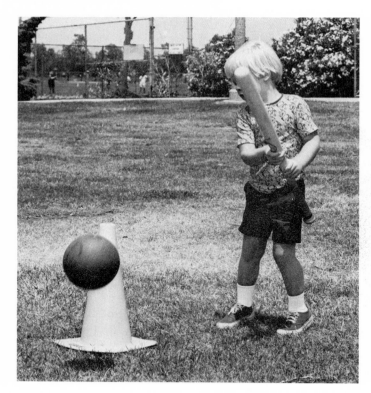

Fig. 5-6. Sidearm striking with a bat is a skill that does not usually appear until a child is 4½ or 5 years of age.

well-defined sequences. As in throwing, the first striking action is with the child facing the object and using only the movement of the arms and hands. Underarm and sidearm striking replaces the overarm method but is highly dependent on the position of the object in relation to the child. It appears that by the time the child reaches 3 years of age, sidearm striking can be initiated with one arm. More difficult patterns of striking that employ both arms, such as batting or golfing, must wait until 4½ to 5 years of age (Fig. 5-6). In general, striking develops sequentially in much the same manner as throwing and in much the same time frame if the opportunities are available to the child and if the striking implements are of the proper size and weight.[15]

PERCEPTUAL DEVELOPMENT

As discussed in Chapter 4, that which gives meaning to the information that comes from within the body or from without the body by way of the various sense organs is known as perception. In general, the acquisition of perceptual information is determined by growth and maturation and by which areas of development are strongest at the time. For example, the first 2 years of life are concerned with perceptual-motor development, with major emphasis placed on the organization of posture and locomotor skills. Perceptual development, during the first years after birth is centered on the functions of touch and movement. As maturation occurs there is a gradual shift to the sense modalities of hearing and seeing.[16] Because of their gaining of both gross and fine motor control, children between the ages of 2 and 4 years are beginning to receive and organize a continuous flow of perceptual information. One should note that before children can effectively perceive and respond to different stimuli, they must become physi-

Table 5-2. Normal developmental characteristics: small muscle and visual perceptual behavior

Age*	Major events
27 months	Builds tower of eight 1-inch cubes. Turns doorknob, Unscrews lid of jar.
30 months	Holds pencil. Loosens shoelaces. Drinks from straw. Copies circle. Knows difference between vertical and horizontal lines.
36 months	Builds tower of ten 1-inch cubes. Holds pencil like adult. Draws vertical line. Strings four beads in 2 minutes. Cuts with scissors.
42 months	Traces diamond. Puts half-inch pegs into pegboard.
48 months	Draws man with three parts. Copies cross. Laces own shoes. Strings seven beads in 2 minutes. Buttons large button. Draws recognizable picture.
5 years	Copies square. Draws man with six parts. Knows difference between horizontal and vertical lines.

Adapted from Arnheim, D. D., Auxter, D., and Crowe, W.: Principles and methods of adapted physical education and recreation, ed. 3, St. Louis, 1977, The C. V. Mosby Co.

*The ages at which the major events noted here occur are approximate.

cally organized. As the human organism becomes refined and organized in all of its functions and processes, it becomes increasingly able to perceive the subtleties of both the external and internal environment (Table 5-2). The young child gradually develops the ability to filter out extraneous stimuli and actively seeks the desired stimulation.

BECOMING A PERSON

The period from 2 to 5 years of age is that time in which the young child changes into a truly unique personality. Having gone through a stage of complete dependency as an infant and the important stage of gaining locomotor skills, the child is now ready to embark on a quest for personal independence. Communicating, socializing, and exploring now become uppermost in the life of the child.

Social development and play

Many theories have been put forth as to why children play. Some authorities consider play as the "work of children" others consider it as satisfying an internal drive toward effectively dealing with environment, while still others consider it as the inherent joy of mastery.[12] In most instances, play is really caused by many factors. It allows for free expression to act out the deep emotions of love, hate, jealousy, happiness, and fear. It provides opportunities for dominating situations, controlling things and people, and imitating the life that surrounds the child. Through play, the complicated world of the young child becomes manageable.

As children become more and more independent in moving about their surroundings, they begin to interact to a greater extent with those people around them. During the first 2 years of life, social development has been determined mainly by the parents. A 2-year-old child is the center of his or her own universe because for the first 2 years after birth the child is for the most part completely dependent on the caretakers in his or her world. The efforts of the 2-year-old child to become independent have often been called the "terrible twos" by par-

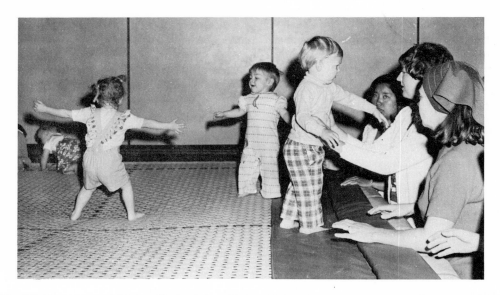

Fig. 5-7. Very young children will often play side by side but normally require very close supervision by adults.

Table 5-3. Normal developmental characteristics: social and adaptive behavior

Age*	Major event
27 months	Imitates other children's play. Eats with fork. Unbuttons large buttons. Indicates need to go to toilet.
30 months	Dresses with help. Avoids specified dangers.
36 months	Takes turns. Feeds self with spoon and fork.
42 months	Puts on shoes. Functions independently in toileting. Plays with another child.
48 months	Plays highly structured games. May have imaginary playmate. Is very aggressive in play. Dresses self. Washes and dries hands. Cooperates in play.
5 years	Dresses without help. Plays in group of three.

Adapted from Arnheim, D. D., Auxter, D., and Crowe, W.: Principles and methods of adapted physical education and recreation, ed. 3, St. Louis, 1977, The C. V. Mosby Co.
*The ages at which the major events noted here occur are approximate.

ents. At this time the child often is stubborn, is negative when asked to cooperate, and shows fear by hiding when strangers are present. The 2-year-old child prefers to engage in solitary play and has very special interests in cuddly stuffed animals, pull toys that make noise, large building blocks, and picture books. He or she likes to imitate family activities like sweeping the floor, brushing the hair, and shaving like daddy.

Gradually, by age 2½ years, the child changes from playing alone to parallel type play, in which activities are engaged in beside another child but with little

Table 5-4. Normal developmental characteristics: language and communication

Age*	Major events
27 months	Repeats two numbers. Knows three prepositions. Names most common objects in home. Uses plurals.
30 months	Identifies objects by use. Knows the number "one." Knows simple songs and rhymes.
36 months	Gives full name. Knows own sex. Identifies at least two objects from picture. Answers simple questions. Talks in simple sentences.
42 months	Counts to three. Follows simple verbal directions. Knows the concepts of longer and heavier. Can tell a story.
48 months	Uses conjunctions. Understands prepositions. Makes five- and six-word sentences. Names the colors "red," "blue," and "yellow." Possesses 800-word vocabulary. Gestures with entire body. Forms sentences.
5 years	Expresses mature articulation. Asks "Why?" Can define six words. Explains composition of materials.

From Arnheim, D. D., Auxter, D., and Crowe, W.: Principles and methods of adapted physical education and recreation, ed. 3, St. Louis, 1977, The C. V. Mosby Co.
*The ages at which the major events noted here occur are approximate.

interaction with that child. The parallel play period is a time when the child believes that "everything is mine, "with toy snatching and even fighting a common practice, often requiring very close adult supervision (Fig. 5-7). A gradual change occurs in the child's acceptance of other children in his or her world. By the time children reach 3 years of age they are much easier to get along with and can even be taught to take turns. They often like to imitate all kinds of things, such as cars, planes, and animals. Making things with the hands, like drawing crayon pictures, finger painting, and making things with large building blocks, becomes fun. At 4 years of age children commonly begin to engage in associative play, in which there occurs some cooperation; in fact, some children of this age may even seek out some special friend or, if one is not available, may invent an imaginary playmate. By the time the child has reached 5 years of age, he or she is a good player and is easy to get along with. Many parents of 5-year-old children state that "they are now a real joy to be around." The 5-year-old child continually seeks out children to play with and deeply enjoys competition in a vast array of large and small muscle activities (Table 5-3).

Communication and learning

All the events in the development of a child are interwoven. The highly complex areas of communication and learning are closely associated with motor and perceptual development, especially during the first 2 years of life. Piaget calls this time span the sensorimotor period, when mental activity is associated primarily with the development of basic movement patterns and with physically active interaction with the environment.[9] In other words, learning is directly associated with moving. Little so-called intellectualizing takes place in the child until the end of the sensorimotor period when Piaget's second broad stage occurs, extending approximately to age 7 years. This second period of cognitive development is called the preoperational period and is characterized by the child learning to use symbols as representatives of something else. Between the ages of 2 and 4 years, the child develops imagination and indulges in symbolic play, wherein one object becomes another object, such as a block of wood, a car or a stick, an airplane. From 2 to 5 years of age, the child develops many perceptual and cognitive concepts, such as shape, distance, length, number, weight, and time; these, along with the development of symbolism through words, assist further to develop the child's mental capacities.

Language must be considered one of early childhood's finest accomplishments. The child, from earliest infancy, learns to communicate thoughts and feelings, first through gestures and then gradually through words. By the end of the second year after birth, the typical child has a vocabulary of between 100 and 200 words; by 3 years of age, about 500 words; and by 4 years of age, as many as 1000 words. By 5 years of age the child is extremely proficient in language, using compound sentences to express feelings and thoughts (Table 5-4).

PHYSICAL EDUCATION AND PRESCHOOL EDUCATION

As discussed in the beginning of this chapter, the early childhood period is a time for building many complex patterns of behavior. The total developmental process during this period is directed toward independence and environmental adaptation. Preschool children have an unquenchable thirst for knowledge, for exploration, and for testing themselves against themselves and their surroundings—in essence, for experiencing all there is to experience. This is a crucial time for children to build confidence and self-esteem and to learn to trust the world about them. Successes at this time must be maximized and failures minimized in order for children to develop the courage necessary to welcome and attempt new challenges.

Physical education within the pre-

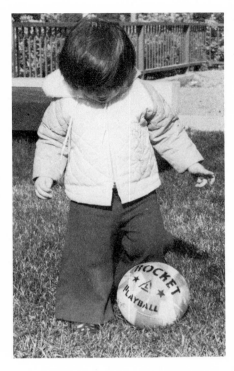

Fig. 5-8. Physical education in preschool must encourage self-discovery.

school or nursery school setting must be concerned with three major factors: the role of the teacher, the curriculum, and the environment. It is essential that the teacher not engage in a highly structured and directive type of teaching. The teacher must assume the roles of guide, encourager, and stager and, at all costs, must avoid stultifying the children's natural inclination to move by too formalized instruction. The normal joy of movement must be maintained and enhanced through self-discovery (Fig. 5-8). The movement curriculum should follow closely the precepts of movement education, in which process and quality become the most important goals (see Chapter 9, Movement education). In many ways the extent to which a child experiences a wide variety of movement opportunities is contingent on the richness of the play environment. to ensure full physical, mental, and emotional development, the play environment should provide an infinite number of ways for the child to participate in large muscle and gross motor activities, particularly those concerned with locomotor skills. There should also be opportunities for fine motor development with priority given to development of manipulative skills and hand-eye coordination. Physical education must provide the child with opportunities to express imaginative play and to freely experience both the perceptual and cognitive domains of learning through the medium of movement activities.

CLASS ACTIVITIES

1. Demonstrate the developmental steps a young child goes through in learning to jump from a height.
2. Demonstrate the developmental steps in learning to ascend and descend stairs.
3. Teach a child to gallop and/or skip by going through all the major developmental events leading up to the skill.
4. Using the developmental concept, teach a child to throw, catch, strike, and kick.
5. Visit a preschool and evaluate its motor development program based on the developmental principles expressed in this chapter.

REFERENCES

1. Arnheim, D. D., and Sinclair, W. A.: The clumsy child, St. Louis, 1975, The C. V. Mosby Co.
2. Bayley, N. A.: The development of motor abilities during the first three years, Soc. Res. Child Dev. 1(1):1-16, 1935.
3. Breckenridge, M., and Vincent, L.: Child development, ed. 3, Philadelphia, 1955, W. B. Saunders Co.
4. Cratty, B. J.: Perceptual and motor development in infants and children, New York, 1970, The Macmillan Co.
5. Eckert, H. M.: Age changes in motor skills. In Rarick, G. L., editor: Physical activity: human growth and development, New York, 1973, Academic Press, Inc.
6. Espenshade, A. S., and Eckert, H. M.: Motor development, Columbus, Ohio, 1967, Charles E. Merrill Publishing Co.
7. Gutteridge, M. V.: A study of motor achievements of young children, Arch. Psychol. 244:1, 1939.
8. Hottinger, W. L.: Motor development: conception to age five. In Corbin, C. B., editor: A textbook of motor development, Dubuque, Iowa, 1973, William C. Brown Co., Publishers.
9. Kaluger, G., and Kaluger, M. F.: Human development, St. Louis, 1974, The C. V. Mosby Co.
10. Knobloch, H., and Pasamanick, B., editors: Gesell and Armatruda's developmental diagnosis, ed. 3, New York, 1974, Harper & Row, Publishers, Inc.
11. McGraw, M. B.: The neuromuscular maturation of the human infant, New York, 1966, Hafner Publishing Co.
12. Piaget, J.: Play, dreams and imitation in childhood, London, 1951, William Heinemann Medical Books Ltd.
13. Stoddard, M.: For a more perfect baby, Twin Falls, Idaho, 1972, Standard Printers Co.
14. Wellman, B. L.: Motor achievement of preschool children, Child Ed. 13:311-316, 1937.
15. Wickstrom, R. L.: Fundamental motor patterns, Philadelphia, 1970, Lea & Febiger.
16. Williams, H. G.: Perceptual-motor development in children. In Corbin, D. B., editor: A textbook of motor development, Dubuque, Iowa, 1973, William C. Brown Co., Publishers.

RECOMMENDED READINGS

Cochran, N. A., Wilkinson, L. C., and Furlow, J. J.: Learning on the move, Dubuque, Iowa, 1975, Kendall/Hunt Publishing Co.
Dauer, V. P.: Essential movement experiences for preschool and primary children, Minneapolis, 1971, Burgess Publishing Co.
Flinchum, B. M.: Motor development in early childhood, St. Louis, 1975, The C. V. Mosby Co.
Gallahue, D. L., and Meadors, W. J.: Let's move, Dubuque, Iowa, 1974, Kendall/Hunt Publishing Co.
Hendrick, J.: The whole child, St. Louis, 1975, The C. V. Mosby Co.

6

Expanding: from 6 to 8 years of age

The primary school years, or middle childhood period, are a time of great enthusiasm, imagination, eagerness to learn, bubbling personality, and bountiful exuberance for living. These years are a time when children seek to expand their horizons beyond their own homes to the homes of friends and to school. Middle childhood is an ambivalent period of both being dependent on parental guidance and wanting desperately to spread the wings but still being too timid to venture far from the protection of home. Sitting still for 10 minutes seems to last a lifetime, and play and lunch periods are the child's favorite times of the school day. In general, the child between 6 and 8 years of age has three major characteristics: changes from a primarily family-dominated social environment to one that is dominated by peers, moves into a world of games and physical activities that require a prescribed level of motor ability, and moves into the world of highly sophisticated abstract symbols and communication skills necessary for reading, writing, and arithmetic.[5] Children now begin to compare themselves to other children; they are no longer the centers of their universes but must learn to cooperate, to take turns, and to be aware that some children can do some things better than they can and, conversely, that they are better than others at doing some things.

PHYSICAL GROWTH CHARACTERISTICS

As discussed earlier, the physical growth period from 2 to 5 years is one of leveling off from the rapid growth of infancy. Between 6 and 8 years growth is slow but constant, with height increasing from 2 to 3 inches and weight from 3 to 6 pounds each year.[7] Limbs continue to grow faster than the trunk, and the body's babyish roundness steadily gives way to a more linear, flat appearance.[4] Baby fat becomes less obvious and is replaced by muscle tissue. The face of the primary school age child lengthens and the baby teeth begin to be lost and replaced by permanent ones. A very important change occurs in vision when the basically farsighted child gradually develops the ability to accommodate nearer images, a necessity for close work in the classroom (Table 6-1).

PHYSICAL DEVELOPMENT

The primary school years are ones of physical stabilization and gradual change. This is a time for perfecting the basic movement patterns established during infancy and early childhood and using them as foundations for the acquisition of a backlog of motor skills.[4] The physiological factors necessary in skill development during the period from 6 to 8 years are numerous. For example, the myelination of nerves is for the most part completed by 8 years of age, allowing for greater strength and accuracy of movement. The average youngster of 8 years has muscles that comprise about one fourth of his or her total body.[9] As muscle tissue increases so does strength. Strength in the young child can best be measured by grip strength. From 6 to 8 years of age there is a gradual increase in grip strength averaging about 2 pounds per year.[1] Flexibility, in contrast to strength, is more variable, depending upon the use children make of their bodies. Girls tend to be more flexible than boys, but although girls have been shown to steadily increase their flexibility up to age 12 years, the ability of various body regions to stretch or bend is extremely specific and is dependent upon the types of activities engaged in habitually.[6] The ability to respond to a stimulus, or reaction time, is another very important factor of motor skill development. As each child matures, speed of reaction to some specific stimulation coming to the child through various senses increases. For example, a 5-year-old child generally reacts two times slower than an adult.[1] Combined with the lengthening of limbs, the increasing of strength and speed of reaction time enables the child to become more effective in dealing with the requirements of complex movement patterns.

During this middle childhood period, children also achieve relative stability in both dynamic and static balance. The 6-year-old child walks a 2-inch wide beam but has difficulty in walking a beam that is 1 inch in width (Fig. 6-1). Five-year-old children can stand on their preferred foot for 5 seconds with their eyes open and arms out to the side, whereas 8-year-old children can perform static balancing on the preferred foot with eyes open and arms folded across the chest for 5 seconds.[1] If the arms are not folded, the 8-year-old child can even balance with eyes closed for 5 seconds.

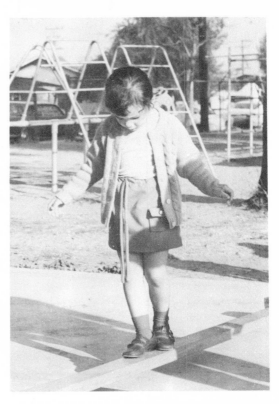

Fig. 6-1. A 6-year-old child attempting to walk the length of a 4-inch wide beam.

Locomotor skills during the middle childhood period display more mature patterns of behavior. There is a steady increase in the ability to perform rhythmical movements such as hopping on one foot and then the other. By age 8 years, the majority of girls and boys can demonstrate two hops on each foot alternately.[8] Jumping vertically increases from an average of 7 inches at age 7 years to over 8 inches by age 8 years. In contrast, horizontal jumping progresses about 1½ inch per year, with 5-year-old children jumping approximately 10 inches and 8-year-old children as far as 14 inches.[2]

Middle childhood is a continuation of the final stage in the development of eye-hand and eye-foot coordination, which began at about 40 weeks of age. In this last stage, the child acquires a more refined control of small muscles. Although

Table 6-1. Physical characteristics*

5 to 6 years	6 to 7 years	7 to 8 years	8 to 9 years
GENERAL DEVELOPMENT			
1. Child sleeps an average of 11 hours 19 minutes.	1. Child sleeps an average of 11 hours 14 minutes.	1. Child sleeps average of 10 hours 58 minutes.	1. Attention span is longer but still short.
2. Attention at play is 12 to 14 minutes.	2. Child has low resistance to disease.	2. Child freely uses language but is still immature.	2. Vocabulary contains 3600 words.
3. Child susceptible to contagious diseases.	3. Vocabulary consists of over 2500 words.	3. Child becomes a good listener.	3. Speech is immature.
4. Vocabulary contains over 2000 words.	4. First baby teeth are lost; six year molars come in.	4. Attention span lengthens.	4. Ten or 11 pernent teeth are in.
5. Child uses 5-word sentences.		5. Permanent teeth appear rapidly.	
6. Girls have larger vocabulary than boys.			

*The ages at which the physical characteristics noted here occur are approximate.

still primarily dominated by gross motor behavior, hand and foot movements, guided by the eyes, assist the child in developing a wide repertoire of skills, such as tying bows, cutting with scissors, drawing with crayons, beginning cursive writing, and projecting objects accurately through the air by kicking and throwing.[10]

Sex differences

Teachers of children in the early childhood and middle childhood periods should be aware of the differences between boys and girls in terms of physical and motor development. Although highly variable, there are sexual differences from the time of birth that may alter the behavior of the individual. In general, girls mature faster than boys. In early childhood, girls, although usually smaller than boys, have relatively longer legs and more narrow hips than boys, a characteristic that gradually reverses in the preadolescent period. The early matura-

tion of girls is also exemplified by the earlier appearance of first and second sets of teeth.

Girls tend to achieve motor coordination sooner than boys, as expressed by their ability to walk sooner (Fig. 6-2). Throughout their lives, boys are, as a rule, stronger than girls, except when girls start into their preadolescent period between 9 and 10 years of age. At this time, girls exceed boys of the same age in strength for a short period of time until the boys reach their prepubertal period between 11 and 12 years of age. However, in other physical attributes, such as balance and flexibility, girls often appear slightly better than boys up to adolescence (Fig. 6-3). Generally, boys between the ages of 2 and 7 years perform activities requiring strength and power, such as throwing, jumping, and kicking, better than girls. On the other hand, girls are usually better at activities requiring small muscle coordination, such as hand skills, rhythm, accuracy, agility, hopping, galloping, and

Table 6-1. Physical characteristics—cont'd

5 to 6 years	6 to 7 years	7 to 8 years	8 to 9 years
GROWTH			
1. Skeletal growth is slow and at a steady rate.	1. Girls are about a year more mature than boys.	1. More growth differences are apparent between the sexes.	1. Different growth between sexes is apparent.
2. Infant top-heaviness is lost and more adultlike proportions emerge.	2. Height is two thirds of adult height.	2. Growth occurs at steady rate.	2. Growth occurs at a slower rate.
3. Head is adult size.	3. Yearly height gain is 1 to 2 inches.	3. Fatigue sets in easily.	3. Motor skills and body control are improving rapidly.
4. Child needs to be active.	4. Yearly weight gain is about 3 to 5 pounds.	4. Child needs large muscle activity.	4. Arm and leg strength is underdeveloped.
5. Large muscles are most used.	5. Knock-knees and protruding abdomen are common.	5. Child enjoys very strenuous activity.	5. Writing is still difficult.
6. Child feeds and dresses self.	6. Most basic skills are acquired.	6. Creative rhythms are fun.	6. Child enjoys vigorous body activities.
7. Child begins to jump rope.	7. Child needs strenuous activity.	7. Child independently dresses self.	7. Tag is enjoyed.
8. Rhythm increases.	8. Child has better rhythm.	8. Child can focus on near object for a longer time.	8. Balancing is better.
9. Child may gallop or skip.	9. Eye-hand coordination is poor.	9. Eye-hand coordination is well established.	9. More difficult large muscle skills can be learned.
10. Handedness is established.	10. Child is better judge of distance.		10. Child has more interest in games requiring small muscle control.
11. Child is nearsighted.	11. Cursive writing is difficult.		
12. Child begins to use more dextrous movements.	12. Child can usually learn to read and write.		

skipping. It should be noted, however, that stereotyping of either sex into specific ability groupings should be avoided.

BODY PERCEPTION AND SPACE AWARENESS

Middle childhood represents a time when the child has established a relatively sophisticated perception of the body and the space in which it functions. From birth, perhaps even from the embryonic phase of life, body and space perceptions are being learned. Although there are many unsubstantiated ideas about the importance of body awareness and cognitive learning, there is a general consensus that they are integral parts of a a child's total development. Cratty depicts a child's body image as including all

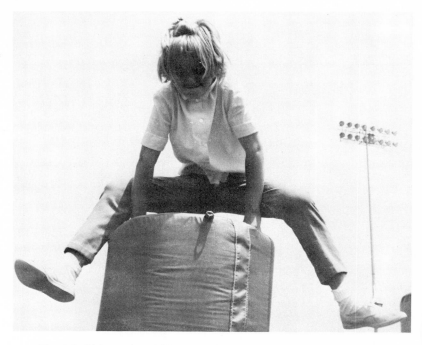

Fig. 6-2. Girls tend to achieve motor coordination sooner than boys.

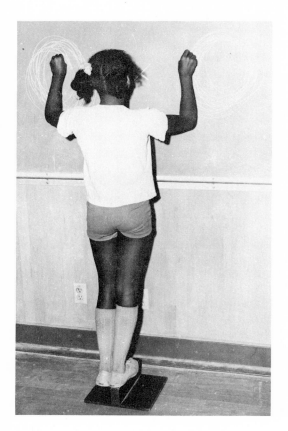

Fig. 6-3. Girls tend to be slightly better than boys in the area of balance up to the time of adolescence.

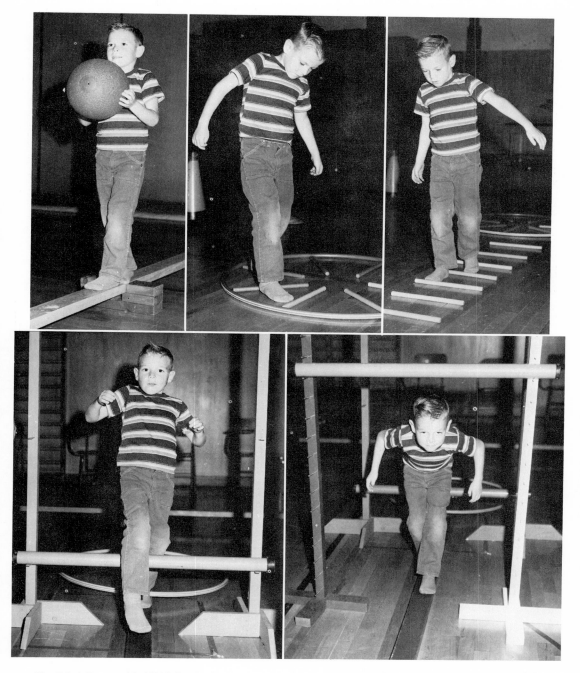

Fig. 6-4. A 7-year-old child is beginning to develop a keen awareness of the body as it relates to spatial problems.

Table 6-2. Emotional characteristics*

5 to 6 years	6 to 7 years	7 to 8 years	8 to 9 years
1. Is very serious	1. Is more stable and less impulsive	1. Depresses easily and displays sulking and sadness	1. Is more sensitive to criticism
2. Fluctuates between dependence and independence	2. Displays extremes of emotion; laughs and cries easily	2. Cries easily	2. May cry easily
3. Shows affection toward others	3. May be loving one minute and hostile the next	3. Gives affection but is restrained	3. Is happy when praised for achievement
4. May have fear and apprehension toward school	4. Is very excitable	4. Wants to be liked	4. Is calmer than before
5. May display temper tantrums	5. Readily shows affection	5. Has deep worries, such as war, burglars, etc.	5. Is more self-reliant and less demanding of parents
	6. Seeks independence but fears it	6. Has fear of being embarrassed	6. Has greater sense of humor
	7. May fear things like ghosts, thunder and lightning, and animals	7. Has less outbursts of anger and less tantrums and fighting	7. Demonstrates less affection
	8. Still may display tantrums	8. Displays jealousy over parent; girls may become jealous of father's attention to mother	8. Still has many fears
	9. May express anger by kicking, hitting, and biting		9. Still fights (boys)
	10. Has quick and violent outbursts of emotion		10. Has less outbursts of anger
	11. Frustrates easily when unable to perform a small motor task		11. May still have jealousy over parent

*The ages at which the emotional characteristics noted occur are approximate.

measurable responses relative to "body size, shape, components [of body parts], perceived capacities for movement, and interactions with the environment."[1]

By the time 5 years of age has been reached, children are definitely aware that there are two sides of the body and are able to locate themselves in relation to other objects. At 8 years of age, laterality is well established and children not only can accurately name their left and right body parts but also are able to identify the left and right parts of other persons.[1] As growth, maturation, and movement experiences progress the 7-year-old child gradually becomes less dependent on vision to determine where the body is in space (Fig. 6-4).

SOCIAL, EMOTIONAL, AND PLAY CHARACTERISTICS

The period from 6 to 8 years of age is one in which a child's world rapidly expands to the world outside of the home. The child's life begins to focus on school and outside activities (Table 6-2). Friends become very important. Middle childhood is the time when each child reaches out for independence but at the same time needs reassurance from the mother and father. This combination of the drive to be autonomous plus the need for dependency creates stresses within the child that produce emotional ups and downs; one minute the child is laughing, the next, crying. Between 5 and 7 years of age, friendships are important, but allegiance to one friend is often weak. At this time the loss of a friend is quickly forgotten, and a new friend is immediately sought; however, at 8 years of age, there develops a greater loyalty to peers than to adults. The 7-year-old child becomes very self-critical, mainly because there is a growing realization that people are different and have strengths and weaknesses. As a result of this expanding self-awareness, criticism from both adults and peers take on added importance. Middle childhood is a crucial period for children to verify that they are worthwhile persons. Being a "good player" is basic to the child's development of a positive self-concept.

Play now becomes more purposeful and less spontaneous. Many personality and social changes occur during the middle childhood period including sex changes and the development of rules and leadership roles (Table 6-3). Children begin to play in small groups of three and four. Whereas the kindergarten child had relatively simple rules of play, 7- and 8-year-old children now have more complex rules and produce greater cooperation between participants.[3] Imagination and exploration reach their peaks between 4 and 6 years of age. The span between 6 and 12 years of age is considered to be one in which there is dedication to testing one's own abilities. Common games of the kindergarten child might be tag, chase, and hide and seek, but when the child reaches 6 or 7 years the games of choice are usually dodge ball, kick ball, hopscotch and rope jumping.[7] Many children of this age enjoy sit-down games like Monopoly or Parchesi or simple card games like Hearts.[7] In the past girls seemed to prefer less physically vigorous games than did boys; however, with cultural changes, many girls play as vigorously as boys do. At all ages girls enjoy playing with boys; however, after the age of 8 years, boys prefer playing with members of their own sex. Because play is often considered a microcosm of the society, it behooves one not to overrationalize reasons for game preference based on sex. It might be speculated that the rapid changes in American sex roles will soon be reflected by changes in current game choices between girls and boys.

Other factors that affect play and that emerge during the middle childhood period are physique and leadership. Earlier-maturing children initially are often more skilled in physically vigorous games and, therefore, achieve a some-

Table 6-3. Typical social play characteristics*

5 to 6 years	6 to 7 years	7 to 8 years	8 to 9 years
RELATION WITH ADULTS			
1. Child is staunch family member. 2. Child wants to help. 3. Child wants to show independence.	1. Child wants to be close. 2. Child seeks praise. 3. Child will take orders. 4. Child dislikes criticism. 5. Child talks freely. 6. Child is very friendly. 7. Child not always sure. 8. Father is more important. 9. Teacher becomes important. 10. Mother is less important.	1. Child talks back. 2. Child questions everything. 3. Child nags. 4. Child is aware of other feelings. 5. Child is very friendly. 6. Child seeks approval. 7. Child wants to to help members of family. 8. Boys get closer to father. 9. Girls more sensitive to father. 10. Teacher is very important.	1. Child identifies with parent. 2. Child copies adult standards. 3. Child challenges parents with "why" and "no." 4. Child demands praise. 5. Child admits doing wrong. 6. Child is dependent on mother. 7. Child seeks teacher's praise. 8. Father is less important.
PEER RELATIONSHIPS			
1. Play is solitary or parallel. 2. Occasionally there is cooperative play. 3. Child prefers a group of three. 4. Affection more than aggression is displayed toward peers. 5. Child begins to enjoy competition. 6. Child is impatient for turns. 7. Child poor group member; he or she grabs and takes and is a tattletale. 8. Sex is ignored in game playing.	1. Child likes small group activity. 2. Child likes loose organization. 3. Leaders develop in small group. 4. Child is still impatient about waiting turn. 5. Child is poor group member. 6. Child is aware of others' rights. 7. Sex differences are ignored. 8. Child may imitate older children. 9. Child domineers and calls names.	1. Real group play occurs. 2. There is better cooperation in group. 3. Child has less impatience about getting turn. 4. Competition increases. 5. Child is poor loser. 6. Child still bosses and calls names. 7. Girls and boys begin to play own games. 8. Child starts to have a best friend.	1. Peer is more important than family. 2. Spontaneous groupings lasting a short while occur. 3. Child will abide by group decisions. 4. There is constant bickering. 5. Games must have rules. 6. A best friend is essential. 7. Boys and girls play less with one another.

*The ages at which the social play characteristics noted occur are approximate.

what higher level of peer acceptance and success. The physically gifted child is also commonly looked upon as a leader more than the less physically gifted.

PHYSICAL EDUCATION AND PRIMARY CHILDREN

Physical education during middle childhood and the primary school years should be directed toward helping children acquire as many movement experiences as possible. Every opportunity must be given the child to explore the environment through all major sense channels. This is an excellent time for employing the basic concepts of movement education in which children become aware of the process and quality inherent in all motor responses (see Chapter 9). Movement education provides the primary child with opportunities to develop keen perceptual-motor awareness of time and space and also to begin to integrate new patterns of move-

ment into imaginative and creative expressions. This is also a time when the child responds well to activities concerned with basic body management through perceptual-motor training (see Chapter 8).

Primary level children like to and need to continually engage in large muscle activities. They respond well to activities that allow them to chase and be chased, to push and pull one another, and to be rough and tumble. This is a time when children are eager to learn basic stunts and activities that test their abilities in movement. Varied gymnastic challenges give the young performer a chance to increase physical efficiency, especially in the realm of strength and muscular control. Games and play should prepare the child for those sports skills that he or she will participate in in later childhood and should offer special opportunities for the development of eye-hand and eye-foot coordination, while at the same time encouraging cooperation under the guid-

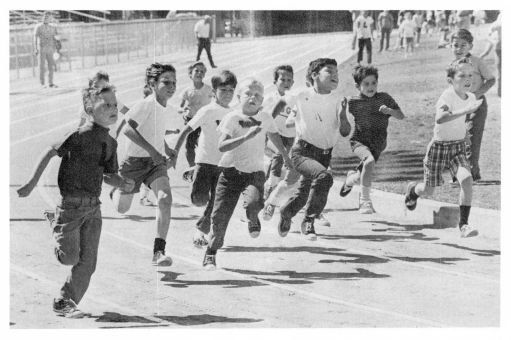

Fig. 6-5. Eight- and 9-year-old boys enjoy testing their speed in running. (Courtesy Jim McCormick.)

ance of simple regulations. In essence, physical education during this period should emphasize accuracy and efficiency in basic movement skills as well as assist the child to perform under relatively simple rules that help to express the values of sportsmanship and fair play.

Besides experiencing lead-up game activities, the child should have rich experiences in rhythm. Rhythmical activities must be considered one of the most important physical education areas for the primary level child. Rhythm education through the means of singing games, creative dancing, and folk dancing offers each child the opportunity to order movement in a prescribed manner. Primary level school children are truly expanding in all aspects of their lives: physically, emotionally, and intellectually. Physical education must be considered a major influence in this development.

CLASS ACTIVITIES

1. Observe a primary level class at play and attempt to pick out those children who appear to need remediation and those who appear to be precocious in motor development.
2. Visit a playground and observe the play behavior of children. Determine what play level of development each child portrays and whether or not it is in line with chronological age.
3. Using a dynamometer, compare the grip strength of the preferred hands of girls and boys in a primary class. Do boys or girls have the greater strength?
4. Selecting two or three measures of motor ability, such as vertical jumping, standing broad jump, or sprinting 25 yards, compare the performance of both girls and boys. Are there children who are below or above normal standards of performance?
5. Identify the motor skills that are common to the lead-up sports acitvities in primary school. How do they progressively become the skills necessary to play regular sports?

REFERENCES

1. Cratty, B. J., and Martin, M. M.: Perceptual motor efficiency in children, Philadelphia, 1969, Lea & Febiger.
2. Cowan, E., and Pratt, B.: The hurdle jump as a developmental and diagnostic test, Child. Dev. **5:**107-121, 1934.
3. Daume, W.: The main features of present-day society. In Abinson, J. G., and Andrew, G. M., editors: Child in sport and physical activity, Baltimore, 1976, University Park Press.
4. Epenshade, A. S., and Eckert, H.: Motor development, Columbus, Ohio, 1967, Charles E. Merrill Publishing Co.
5. Havighurst, R. J.: Developmental tasks and education, New York, 1950, Longman, Inc.
6. Hupprick, F. L., and Sigerseth, P. O.: The specificity of flexibility in girls, Res. Q. Am. Assoc. Health Phys. Educ. **21:** 25-33, 1950.
7. Kaluger, G., and Kaluger, M. F.: Human development, St. Louis, 1974, The C. V. Mosby Co.
8. Keogh, J. F.: A rhythmical hopping task as an assessment of motor deficiency. Presented at the Second International Congress of Sports Psychology, 1968, Washington, D.C.
9. Mathews, D. K., Kruse, R., and Shaw, V.: The science of physical education for handicapped children, New York, 1962, Harper & Row, Publishers, Inc.
10. Williams, H. G.: Body awareness characteristics in perceptual motor development. In Corbin, C. G., editor: A textbook of motor development, Dubuque, Iowa, 1973, William C. Brown Co., Publishers.

RECOMMENDED READINGS

Hacaen, H., and de Ajuriaguerra, J.: Left-handedness, manual superiority and cerebral dominance, New York, 1964, Grune & Stratton, Inc.

Keogh, J. F.: Motor performance of elementary school children, Los Angeles, 1965, University of California Physical Education Department.

Latchaw, M., and Egstrom, G.: Human movement, Englewood Cliffs, N.J., 1969, Prentice-Hall, Inc.

7

Refining: from 9 to 12 years of age

The period from 9 to 12 years of age is commonly known as late childhood. This is a time when the child is often exuberant and excited about the vast wonders of life. There is a desire to learn all there is to know about the world; often there is great impatience when learning comes with some difficulty. The child of this age commonly sleeps 9 to 10 hours per night and eats everything in sight. Girls may excel in a wide variety of motor skills when compared to boys of the same age. Girls are taller and are often heavier and stronger than boys. Late childhood is a time when heroes and heroines become very important. Strong attachments may be made to those persons who have received great acclaim in sports, the sciences, or the world of the arts. Emotions may be high one minute and low the next. What friends think and do is everything, and close friendships are made that tend to exclude so-called outsiders. Cliques and clubs representing special interests take up a major amount of the child's interests and energies. Recess becomes a time to band together. What is fair and not fair often becomes a consuming thought. Because conformity to one's own group's standard of behavior is uppermost, adult interference in that code may be tolerated but usually with some disdain.

PHYSICAL DEVELOPMENT

Late childhood, or the prepubescent period, must be looked upon as the bridge between middle childhood and adolescence. It is a time of transition.

Growth factors

As in the middle childhood period, growth is relatively slow and uniform. A gradual gain occurs in bodily measurements as well as in the aptitude for more complex physical activities. It must be understood that children may vary a great deal in their individual patterns of growth and development and still be considered to be in a normal range. Even though children may vary in height and weight, they usually follow a consistent pattern from birth to maturity. The Meredith method of evaluating a child's growth is a way of using age, height, and weight to plot normal channels of development (Fig. 7-1). A child generally will follow one channel until full maturity has been attained. Differences in growth in late childhood seem to be more apparent than in the earlier stages of development. Late childhood is a period when some children, obviously more immature than many of their peers, may acquire severe feelings of physical inadequacy.

The prepubescent stage of development is that period just prior to adolescence. The prepubescent child may display a decided weight and height increase along with a marked increase in muscle strength (Table 7-1). The age of 12 years for girls and 14 years for boys represent the usual times that adoles-

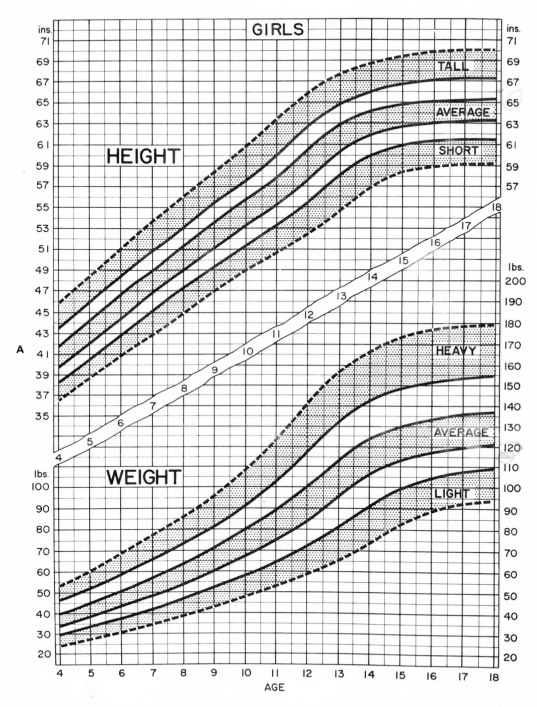

Fig. 7-1. Growth of girls and boys. (Reprinted with permission of the Joint Committee on Health Problems in Education of the National Education Association and the American Medical Association.)

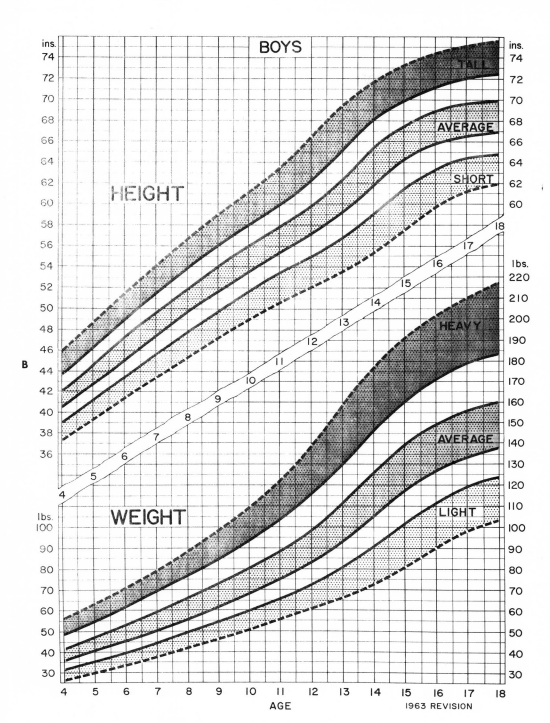

B

Fig. 7-1, cont'd. For legend see opposite page.

Table 7-1. Physical characteristics*

9 to 10 years	10 to 11 years	11 to 12 years
1. Growth is gradual and steady.	1. Boys weigh 74.8 pounds.	1. Boy's height is 57.0 inches.
2. Muscle growth is accelerated.	2. Girls are 56 inches tall.	2. Girl's height is 58.3 inches.
3. Average height for boys is 53.3 inches.	3. This is a very healthy time.	3. Growth is 2 inches per year.
4. Average height for girls is 52.3 inches.	4. Boys like daring activities.	4. Boy's weight 77.2 pounds.
5. A gain in height of 1 inch per year is normal.	5. Follow the leader is fun.	5. Girl's weight 78.3 pounds.
6. Average weight for boys is 66 pounds.	6. Balancing on a narrow fence is a challenge.	6. Tall girls may feel very self-conscious.
7. Boys gain 3.7 pounds per year.	7. Some girls may have reached puberty.	7. Small boys may feel very self-conscious.
8. Average weight for girls is 63.8 pounds.	8. There are obvious differences between fast- and slow-maturing girls.	8. Most permanent teeth are in.
9. Girls gain 4.8 pounds per year.	9. Girls may be self-conscious of breast development.	
10. This is a very healthy time.		
11. There is an improvement in ability to manipulate small objects.		
12. Eye-hand coordination is good.		
13. This is a time for crafts and using tools.		
14. Child has great energy.		
15. This is the beginning of team games.		
16. Activities that test individual abilities are important.		
17. Child may make fun of the less able.		

*The ages at which the physical characteristics noted occur are approximate.

cence is reached. Early-maturing boys and girls are generally large in late childhood and often reach their maximum growth in a relatively short time span in adolescence. Children who are comparatively more immature at this time commonly reach their full maturation over a longer period of time and may ultimately become taller than their earlier-maturing peers.

Muscle control

The last stage of childhood is marked by the perfecting of those skills that have been acquired in earlier stages of devel-

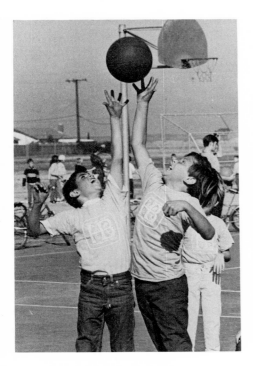

Fig. 7-2. Late childhood is a time when highly complex skills can be effectively engaged in. (Courtesy Jim McCormick.)

opment. The nervous system is now sufficiently mature to allow for small-muscle control and refined coordination[12] (Fig. 7-2). Agility, accuracy, and endurance are improved. The basic motor skills that have been acquired earlier become a springboard to the development of sophisticated skills requiring a much higher level of motor ability. Now children can run faster, throw farther, catch better, and jump and climb with a great deal of proficiency. Children between 9 and 12 years of age appear to be in constant motion and at times have almost boundless energy that may quickly turn into profound fatigue. Their energy often drives adults to distraction. Although there is considerable improvement in small-muscle control, vigorous large-muscle activity is usually preferred over less strenuous, fine motor activities. Boys traditionally become involved in the more physically active games and sports that test the

qualities of daring and courage, although today many girls are using this same mode of expression.

Late childhood is an ideal time in which to assist children in learning complex motor tasks. Children at this age are usually eager to perfect skills that are challenging. This child now profits greatly from sports and games that are well organized and well structured. Lockhart states that during late childhood "a broad array of activities, increasingly complex in nature should be planned so that strength, balance and flexibility and the specific coordination and timings of specific skills can be developed."[8]

In terms of motor ability there occur even greater sexual differences in late childhood than in the earlier stages of development. Girls in the prepubescence period may exceed boys of the same chronological age in activities requiring strength and endurance; however, when boys enter their prepubescent stage of development, they will generally surpass girls in strength and physical size. It seems that the only major difference between the sexes in potential for physical activity is the male's greater potential for strength and endurance. There is, in reality, a great deal of overlapping in the ability of both sexes to learn skills. It can be speculated that the major difference between girls and boys during this time is really not one of physical capacity but one of culturalization, which has produced preconceived attitudes about which sex should engage in vigorous physical activity.[8]

SOCIAL AND EMOTIONAL DEVELOPMENT

By the time children reach their ninth birthday they have, for the most part, changed from orientation to the family setting to interests that are mainly peer centered (Table 7-2). Peers begin to have deep influences on the life of the child; personal attitudes, goals, and general be-

Table 7-2. Social characteristics*

9 to 10 years	10 to 11 years	11 to 12 years
1. Child is peer oriented.	1. Girls would like to play with boys.	1. Belonging to well-organized groups is important.
2. Child is loyal to group or gang of same sex.	2. Girl groups are tightly knit.	2. Boys and girls are admired for their sports ability.
3. Child seems to reject adult standards.	3. Some bickering exists between boys and girls.	3. Boys may gain prestige by being masculine.
4. Boys begin to show masculinity.	4. Girls may gain prestige by being feminine.	
5. Children have secret places to meet.	5. Children are critics of adult behavior.	
6. Child prefers to be with more than two peers.		
7. Boys exclude girls.		
8. Boys tease girls.		
9. Fathers have greater importance.		

*The ages at which the social characteristics noted here occur are approximate.

havior are dominated by the peer group, a trend that will continue throughout adolescence. A tremendous loyalty develops toward one's group or gang, often with rejection of the once accepted adult standards of behavior. Doing things with the family now becomes a "drag," and being with a member of one's own sex is the thing to do. Boys have a stronger inclination toward wanting to be with members of their own sex than do girls.

It is truly crucially important for children to be accepted by their peers. To know that one is accepted by friends is to have feelings of self-worth and importance. Children who are different in some way or who play poorly may find they are rejected by the group, a situation that could cause irreparable emotional damage, eventually requiring professional psychological intervention. Late childhood is when children seek mutual support from one another. It is a time when children have a secret hiding place, a secret code, a secret password, or a special handshake. To know a secret and be able

to say, "I won't tell you because you are not in our club" gives a degree of importance to the bearer of the secret as well as a sense of exclusion to the one not in the group.

Loosely organized groups are developed when children are between the ages of 9 and 10 years. When children reach 11 or 12 years of age, they commonly want to participate in more structured environments, such as formalized clubs or organizations.[5]

Social expectations as related to sexual differences now become highly significant (Table 7-3). Social pressure may be applied to cause boys and girls to behave in a prescribed manner. Boys, for example, may be encouraged to acquire the so-called macho mystique to express masculinity. It may become important to be a he-man; to be tough, strong, and daring; and to be able to have an "I won't cry no matter what happens to me" attitude. Girls, on the other hand, often may be expected to be less vigorous and aggressive than boys; however, in most parts of

Table 7-3. Emotional characteristics*

9 to 10 years	10 to 11 years	11 to 12 years
1. Child giggles and squirms.	1. Child seldom cries.	1. Child constantly worries.
2. Child shows temper over frustrations.	2. Child is slow to anger.	2. Child fears many things.
3. Boys become sullen and sulk.	3. Noise is pleasurable.	3. Anger is more easily aroused.
4. Girls cry and have temper outbursts.	4. Child has few worries or fears.	4. Child can control outbursts of emotion.
5. Child has fear of being different.	5. Child usually respects school rules.	5. Child may verbalize discontent with bad language.
6. Anxiety is common.	6. Child may feel no one likes him or her.	6. Boys want to display their strength.
	7. Child needs to have ego bolstered constantly.	7. Emotions sweep between love and hate.

*The ages at which the emotional characteristics noted here occur are approximate.

the United States, vigorous activity is now accepted for both sexes. Girls' acceptance by adults commonly requires that they be friendly, sensitive, clean, tidy, courteous, kind, emotional, attractive, and more grown-up than boys of the same age.[6] Although it varies a great deal throughout the United States, there is a welcome trend toward encouraging boys to openly show their emotions honestly and girls to become more assertive in pursuing vigorous physical activities if they so desire.[3]

To children on the verge of adolescence, gender identification takes on increased meaning. Children of 7 or 8 years of age usually identify with the parent of the same sex but are still dependent on their mothers for many of their personal needs. For both boys and girls during late childhood, the father increases in influence within the family. It has been suggested that influence increases because the father often has the freedom of action that the child of this age would like to have. In the traditional role the father

seems to the child to be free to move about in the world without the apparent constraints of home ties that the mother has. As children normally model a parent of the same sex, they also engage in games and sports activities that they consider to have a feminine or masculine connotation.[3]

The emotions of a child between the ages of 9 and 12 years, like all other developing characteristics, are in a process of transition and refinement. The 9-year-old child may sulk, cry a lot, and have unexplainable outbursts of emotions. The 10-year-old child is typically easygoing and predictable, while the 11-year-old child may display vague fears and worry a great deal about seemingly minor things and have large swings of emotion between sad and happy, a trend that continues throughout adolescence.

Kaluger has summarized Bernard's list of the major developmental tasks to be accomplished by the child between the ages of 9 and 12 years as:

1. Gaining freedom from primary iden-

tification with adults by learning to become self-reliant.

2. Developing social competency in forming and maintaining friendships with peers.
3. Learning to live in the adult world by getting a clearer perspective on one's peer group role or place in that world.
4. Developing a moral code of conduct based on principles rather than specifics.
5. Consolidating the identification made with one's sex role.
6. Integrating and refining motor patterns to a higher level of efficiency.
7. Learning realistic ways of studying and controlling the physical world.
8. Developing appropriate symbol systems and conceptual abilities for learning, communicating, and reasoning.
9. Evolving and understanding self and the world.[2,5]

PHYSICAL EDUCATION IN THE LATE CHILDHOOD PERIOD

Late childhood is marked by a steady increase in growth and development. The child is preparing to become an adolescent in all ways. Although there is steady growth, differences in rates of maturational growth become more obvious during this time than in previous periods. Physical education becomes one of the most important components in the total education program and an essential force in helping children bridge the gap between middle childhood and adolescence.

All older children should continue to have the opportunity to participate in well-planned and well-conducted physical education programs. Such programs should promote maximum movement opportunities through a wide range of activities. If children have a good background of sound movement experiences

and have sufficient innate potential, they can now be instructed in some of the most difficult patterns of movement. It may be said that children between 9 and 12 years of age are as capable of learning skills requiring intricate patterns of coordination as they are at any time in their lives. Children, at this age, have the ability to learn lifetime sports such as golf and tennis.

Program offerings during this period should be advanced gymnastics and sport skills (Fig. 7-3). At this time, children should refine their abilities in throwing, catching, kicking, and striking as well as in the basic transport skills of running and jumping. There should be opportunities for the child to increase balance abilities through a wide variety of airborne and apparatus activities. Games and sports activities that require a high level of physical proficiency, such as soccer, softball, hockey, and basketball, are appropriate at this time (Fig. 7-4). Children who are developmentally ready should be taught those skills necessary for participation in these activities. Rhythms, in the form of dance, should continue to be offered as one of the most important areas within the physical education curriculum. Contemporary dance and round and square dances, which provide excellent avenues for self-expression and socialization, should be encouraged for both girls and boys. Although physical fitness should be an inherent part of the physical education curriculum at every level of development, it should be emphasized in late childhood education by having each child perform specific physical fitness exercises. Emphasis at this time must be given over to the fitness components of strength, joint flexibility, and muscle and cardiorespiratory endurance as well as to learning the important skill of relaxing muscle tension at will. Although we consider late childhood to be a time in which teacher-directed instruction is appropriate for high-level skill development, we also believe that movement education

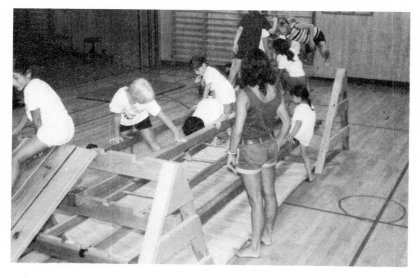

Fig. 7-3. Children exploring movement potential on a piece of apparatus.

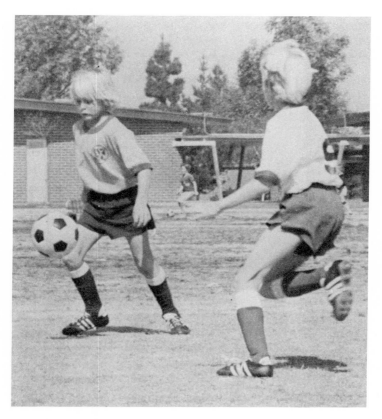

Fig. 7-4. Soccer, which requires a great deal of physical proficiency, is becoming increasingly popular among elementary school children.

techniques employing the exploration of new ways to move, especially in the relationship of the body to large and small apparatus, are a valuable addition to the well-rounded physical education program.

A TIME FOR STRATEGY AND TACTICS

One must be reminded that the child between the ages of 9 and 12 years, besides developing physically, has grown in the ability to perform more difficult intellectual tasks.[5] Paralleling the increased capacity to think logically and to solve mental problems is the beginning of effective employing of strategy and tactics in games and sports activities. Sports strategy may be defined as the planning of the means by which a fair advantage can be taken of an opponent, while tactics must be considered as the actual carrying out of the strategy. When a child has gained the ability to effectively perform

well the motor factors of a particular activity, then ways to gain the "upper hand" over his or her opponent can be developed.[10] Children in middle childhood may use rudimentary strategies and tactics in their games; for example, in dodge ball the child who is "it" may learn to fake a movement in one direction but move in another, and in playing the game of kick ball, children soon learn various techniques, such as faking a pitch to jockey an opponent off base. The process of learning to outwit an opponent can be carried over to the highest level of competitive endeavor. Children who play organized sports are taught how to employ strategy and tactics; however, this is never really effective until the performers can think less about executing the skills of the game and more about the strengths and weaknesses of their opponents. The child between the ages of 9 and 12 years is usually concerned more with immediate rather than future events. Common tactics that can easily be taught at this age are to fake

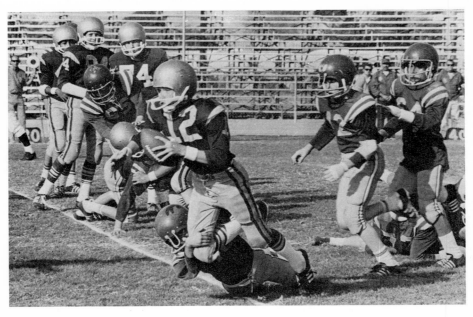

Fig. 7-5. With proper adult supervision, football provides outstanding opportunities for the use of strategy against an opponent. (Courtesy Jim McCormick.)

an opponent out of position, to vary the speed of play, or to make fair use of psychological pressure to force opponents into mistakes.

A teacher of elementary physical education must be cognizant of the fact that there is a moral side to the use of strategies and tactics. The child between the ages of 9 and 12 years is beginning to clearly understand right and wrong and what is fair and unfair. Although children generally reject adult standards of behavior, proper rules of conduct are still very important within the peer group. Both teachers and coaches have a deep moral obligation to help their charges to clearly discern between tactics that reflect sportsmanlike and tactics that reflect unsportsman-like behavior. Engaging in sports will not automatically develop sportsmanlike conduct; sportsmanship must be carefully planned and taught to the young performer. Too often elementary school teachers and lay coaches attempt to emulate what they believe to be the attitude of coaches of university and professional teams—that winning is the most important aspect of playing sports. The attitude that one should win by any means possible is deplorable.[14]

COMPETITION IN LATE CHILDHOOD—PROS AND CONS

There has long been a controversy among parents, lay coaches, professional coaches, educators, behavioral scientists, and the medical profession as to whether or not competitive sports are advisable for the physically and emotionally immature child. Generally, parents, especially those who are actively involved in youth sports, and coaches consider that the benefits of such activities far outweigh the liabilities. On the other hand, many educators, psychologists, and physicians are somewhat skeptical that sports competition, especially that which is outside the jurisdiction of the school, is really beneficial to the young participants, be-

lieving that intense competition and training may be harmful to the physical and emotional health of the young performer. However, if properly managed, age group competition can be beneficial to children who are physically and emotionally mature.

Are injuries really a problem?

There is a lack of in-depth accident statistics related with children in sports participation. From the information available there is an indication that unsupervised play is far more dangerous than that which is organized. Children participating in supervised play activities, such as physical education or intramural or interscholastic competition, appear to have relatively few injuries that require medical attention or that result in loss of school days.[9] The extracurricular sport that has been studied most extensively is Little League baseball. It was found that the greatest number of serious medical problems occurring to the players was caused by hard repetitive throwing of the baseball.[13] Although the results are inconclusive, organized tackle football was found to produce very few serious injuries even though there are large numbers of children playing throughout the country.[9]

Immature bony structure

Many physicians are concerned because children who engage in highly competitive sports activities have skeletal structures that are relatively immature. The human skeleton at birth is mainly composed of a firm but flexible substance known as cartilage, which is gradually replaced by hard bony tissue as maturation takes place. The degree of maturation is commonly measured by the extent of skeletal ossification.[7] The growth centers of the skeleton are composed of cartilaginous material, remaining so until growth is terminated. A completely mature skeleton may not be present until the individual reaches early adulthood. For example, the thigh bone usually continues to grow and does not become completely ossified until around 19 years of age. The main concern of opponents of a highly competitive and physically vigorous sports program, especially the contact or collision variety, is that injury to the immature skeleton may cause a premature cessation of growth in that bone.[6] The injury most cited as directly sustained from sports participation is fracture of the growth centers of the elbow. This condition has been called "Little League elbow" and is attributed to pitching or repeated hard throwing of a baseball. When one considers that a boy 11 or 12 years old can throw a baseball with a force of 70 miles per hour, it is no wonder that trauma may occur to the immature elbow.[5] However, out of the more than 2 million boys playing Little League baseball, ranging between the ages of 8 and 12 years, the incidence of acute injury requiring medical attention is insignificant. Of more important concern to many physicians is the repeated microtraumas that occur over a period of time and that may produce chronic or even degenerative conditions in the young athlete's immature bony structure. Besides the elbows, the hips, the knees, and the spine are common sites for chronic and degenerative problems to occur to children in the late childhood period. These conditions may or may not be attributed to physical activity.

Even though many people have verbalized their antagonism toward the more vigorous contact or collision sports for youngsters, there appears to be little available information that substantiates such concerns. In fact, such endeavors as ballet dancing may place greater stresses on the growing child than does the contact sport of tackle football. Reputable and well-informed teachers of ballet are extremely cautious about allowing a young dancer to go en pointe. A girl must be at least 7 or 8 years of age, when the major growth centers of the feet have matured, before dancing en pointe can be permitted.[1]

Needless to say, immature skeletons must be protected against violent and repetitive stress in order to avoid permanent growth problems and the possibility of acquiring some chronic or degenerative condition that could adversely affect the child for the rest of his or her life.

Psyche

Also of major concern is the possibility that high-level sports competition may be psychologically harmful to the emotionally immature. Will a child who is placed under constant competitive pressures, such as playing in all-star games, championships, or play-offs, develop emotional problems (Fig. 7-6)? It is not easy to answer this question. Some studies express the opinion that no harm occurs,

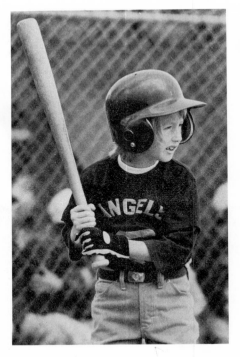

Fig. 7-6. Little League baseball, if properly conducted and supervised, can be a rewarding experience for the child. (Courtesy Jim McCormick.)

while others indicate that undesirable behaviors may stem from the emotional stress of high-level competition over an extended period of time.[11] One can gather from the available information that emotional problems stemming from competition are directly related to the values parents and adult leaders place on competition. Many problems may be averted by educating parents that the joy of participation is the important thing, rather than winning at all costs. This is not to say that winning is not important, but it should be viewed as a reward for successful participation. It is important that adult leaders be recruited who are sensitive to the emotions of children and who will attempt to develop a positive self-concept within each child.[15]

How hard should children train?

There have long been questions as to how hard children should engage in physical training, whether training would physically harm the immature person, and what effect training would have on the child's skeleton, musculature, heart, and lungs. The answers. to these questions can be either positive or negative, depending on the type and intensity of the physical training. One must remember that exercise is essential for normal growth and development. Children who are in some way deprived of proper physical activity will fail to reach their full growth potential and will often be smaller and less physically able than more active children of the same age. In fact, children who engage in physical

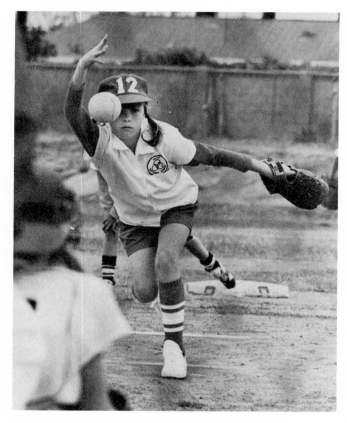

Fig. 7-7. Children can engage in hard physical training without adverse effects if it is properly conducted and controlled. (Courtesy Jim McCormick.)

training as a prerequisite for a particular sport have often been found to have wider and stronger bones than less-active children[15] (Fig. 7-7). However, if training is carried to the point of overstressing the child's body, injuries can result, especially to the immature skeleton.

Another common question that arises is whether or not the child between the ages of 9 and 12 years should train against a heavy resistance in order to increase strength. Heavy resistance, such as lifting weights, has been found, in many cases, to positively affect the skeletal structure by increasing its width and density. However, it can be speculated that even though the incidence of injury is apparently low, because of a lack of current data, it would seem advisable not to allow the growing child to be overly stressed through heavy resistance type training programs. If resistance exercises are considered necessary for a given sport, the safest approach is to either employ a program of low weight and high repetition through a full range of joint movement or use an isokinetic method whereby the resistance that is imparted matches the force that the child is able to apply.[15] Teachers or coaches using resistance techniques to increase strength in their young charges should avoid having the child overspecialize selected muscle groups but should encourage an equal amount of exercise to the entire body. Exercise specialization should be avoided because the individual in late childhood is highly susceptible to postural imbalances. Specialization of strength training to those muscles that are concerned with the specific sports activity ultimately can result in serious postural problems.

Another area of contention in the conditioning of youngsters between the ages of 9 and 12 years is the amount of stress that can be safely placed on the heart and lungs. The human body at all ages has a great capacity to adapt to cardiorespiratory stress. There is no information to date that indicates that training designed to improve heart and lung capacity will be detrimental to a growing child (see Chapter 16). It is our contention, however, that schools pay too little attention to helping children develop their hearts and lungs and should place more emphasis on this fitness component.

• • •

To summarize, competition is a human characteristic that often becomes apparent as early as the first year of life and is generally well established by 7 years of age. It is seen in both sexes but, because of cultural influences, becomes more pronounced in males. In itself, competition is not harmful, but it becomes so when stresses are applied that exceed the individual child's physical and emotional limits. All children should have the opportunity to compete but only if the competition is in keeping with each child's physical and emotional level. Children who are physically gifted should be encouraged to develop their potential in games and sports (see Chapter 16). One should be aware that if competition or training methods have some deleterious effect on the children, it usually results from some external factor rather than from a factor within the children themselves. The pressures that are placed on the children by parents and adult leaders to exceed their limits are probably the main reason children are injured. It is, therefore, essential that children be directed and guided by highly responsible adults who care only for their well-being.

CLASS ACTIVITIES

1. Determine the practices in a youth sport that do or do not equalize the play of all children.
2. Study an organized sport for youth for precautions taken to prevent exceeding maturity levels.
3. Attend a youth sports event and observe the behavior of parents, coaches, and participants.
4. Interview an orthopedic surgeon, preferably one who treats children. Ask the physician for his or her feelings about children competing in athletics.
5. Research how bones grow.

REFERENCES

1. Ballet dancers' injuries pose sportsmedicine challenge, The Physical Physician and Sportsmedicine 4(11):44, 1976.
2. Bernard, H. W.: Human development in western culture, ed. 2, Boston, 1966, Allyn & Bacon, Inc.
3. Cratty, B. J.: Perceptual and motor development in infants and children, New York, 1970, The Macmillan Co.
4. Guggenheim, J. J., and others: Little League survey: the Houston study, Am. J. Sports Med. 4(5):189, 1976.
5. Kaluger, G., and Kaluger, M. F.: Human development: the span of life, St. Louis, 1974, The C. V. Mosby Co.
6. Larson, R. L.: Physical activity and the growth and development of bone and joint structures. In Rarick, G. L., editor: Physical activity: human growth and development, New York, 1973, Academic Press, Inc.
7. Larson, R. L., and others: Little League survey: the Eugene study, Am. J. Sports Med. 4(5):201, 1976.
8. Lockhart, A. S.: Highlights of total development. In Corbin, C. B., editor: A textbook of motor development, Dubuque, Iowa, 1973, William C. Brown Co., Publishers.
9. National Safety Council: Accident facts, 1976, The Council.
10. Pestolesi, R. A.: The strategies. In Hall, J. T., editor: Fundamentals of physical education, Santa Monica, Calif., 1969, Goodyear Publishing Co., Inc.
11. Sherif, M., and others: Intergroup conflict and cooperation: the Robber's Cave experiment, Norman, Okla., 1961, University of Oklahoma Press.
12. Singer, R. N.: Motor learning as a function of age and sex. In Rarick, G. L., editor: Physical activity: human growth and development, New York, 1973, Academic Press, Inc.
13. Torg, B. G., and Torg, J. S.: Sex and the Little League, The Physician and Sportsmedicine 2(5):45-50, 1974.
14. Tutko, T., and Bruns, B.: Winning is everything and other American myths, New York, 1976, The Macmillan Co.
15. Wilmore, J. H.: Athletic training and physical fitness, Boston, 1976, Allyn & Bacon, Inc.

RECOMMENDED READINGS

Bucher, C. A.: Foundations of physical education, ed. 7, St. Louis, 1975, The C. V. Mosby Co.
Jones, M. C., and N. Nancy: Physical maturing among boys as related to behavior, J. Educ. Psychol. 41:129-148, 1950.
Wickstrom, R. L.: Fundamental motor patterns, Philadelphia, 1970, Lea & Febiger.

INSTRUCTIONAL FOUNDATIONS

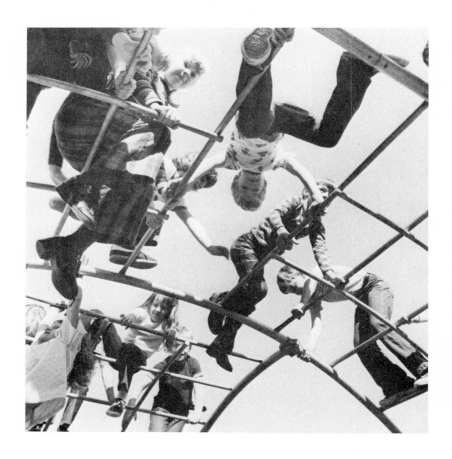

Part Three provides detailed discussions of concepts, methods, and principal curricular approaches commonly found in elementary physical education. It presents both theoretical and practical applications in the areas of basic body management through perceptual-motor training, movement education, physical fitness, integrated learning and classroom activities, and the exceptional child.

8

Basic body management through perceptual-motor training

This chapter is concerned with basic body management through perceptual-motor training, employing tasks of increasing difficulty. It is directed toward the acquisition of proficient motor skills rather than the development of competency in cognitive skills, such as those represented in reading and arithmetic.

In the last decade there has been a decided trend toward teacher/administrator accountability to the main consumer of education—the learner. This trend has come about, at least in part, from a dissatisfaction with low test scores demonstrated by children throughout the country in reading and arithmetic as well as from parents' growing displeasure with large, overcrowded, and impersonalized classrooms and their desire for individualization of instruction. One might also speculate that programs such as those dedicated to perceptual motor development have led parents to believe that the best education is that which provides the child with individual instruction.

Competency-based or programmed instruction, which follows many of the concepts put forth by computer science, made educators throughout the United States responsible for their programs. The programmed instructional approach is often applied when prescriptive or individualized teaching is appropriate, as in a remedial setting for children who may be functioning at the preschool or primary school level.

WHAT ARE MOVEMENT SKILLS AND TASKS?

The term *skill* is used grammatically in two ways. It refers to a specific motor task to be demonstrated. A skill that has been performed in its entirety is considered a completed *task;* however, to execute a task skillfully may take many additional practice hours. Skill may also be described as "the learned ability to bring about predetermined results with maximum certainty, often with minimum outlay of time or energy, or both."[12]

A series of tasks or skills directed toward some external goal is said to be a *motor pattern.*[8] Many patterns of movement combined in such a manner that they do not vary and are highly predictable are considered a *routine,* such as one might perform in dance or gymnastics. For example, Godfrey[8] describes walking as a motor skill that requires very limited movement precision, while locomotion, a motor pattern, may include a variety of actions, such as walking, running, leaping, and even jumping. A complicated movement skill may be a composite of many lesser, but increasingly difficult skills.

Task progressions and learning

A hierarchy is a continuum of ordered events. In reference to motor learning, a hierarchy refers to a task of less difficulty being a prerequisite for the learning of a task or skill of greater difficulty. If a hierarchy of tasks is to be learned, the tasks must be joined to one another by a logical sequence of events in a close enough time period so that the relationship of each part can be easily understood by the learner; this is particularly true when perceptual-motor tasks are presented. *One should note that tasks that are performed without any obvious relationship to one another become disjointed and eventually splintered skills.*

LEARNING PERCEPTUAL-MOTOR SKILLS

Since the late 1950s, educators have been concerned with enhancing learning and favorably affecting perceptual-motor behavior. Programs designed to assist children's perception have been variously titled movement education, educa-

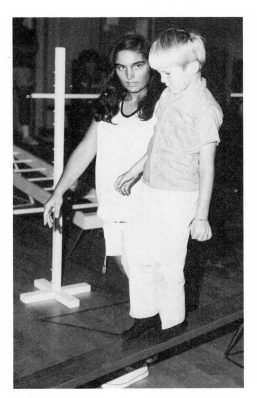

Fig. 8-1. Many perceptual-motor programs purport to assist children in their cognitive domain.

tional gymnastics, perceptual-motor training, sensorimotor training, and psychomotor training (Fig. 8-1). Although often varied in their approaches, these programs were based on developmental principles and were concerned with assisting children in learning through the cognitive domain. Gradually through the years, these programs have been found useful as remedial programs for children with special learning problems or as programs to enhance learning at the preschool or primary levels.

A current dilemma

The popularity of the perceptual-motor development program in the 1960s is beginning to wane, as do so many trends in education.[7] This decrease in interest has been caused, in part, by a lack of research that substantiates the fact that academic achievement can be improved significantly through a perceptual-motor training program. In a review of a large number of studies on the effect of perceptual-motor activities on academic achievement, Humphrey[9] found that approximately one third of the studies showed a positive correlation, while two thirds did not and were doubtful of the effect of perceptual-motor activities on learners, especially those with no obvious learning problems. Of those studies that supported perceptual-motor training as a means of enhancing academic achievement, many indicated that positive changes may have been attributed to better attitudes toward learning rather than an enhancement of intellectual abilities.[14] Recent studies, however, show some relationship among eye-motor control, perception and motor ability, and comprehension.[1,16] Perceptual-motor training, therefore, should be considered one approach to assisting the developmentally very immature child or a child requiring special remediation in the area of processing information both in the psychomotor and cognitive domains.

The perceptual-motor process and skill development

The perceptual-motor process is simply defined as the managing of information coming to the individual through the senses, the processing of the information, and then the reacting to the information in terms of some behavior (Fig. 8-2). Although simply stated, in reality the perceptual-motor process is extremely complex, requiring many interrelationships of abilities on the part of the processor. Sensory information is first recognized, discriminated, and selectively carried through nerve pathways to various levels of the brain. The initial reception of information is conducted through the primary channels, commonly known as the senses. The sensory information must then be processed for current or future use. All information is compared, integrated, and stored within the brain on the basis of previous experience of the individual and may be used by the individual as a means of adjusting current or future movement behavior.

Perception cannot be separated from the cognitive or psychomotor domain of human behavior; it must be considered inseparable and dependent as well as reciprocal. To think or move purposefully, a person must receive and perceive hundreds upon thousands of impulses from external and/or internal stimuli. From the time of conception the individual is perceiving and reacting to the environment through the perceptual-motor process.

A breakdown at any point along the perceptual chain of events can lead to dysfunction, such as difficulty in information retrieval or the inability to differentiate between stimuli.[4] In physical education the child must rely on numerous perceptions in order to perform skilled movements. Children who are observed to be awkward on the playground may in reality be developmentally younger than their chronological age, may lack specific play experiences, or may have some perceptual dysfunction.[2] These same children may also be unable to cope with the countless discrete perceptual requirements associated with the classroom.

Many classroom and physical education curriculums today depend heavily on the precepts of progressive development. As discussed earlier in this text, maturation basically follows an orderly sequence of events characteristic of all human beings and yet unique for each

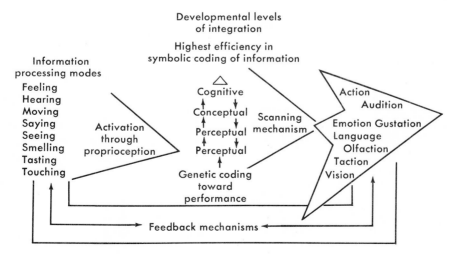

Fig. 8-2. Conceptual model of a functional learning system. (From Sheldon R. Rappaport, Effective Educational Systems, Inc., Onancock, Va.)

person. In observing orderly development, human beings have created labels to identify developmental milestones and periods. The development of the emergent human organism is carefully plotted, scheduled, and staged according to what is considered a normal chronology of sequential development, with those who fall outside the normal pattern of development thought to be atypical.

Generally speaking, perception is the process of interpreting stimuli through the senses according to past experiences. Perception must, therefore, be considered a function that can be learned and modified by varying the environment. Physical education can aid the child in accurately interpreting sensations that come from the surroundings. A teacher concerned with a child's perceptual-motor development will maximize experiences perceivable through the various sense channels.

Following is a discussion of important perceptual factors related to movement processes through specific sense channels.

Visual-motor skills

Vision is highly complex and involves much more than the sharpness of sight called visual acuity. Oxendine said, "What an individual sees is the result of a psychophysical process which integrates gravitational forces, conceptual ideation, spatial-perceptual orientation, and language functions."[13] For learning through vision to occur efficiently, the eyes must focus readily on the intended object and must function symmetrically.

Visual acuity. Visual acuity refers to an ability to discriminate between symbols or objects within a personal field of vision. Normal visual acuity is considered to be 20/20, or what the average person can see at a distance of 20 feet. A child indicating difficulty in seeing details clearly at a distance may squint in an effort to see more distinctly or may prefer

near-point indoor activities to outdoor playing. Blurred vision, eye fatigue, headaches, and dizziness are often complaints of children having defects in visual acuity. Although visual acuity is within the eye proper and not in the brain, it nevertheless affects the clarity of perceptual experiences.

Visual coordination. Visual coordination, or ocular control, is binocularity of vision, such as is used in the teaming of the eyes when reading or visually pursuing an object in space. Oculomotor coordination involves the following important functions:

1. *Fixation.* The ability to accurately direct the eyes toward a specific point. Ideally, the child should be able to make rapid visual adjustments or accommodations between near-point and far-point objects, such as in focusing on an incoming ball and then throwing the ball accurately to a partner a distance away.
2. *Visual pursuit.* The ability to accurately track objects moving in space.
3. *Convergence.* The turning inward of the two eyes toward the nose as they focus on objects at different distances from the face. The two eyes increasingly turn equally inward as objects come nearer to the viewer.

Coordinated eye movement is essential for success in symbolic learning situations, particularly in reading and writing, as well as for success on the playground, where object management is so critical in games and sports activities.

Visual-motor form discrimination. Visual-motor form discrimination is the ability to recognize differences in shapes and symbols found in the environment. Children having this ability are able to match or clearly differentiate like and unlike symbols, designs, letters, and eventually words through visual cues. This is a factor necessary for classroom motor skills to be learned. It also involves discrimination of three-dimensional forms in space through the sensory input of sight and feel. The child is capable of matching solid objects by both seeing and feeling them. Although less obvious in play situations, visual form discrimination is a requirement for the recognition and management of objects in space, such as in catching a thrown ball or kicking a moving ball.

Visual figure-ground discrimination. Visual figure-ground discrimination is the recognition of meaningful differences in objects with varying foregrounds and backgrounds. This perceptual skill requires the child to be able to concentrate and focus attention on a visual stimulus. Without it, the child is unable to pick out or select pertinent symbols from the environment. Dysfunction in this area is reflected in physical education when a child is unable to catch, bat, strike, or kick a moving object consistently because it is

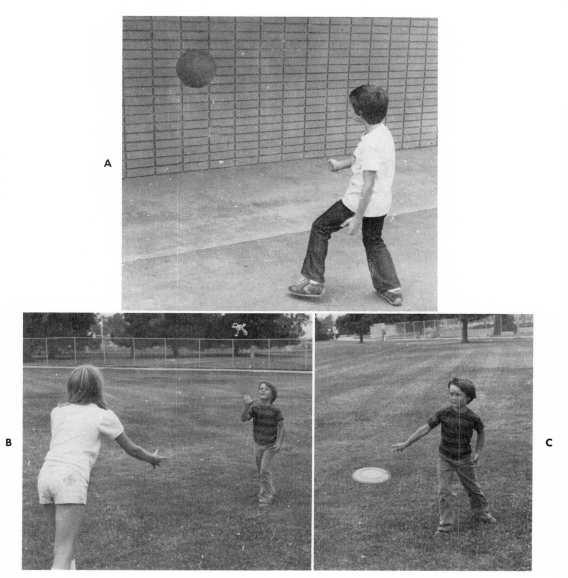

Fig. 8-3. Projecting objects accurately requires a high level of visual guidance.

lost in the varied backgrounds of sky, trees, and buildings.

Visual memory. Visual memory, or retention, is the ability to retain and accurately recall visual experiences after a time period has elapsed. Visual memory is determined by how well the child is able to retrieve stored information when provided with a set of visual cues. The capability of translating the process of visual memorization into some motor act, such as throwing a ball or writing a letter, is known as the combined skill of visual-motor retention. It allows the child to recall learned visual experiences and respond through movement with a logically ordered series of acts. Complex play situations involving many different patterns of movement performed in a prescribed manner require children to retrieve the correct responses from their visual memory bank. Children having difficulty in visual memory will be unable to participate in complex games, sports, or dances.

Visual-motor and eye-hand and eye-foot coordination. Visual-motor and eye-hand and eye-foot coordination is essential for manipulative tasks as well as for game playing involving different projectiles. Motor tasks requiring detail or accuracy involve the synchronization of many small muscles of the hand and foot, which in turn are coordinated with vision. Such varied skills as lacing shoes, stringing beads, throwing at a target, and kicking a rolled ball require the synchronization of small and large skeletal muscles along with visual guidance (Fig. 8-3). Also to effectively play a game of softball or kickball, children must be able to accurately perceive the speed of the moving ball, the distance between players, the amount of force that must be applied to the ball, the direction in which the ball is projected, and how hard a ball has been hit or kicked.

Visual-motor integration. Visual-motor integration is the utilization of all visual-motor factors in a highly coordinated manner. With visual-motor integration the child is able to solve a multitude of complex visual-motor problems, perform effectively in the classroom, and play games and sports that involve a high degree of coordination between eyes, hands, feet, and large and small muscles. The child can play ball-handling games and team sports as well as draw and reproduce symbols accurately with pencil and paper. In addition, the visually well-integrated person is able to effectively perform *eidetic imagery,* or see with the mind's eye. In other words, the child learns to reproduce within the mind a picture that is based on past movement experiences and used for current or future action. Eidetic imagery is a means of mentally practicing an act and serves as a means of eliminating past errors in some movement sequence.

Auditory perceptual-motor skills

Audition, like vision, requires a number of discrete perceptual abilities, some of which are auditory acuity, auditory-motor discrimination, auditory-motor rhythm perception, auditory memory and sequencing, and auditory integration.

Auditory acuity. Auditory acuity is the ability to hear, to discern auditory stimuli. Two important factors in auditory acuity are the ability to attend, or listen, and the ability to locate where sound is coming from, or determine sound direction. Auditory acuity is important in physical education when activity directions must be given by the teacher or peer and is an integral part of many games, sports, and dances. Although secondary in importance when compared to sight, auditory acuity often provides information on when an object has been projected, such as when a ball is batted; determines the sequencing of sound such as in rhythms; and provides a means of determining partner relationships, such as the position of a teammate or opponent.

Auditory-motor discrimination. Audi-

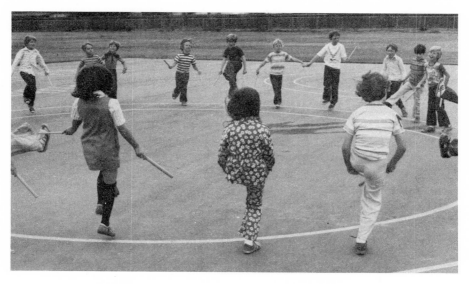

Fig. 8-4. Learning auditory sequencing through rhythmical activities.

tory-motor discrimination is the distinguishing of the difference between meaningful sounds. It includes such abilities as auditory figure-ground discrimination, in which, as in visual figure-ground discrimination, the perceiver is able to pick out specific tones and frequencies from a complex background of sounds.[18] Also auditory discrimination consists of understanding the spoken word and the motor capability of matching and duplicating sounds verbally, such as imitating animal noises or producing rhyming words, which is so important to the preschool and primary school child. Communication is seriously hampered when there is a disturbance in sound discrimination. Directions may be misinterpreted or distorted, making the learning of physical education activities difficult or even impossible. All children, therefore, should be given rich experiences in both interpreting and producing sounds.

Auditory-motor rhythm perception. Auditory-motor rhythm perception involves the recognition of sound patterns that are predictable and organized. It consists of identifying tempo and accent rhythm patterns.[18] Rhythm experiences through the auditory mode are essential to the young child in developing a sense of time, in sequencing an action, and in gaining spatial awareness (Fig. 8-4). Combined with motor responses, such as playing a musical instrument, dancing, or singing, auditory rhythm perception provides a medium for self-expression.

Auditory memory and sequencing. Auditory memory is the retaining and recalling of information. Children must be able to accurately retrieve information when given an auditory stimulus and then express the information by either a verbal or a movement response. Auditory sequencing is the direct extension of auditory memory. The child retains information in a logical order, recalling and expressing it in an accurate, sequential order. Activities like singing songs, telling stories, or carrying out a series of movement instructions require the ability to retain the memory of a sound and then pull it out of the memory bank to relate it to the activity in some meaningful way.

Auditory integration. The dual abilities of hearing and moving are utilized to a great extent in physical education. The child may move to verbal directions by the teacher or may show the paired response of audition and movement that is stimulated by a rhythmical cadence. A well-planned and well-initiated physical education program assists in the integration of the auditory mode in its sensory input and motor output.

Tactile perception

Tactile perception develops early in prenatal development, with touch receptors highly concentrated in and around the mouth, in the fingers and palms of the hands, and in the soles of the feet. Development of touch perception progresses in the usual developmental direction, from the head to the foot and from the midline outward. It is developed through experiencing contrasting surface temperatures, shapes, and textures, such as rough and smooth, hot and cold, sharp and blunt, soft and hard, wet and dry, and sticky and greasy. Identification of shapes usually is developed after surface discrimination. By feel, the child learns to distinguish between basic geometrical shapes, such as circles, squares, and rectangles, and other more complicated forms (Fig. 8-5). Later, the child develops the ability to identify and label a variety of objects without visual assistance, or just by feel.

Physical education can provide a good source of tactile stimulation for the maturing child. Activities such as swimming, crawling, and rolling on different surfaces allow the child to feel the environment through the entire body. A good rule for assisting in the development of touch experiences is to allow the child to play barefoot on surfaces with different textures, such as grass or dirt, or on surfaces that are flat, rough, or hilly.

Kinesthesis

Kinesthesis is perception of movement, or muscle sense. It is the awareness of body movement and of the body's relative position in space. Kinesthesis is primarily based on internal stimuli from sense receptors, called proprioceptors, located in muscles, tendons, and joints and from the vestibular system and semicircular canals in the inner ear. The proprioceptors provide a continuous feedback of information on body orientation and muscle tension levels. Because kinesthesis is a complex of many inde-

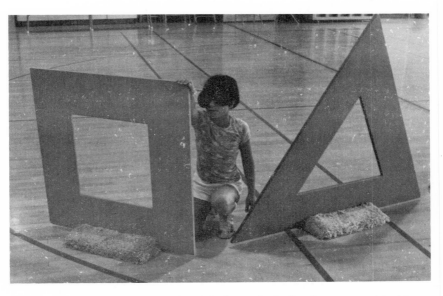

Fig. 8-5. A child can learn to distinguish shapes by feeling large geometrical forms.

pendent and interdependent constituents, it cannot be considered a general trait.[12,17] The so-called body sensation, therefore, is a compilation of many specific abilities. Consequently, the more varied movements and positions a child can engage in the greater the opportunity for acquiring a rich repertoire of kinesthetic, perceptual experiences for future use in learning motor skills.

Balance and posture

Balance and posture are closely associated with kinesthetic awareness. Balance is the ability to maintain equilibrium when moving or not moving. Maintaining a body position or posture requires numerous neurological, anatomical, and physiological perceptions, such as those stemming from vision, the vestibular mechanisms, neck reflexes, the touch senses, and the organs of proprioception, all of which provide an awareness of posture and movement changes and a knowledge of placement, weight, and resistance of objects in relation to the body as a whole.

Together with the internal senses of proprioception and the vestibular system, vision gives external information as to one's position in space. Coordinating with vision, touch, and other proprioceptors, the vestibular apparatus is a major system for the acquisition of balance and postural perceptions.

Recently the theories of Ayres[3] have become increasingly popular among educators and movement specialists concerned with the learning handicapped. Ayres' work shows a possible relationship between brainstem and vestibular dysfunction and some learning deficiencies. Ayres theorizes that by providing the child with special activities that affect the brainstem and vestibular system, one can provide a normalizing effect for the faculties of sensory integration. Whether the motivation is to assist the child in learning or to make the child a better mover, it is essential that every opportunity be afforded the child for experiencing balancing activities.

Perceptual-motor activities of balance and posture are divided into two major categories, each requiring its own set of

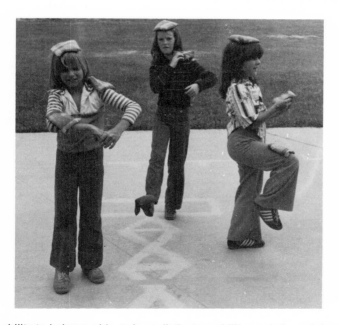

Fig. 8-6. The ability to balance objects is as distinct an ability as static and dynamic balance.

abilities. These are static balance and dynamic balance. A third balance ability that might be added to this list is object balance, or the ability to steadily maintain some external object in balance, such as in walking with a glass of water without spilling it or balancing a beanbag on the head (Fig. 8-6).

Body and space perception

Three areas of perception stand out as being highly important to the developing child: body knowledge, body image, and spatial relationships.

Body knowledge. Body knowledge is the understanding of "who I am." Knowledge of the body begins at birth and continues throughout life. It increases and becomes more detailed as the child grows and matures. First the larger areas of the body are understood, followed by smaller and more discrete parts of the visible body. Often, body planes, such as front and back and top and bottom, are learned, followed by the learning of body movements.

Body image. Body image, like body knowledge and spatial relationships, is slowly acquired from the time of birth and directly associated with maturation and growth. Body image is the feeling that children have about themselves; it occurs as a result of all the perceptions that have been acquired during the child's lifetime. Body image is also the perception of body part relationships to the external world, their relative position in space, and the effect of gravity upon them.

Four factors stand out as being crucial in the development of the body: *kinesthetic awareness,* or the awareness of the movement capability of the body; *laterality,* or the internal awareness of the two sides of the body; *verticality,* or the awareness of the perpendicular alignment of the body segments; and *directionality,* or the projection of laterality outward into the spatial world.

As discussed on pp. 158-159, kinesthetic awareness is the ability to perceive movement. It is a major factor in the awareness of "self" and the image that children have of themselves.

Laterality is an important perceptual ability and is necessary in the structuring of symbols and objects in space. The development of the internal awareness of right and left allows an individual to coordinate reading from left to right and to identify positions of symbols on a page and, in the realm of motor skills, assists in tasks requiring lateral coordination and balance.

Verticality is the essential perceptual awareness of up and down. It is directly associated with the posturing and the internal sense of where the head is in relationship to the feet.

Directionality is a necessary perceptual attribute for spatial references. It allows an individual to relate to objects that are external to the body. Reading and writing skills are dependent on the awareness of right and left, up and down, and back and front. Movement skills in physical education are also dependent upon directionality. Without it children may be clumsy at play or unable to effectively perform games, rhythms, or sports. Inherent in directionality are the perceptions of time, distance, space, and synchrony to name just a few.

In order for children to effectively deal with objects that come to them or that they project, they must be able to perceive the distance, speed, and direction of the object's movement. For example, in a game of dodge ball the persons in the circle must be able to predict how far the ball is thrown, the speed of the throw, and the time the ball will take to reach them, making it necessary to dodge (Fig. 8-7). In dodging the ball the child must also perceive the place the ball will arrive and then move away from that spot. In batting a softball the batter must perceive the distance from the pitcher, the speed of the pitched ball, the position of the ball in

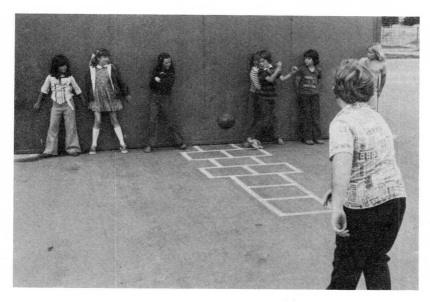

Fig. 8-7. Playing dodge ball effectively requires the child to have high levels of both time and space perceptions.

space, and when to begin swinging the bat in order to hit the ball. The batter must also have some prior perceptual information as to how heavy the bat is and how fast it can be swung. Besides being used in games or sports that use projectiles, directionality is essential in executing stunts in gymnastics and in dance. For example, executing a forward roll requires the perceptual abilities of determining the position of the body in space, the speed of the roll, and the timing of the sequence of movements, such as tucking the head, rounding the back, pushing off from the mat, rolling, and standing up.

Spatial relationships. Spatial relationships have been defined in more detail in Chapter 9 and generally imply that space is that expanse that extends from the body outward in all directions to infinity. The body and all other material objects are contained in space. The body is a reference point for the identification of positions of external objects. The perception of spatial relationships is integrally associated with growth and maturation and, most specifically, with body image and body knowledge. Children must first

have a sense of "self" before they can begin to accurately perceive those things that are outside of themselves.

Perceptual-motor integration

Perceptual-motor integration is the bringing together of all the elements of perception to form a well-coordinated and functioning whole. Perceptual-motor integration may be referred to as perceptual-motor matching in which the child, the perceiver, utilizes a number of senses to establish identity with the environment.[5] In other words, a child learning the concept of round sees it, feels it, and hears the label. All these senses—vision, tactility, and audition—coincide to form accurate perception. In order for children to make comparisons and varied responses to their movements, they must have stored a backlog of perceptual experiences. It is essential that children have in their background a great variety of perceptual-motor experiences derived from play and other general movement activities. With a backlog of these experiences children can engage in *motor*

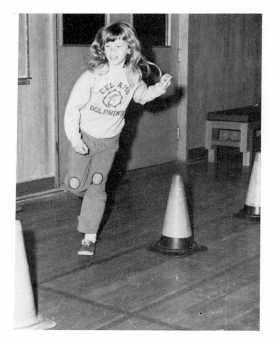

Fig. 8-8. Moving quickly through an obstacle course requires an ability to engage in motor planning. (From Arnheim, D. D., and Sinclair, W. A.: The clumsy child, St. Louis, 1975, The C. V. Mosby Co.)

planning, the using of past movement experiences to solve new movement problems without prior instruction (Fig. 8-8). Ideally, a motorically well-integrated person can make instantaneous perceptual-motor decisions when confronted with unique movement problems.

A wide variety of perceived responses related to past experiences, accurately interpreted and properly stored, provide the learner with information that can be used for solving current or future motor problems. Each set of adequately stored experiences can be selected and retrieved for use in other motor performances. Children must be continually provided with movement problems within their capabilities to solve. Perception develops as the performer struggles for mastery over each movement problem. When the task at hand no longer presents a challenge to the learner, the perceptual

process fails to be stimulated. To aid the child in perceptual development, the teacher must provide movement problems that are outside the immediate motor repertoire but that are similar to previously accomplished tasks. Motivated and challenged by a novel experience, the learner struggles for understanding and mastery and, as a result, develops a backlog of perceptual experiences.

As is every segment of education, physical education is vitally concerned with improving the learning process and the potential of an individual to learn. Perceptual-motor efficiency is highly important for success in active game skills. Children who lack rich backgrounds of movement and perceptual experiences may be impaired not only in their ability to move efficiently but also in their social and emotional development.

THE BASIC BODY MANAGEMENT CURRICULUM

In contrast to the "games approach" used during early childhood, basic body management through perceptual-motor training as a part of physical education is mainly concerned with the child's individual developmental requirements. Historically, children have been assigned games to play without thought to their biological maturity or readiness to learn specific skills. We contend that basic body management and perceptual-motor training cannot be separated from good physical education. They must be considered necessary approaches to physical fitness for young children and for older children in need of specific movement intervention because of a maturational lag or some neurological dysfunction.

Motor development programs designed to enrich the perceptual environment of the young child contain activity opportunities in the large areas of general total body management, object management, and emotional control. Specifically, the program should include logically sequenced task areas that utilize a multisensory approach.

In physical education the sense channels of vision, kinesthesis, and audition are primarily used to accomplish motor skills. Seldom are these sense modes used singularly, but they are interwoven in a complex fashion to accomplish the desired movement. Certain senses may predominate, depending on specific skill requirements. For example, vision may predominate in controlling objects in space, such as in catching a thrown ball, but kinesthesis cannot be discounted in regulating the body position and in initiating the muscle control necessary to actually catch the ball. Kinesthesis may be most important in an activity such as bouncing on a trampoline, but vision is very helpful in maintaining body orientation when the individual is suspended in the air. Audition, on the other hand, is essential for rhythms and the communications required in games and sports.

Important in all motor skill development are the perceptual components of general motor control and general motor skill development. In order to attain general motor control, the child must achieve an individual level of physical efficiency in terms of muscular strength, muscular endurance, joint flexibility, and stamina; the child must also acquire basic motor control, involving coordination in balance, use of large and small muscles, and the combining of eye and hand and eye and foot. General motor skills are acquired through the learning of movement patterns, such as locomotion and regulation of objects, and the development of basic play skills, such as throwing, catching, striking, and kicking.

Creating the program

The basic body management program of perceptual-motor training utilizes a developmental approach in helping children to reach their full potential. Through this approach the teacher has the opportunity to become more aware of the maturity and readiness levels of each individual child. Early identification of children who may have difficulty as physical performers or learners is also possible through this approach. Although the basic body management program is most successful with young children, many of its offerings can be considered helpful for older children who need remedial help.

The basic body management program attempts, through a sequential task-learning process, to assist children in becoming more successful in managing their bodies in a wide variety of movement situations. At the same time it attempts to provide the child with movement experiences that are multisensory in nature. In essence, this program strives to provide children with tasks that are appropriate for their particular maturation and readiness levels while at the same time stimulating integration of the nervous system in order that increasingly more complicated motor activities may be accomplished.

The teacher

Schools vary in how they provide instruction in their basic body management programs. In the self-contained classroom, the teacher is responsible for teaching in this area. Other systems provide a specialist in physical education, and others engage aides, either on a voluntary or on a paid basis. Many elementary schools throughout the nation are enlisting parents to conduct their basic body management programs. In situations in which aides or parents are used, teachers have the final responsibility of making sure that the program is initiated properly. The individual assigned to this program as teacher must be highly enthusiastic and, above all, must become involved both physically and emotionally in the performance of the task.

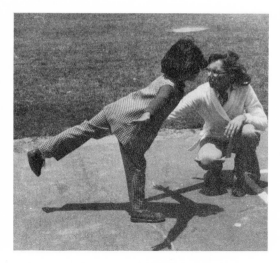

Fig. 8-9. Pretesting and posttesting is essential to determine the progress of each child.

Assessment

Children should be assessed as to their individual ability level before the program is begun. Preprogram assessment identifies children who may need special attention and provides a basis for emphasizing certain specific task areas. Pretesting and posttesting of the child are essential for determining individual progress (Fig. 8-9). Information gained can be used to diagnose perceptual-motor deficits and to provide direction in programming. Children having basic motor deficits can be given special remedial activities. Pretesting and posttesting also give teachers guides to their effectiveness in conducting the program.

Evaluation tools commonly used to determine basic motor effectiveness fall primarily into three categories: motor proficiency tests that attempt to determine motor maturity by definitive measurement, survey tests that use observation for assessment, and scales to determine specific developmental levels. Employment of these tests can be invaluable for the elementary teacher.

It is important that teachers of elementary physical education learn to observe movement critically. The following example of a simple survey assessment provides the teacher with information in five major aspects of body control: relaxation, locomotion, static balance, posture, and body perception.

MOVEMENT OBSERVATION SURVEY

Completion time: The assignment requires 1 hour for a class of 25 students.

Materials needed
1. Exercise mats
2. Firm, flat surface for hopping
3. Stopwatch, watch with a sweep second hand, or clock
4. Device to get the student airborne, such as trampoline, Spring-O-Line, or inner tube
5. Movement observation survey sheet (Fig. 8-10)

Special dress requirements: Students should wear tennis shoes.

Objectives: After completing this survey, the teacher should be able to:
1. Recognize the child's ability to consciously relax a specific body part
2. Determine the child's ability to hop on one foot at a time and to alternately hop on either foot
3. Determine the child's ability to maintain a static balance position
4. Assess the child's ability to maintain body alignment while airborne
5. Assess the child's ability to accurately imitate the body movements of another person

Procedures for conducting the survey: The teacher should:
1. Follow the description of each observation component
2. Observe children in groups of five or six
3. Record the findings for each child on the movement observation survey sheet

Observation components

Relaxation

Factor measured: The ability of a child to let the arm become tensionless.

Materials needed: Mat.

Regulations: While the child is in a back-lying position, the teacher lifts one of the child's hands by the fingers off the mat (approximately 12 inches). The child relaxes the arm completely or as much as possible, allowing

MOVEMENT OBSERVATION SURVEY SHEET

Motor task area	Specific task performance	Write in appropriate score	Comments by the observer
Relaxation	Letting arm go limp 5—Arm falls completely limp 4—Arm falls with very slight tension 3—Arm falls with moderate tension 2—Arm falls stiffly 1—Arm is pulled down		
Locomotion	Hop 5—Hop easily done, alternating from one foot to the other 4—Hops unrhythmically 3—Cannot alternate feet 2—Can hop on one foot but not on the other 1—Unable to hop on either foot		
Balance	Static balance variations (all held for 10 seconds) 5—Stork stand (sole of the raised foot placed on the side of the opposite knee) on each foot, hands approximately 1 foot apart and extended over head 4—Stork stand on each foot, hands on hips 3—Stand on one foot with the other lifted off the floor slightly, hands on hips 2—Stand on one foot, hands down at side 1—Cannot stand on one foot		
Posture control	Spring-O-Line or trampoline 5—Jumps smooth and well coordinated with feet together at top of jump 4—Feet spread at top of jump 3—Jumps stiff 2—Emphasis on one side of body 1—Off balance, arms and legs moving at different times		
Body image	Movement mimicry 5—Imitates accurately and without hesitation 4—Imitates accurately but with some hesitation 3—Imitates accurately but with much hesitation 2—Imitates inaccurately 1—Unable to mimic		
	Score (25 points are possible)		

Additional comments:

Fig. 8-10. Movement observation survey sheet.

it to drop back to the mat. The test is repeated three times.

Locomotion

Factor measured: The ability of a child to hop in place on one foot.

Materials needed: Firm, flat surface.

Regulations: The child hops three times on one foot and then three times on the other foot.

Balance

Factor measured: The ability of a child to maintain a variety of static positions for 10 seconds on one foot.

Materials needed: Firm, flat surface and stopwatch.

Regulations: At a signal, the child takes a balance position and holds it for 10 seconds. Three attempts are allowed at maintaining a balance position. (See score sheet, Fig. 8-10, for suggested balance positions.)

Posture control

Factor measured: The ability of a child to maintain proper postural control while airborne or rebounding.

Materials needed: Any device that will spring the child into the air, such as a Spring-O-Line, a trampoline, or a covered inner tube.

Regulations: The child springs up every time the teacher makes a sound, such as clapping the hands (in a rhythm of 40 to 60 beats per minute). The teacher observes how well the child coordinates body parts in the air and maintains a good balanced position on landing.

Body image

Factor measured: The ability of a child to accurately, smoothly, and decisively imitate unilateral, bilateral, and cross-lateral limb movements.

Materials needed: None.

Regulations: Standing and facing the teacher, the child follows the movements of the teacher exactly, as if looking into a mirror.

Suggested movements: (1) Each limb, singly, is moved to a specific lateral position; (2) both limbs on one side of the body are moved simultaneously to a specific lateral position; (3) an arm and a leg on opposite sides of the body are moved simultaneously to a specific lateral position; (4) one hand is placed on a body part on the opposite side, for example, the right hand is placed on the left shoulder or knee; (5) movement 4 is repeated with the other hand placed on a different body part.

Task categories

Numerous abilities and skills comprise efficient basic body management. Eight have been selected as most representing the movement needs of the developmentally immature child: muscular tension and release, locomotion, body and space perception, functional posture management, balance, rebound and airborne control, management of objects in play, and rhythm management.

All these task categories overlap one another; no task can be considered to be discrete, but each must be thought of as relying on a multitude of cognitive and perceptual-motor processes. The tasks presented here are designed not to splinter or segment the child's attention into the development of unrelated skills, but rather to act as a staircase to a higher order of movement expression.

Muscle tension sensitivity training. The more difficult a movement skill, the greater the need for the ability to relax and contract appropriate muscles at will. Children become familiar with muscular tension levels through a wide variety of movement exploration and play experiences.

Those who work with young children in the classroom and on the playground should assist them in becoming aware of how the body moves and the role muscles play in overcoming resistance. Children should learn the concept that movement is the result of selected muscle tension and relaxation. They must become aware that the reduction of tension is essential for recovering energy and for coordination as well as for good mental and emotional health.[6,15] The teacher should assist the child in becoming aware that the mind and body are inseparable and that worry or mental upset can result in

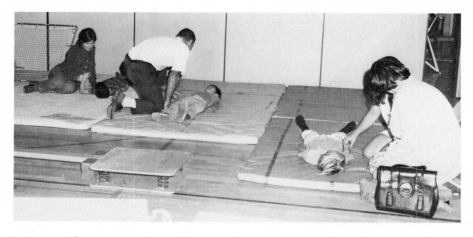

Fig. 8-11. All children should be taught sensitivity to muscle tension and how to reduce tension through relaxation.

muscular tension, and, therefore, children should become sensitive to tension and learn to reduce it through conscious control[10,11] (Fig. 8-11).

A prerequisite to good body coordination and management is the ability to contract and relax muscles at will. Controlled tension and relaxation of opposing muscles allows for coordinated and efficient movement without undue fatigue.

Muscular tension is related directly to an individual's emotional state, so the child who is anxious or psychologically upset will often express anxiety through an increase in muscle tonus. In essence, conscious control of muscle tension provides the child with a better climate for muscular synchronization and emotional control. The main avenues to tension reduction in physical education are rhythmical movement activities, play that drains energies, stretching exercises, and, the most beneficial and lasting means of tension reduction, conscious control by the use of imagery and tension sensitivity training.

A series of guided, relaxation activity progression sessions assists the child in becoming increasingly aware of body tension and how to let these tensions "go" at will. Overt stiffening of the body should be less required as the child becomes more skillful. Although a reclining

position is desirable, the child should be able to let go of tension in any position.

Many factors can be added to assist the teacher in conducting a successful program of relaxation, some of which are a room temperature of 76° F, comfortable loose-fitting clothes for the children, and an exercise mat for each child. Additional factors beneficial to this program are the use of breath control, imagery, and sound, such as music. Controlled breathing assists the child in letting go of tensions, particularly in the beginning of a session. The child is instructed to first inhale slowly and deeply and then to exhale slowly. The teacher instructs each child to become limp as the air is exhaled. As a state of relaxation occurs, breathing will automatically become progressively slower and more shallow.

Imagery should be used by the teacher as part of the approach to tension reduction. Phrases like "melting like an ice cube on a hot day," "limp as a rag," "light as a cloud," and "floating like a kite" may assist children in conceptualizing relaxation and tension. Often the teacher may emphasize abstract imagery by concrete demonstrations. The children may more easily understand if the teacher gives contrasting imagery directions such as "show me what a mechanical man looks like" and "show me what a Raggedy Ann doll looks like" or "show me what a flag on a flagpole looks like when there is no wind."

Children should also become aware that sounds can produce tension and/or relaxation. Soft, slow music produces a soothing effect, or a metronome set at a slow cadence provides a relaxing setting for rhythmical movement; these can also serve as a background for the tension reduction program. One should not discount the teacher's voice as an instrument for relaxing children. A voice that is quiet, low, slow, and distinct tends to reduce anxieties and muscular tension, whereas a voice that is loud, high, rapid, and difficult to understand does not.

The following activities, including imagery and muscle tension sensitivity, are presented according to levels of difficulty.

Relaxation through imagery.* Equipment to enhance imagery might include a radio or record player to play relaxing background music or a metronome set between 48 and 68 beats per minute and a comfortable, quiet, dark place to recline. Lying on a soft mat is ideal; however, imagery can also effectively be carried out in a sitting position. The room should be darkened and the temperature no less than 74° F. If possible, extraneous noise should be held to a minimum so that just the voice of the instructor is heard. Children who have difficulty in keeping their eyes closed may wear blindfolds.

To prepare for imagery the teacher should have the children stare at a spot on the ceiling without blinking until their eyes become tired; then instruct them to slowly allow them to close and have each child take five deep breaths, inhaling and exhaling slowly.

The following is a list of images that can be suggested, depending on the age and interest of the participants.

---

*Adapted from Arnheim, D. D., and Sinclair, W. A.: The clumsy child, 1975, St. Louis, The C. V. Mosby Co.

1. Imagine that your body is very heavy and sinking into the floor or as light as a feather.
2. Imagine you are a pat of butter in a warm frying pan, slowly melting.
3. Imagine yourself floating on a cloud.
4. Imagine yourself in a warm bath.
5. Imagine you are gliding along in a sailboat.
6. Imagine yourself in a warm, soft bed.
7. Imagine yourself lying on the front lawn, with the warm sun beating down, watching the clouds go by.
8. Imagine you are a soft marshmallow melting in a hot cup of cocoa.

It should be noted that for imagery to be most effective, it is important that the child be able to conceptualize the difference between overt tension of the body and the physical release of that tension. To emphasize this point it may be advisable to contrast imagery by having the child become limp as a rag and then become heavy as a big rock or stiff as a board.

Muscle tension sensitivity training exercises

Level I—total body. The purpose of muscle sensitivity training is to assist the child to discover the general feeling of a muscular tension level and to increase or decrease it at will.

To prepare for relaxation the child first goes through some imagery activities. In the first stages of learning the child should obviously stiffen and sag the body to develop the concept of tension and release. As control is gained, less obvious stiffening and sagging are required until finally all that is needed is to think about letting go of tension. The concept of tension recognition must be introduced to the child gradually without a sense of urgency or forcefulness. Depending on the ability of the child to concentrate, the relaxation period should not exceed 15 minutes. The best indication to the teacher that the child is learning to consciously release tension is the absense of resistance when a body part is lifted or moved. In the beginning sessions, resistance testing should automatically follow the relaxation of a given part. With this procedure the child has an immediate feedback as to the success of his or her efforts.

Muscle tensing sequences used in sensitivity training are:

1. Have the child stiffen the entire body for approximately 15 seconds or to the point of fatigue, whichever occurs first.
2. At the end of 15 seconds, have the child gradually decrease the stiffening, and observe the degree of limpness in the body.
3. Talk about how good it feels to be limp and relaxed in contrast to being stiff and tense.
4. When the child is limp, determine the lack of muscle tone in the body by lifting and dropping one arm. If the arm falls loosely to the floor without any visible restriction, then complete relaxation can be assumed to have taken place. If the arm resists falling, then it can be assumed that relaxation is not complete.

Level II—upper- and lower-limb relaxation. Level II can be introduced to the child who is developmentally at least 7 years old. When the child has successfully accomplished imagery and level I, then level II is introduced; it mainly involves both upper and lower limbs.

1. As in level I, the child visibly brings tension into his or her limbs, gradually decreasing it until relaxed limbs occur.
2. The child clenches both hands as hard as possible, tensing the forearms and straightening the elbows until both arms are completely stiff. The child is then instructed to slowly let the upper arms "go loose," then let the forearms relax, and finally open the hands and allow the fingers to become limp.
3. As indicated earlier, stiffening of the limbs becomes less and less obvious

as the concept of conscious tension reduction is learned. In other words, the child develops the ability to mentally control the muscle tone of the various upper and lower limb segments.

4. The legs are stiffened by first curling the toes down, then pointing the feet down, and finally locking the knees by fully extending the legs.
5. Like arm stiffening, leg stiffening is maintained for approximately 30 seconds and is followed by a gradual release of tension in the thigh, knee, lower leg, ankle, and then foot.
6. After he or she can perform the skill in both limbs the child is ready to learn unilateral relaxation.

Level III—unilateral relaxation. Level III is concerned with development of unilateral body control through tension-release methods that normally can be attained by children with a motor development of 9 years of age.

1. Unilateral relaxation consists of controlling the muscular tension levels of only one side of the body, such as tensing the left arm and leg while completely relaxing the right side and then tensing the right arm and leg while relaxing the left side. In this way the child begins to more fully differentiate body parts as well as distinguish between the two sides of the body.
2. Level III should be attempted only after successful execution of levels I and II but, like the first two levels, should be started with stiffening to the point of fatigue or for 15 seconds, whichever occurs first, followed by gradual release of tension to the point of limpness.
3. When the child has learned to successfully control one side of the body, then he or she concentrates on the other.

Level IV—relaxation of specific body parts. Level IV is the relaxation of specific individual body parts. Success in level IV indicates that the child can consciously reduce tension in most of the body's large muscles.

1. Full control of the tension levels of the large muscles normally requires a great deal of skill and is usually not achieved until late childhood or the teens.

2. After the children's early attempts at gaining segmental control by consciously tensing and relaxing, the teacher and class may determine the areas of the body that they have most difficulty in relaxing. Areas that are commonly difficult to reduce tension in are the low back, the neck and shoulders, and the abdominal region.

3. When the children have mastered the ability to consciously relax the major portions of the body, they can concentrate on the more difficult areas rather than going over areas already mastered.

Following is a list of body actions and the areas in which tension will be felt by the child:

Action	Area where tension is felt
1. Curling right toes down	Bottom of toes and foot
2. Curling left toes down	Bottom of toes and foot
3. Curling right toes back	Top of toes and foot
4. Curling left toes back	Top of toes and foot
5. Pointing right foot down (not curling toes)	Bottom of foot, back of calves
6. Pointing left foot down (not curling toes)	Bottom of foot, back of calves
7. Curling right foot back (not curling toes)	Top of foot, top of leg
8. Curling left foot back (not curling toes)	Top of foot, top of leg
9. Extending right knee (straightening knee slightly)	Top of thigh
10. Extending left knee (straightening knee slightly)	Top of thigh
11. Flexing right knee (curling knee slightly)	Back of thigh
12. Flexing left knee (curling knee slightly)	Back of thigh
13. Rotating thighs outward	Outer hip region
14. Rotating thighs inward	Inner hip region
15. Squeezing buttocks together	Buttocks region
16. Tightening abdominal muscles	Lower abdominal region
17. Pressing back against floor	Spinal region
18. Pinching shoulder blades together	Upper back and shoulders
19. Pressing head against floor	Back of neck
20. Gripping right hand	Hand and forearm
21. Gripping left hand	Hand and forearm
22. Gripping right hand and curling wrist and elbow	Front part of arm
23. Gripping left hand and curling wrist and elbow	Front part of arm
24. Gripping right hand and curling it back, and flexing elbow	Back part of arm
25. Gripping left hand and curling it back, and flexing elbow	Back part of arm
26. Shrugging right shoulder	Upper shoulder and side of neck
27. Shrugging left shoulder	Upper shoulder and side of neck
28. Curling neck forward	Front part of neck

Locomotion. The ability to move freely about the terrain is one of humankind's greatest attainments. In the upright posture the hands are free to explore and manipulate things in the environment. Locomotor skills are, therefore, one of the most important areas of basic body management. The task categories that can be assigned to locomotion are rolling, crawling, creeping, climbing, walking, stair climbing, jumping, hopping, skipping, running, and leaping.

Rolling, crawling, creeping, and climbing*—level I. All activities should be executed as precisely as possible, with each activity being performed slowly with a gradual increase in speed as control is gained.

Rolling in a straight line. The children lie on their backs with their bodies fully extended, feet together, and arms held to the side. Each child attempts to roll as straight as possible. The head first turns in the direction of the roll, followed by the hips. The trunk is twisted, the shoulders lifted, and one thigh rotated inward and over the other thigh. In this manner, all segments of the body are aligned and maintained in good control. When the child is able to roll effectively in one direction, then rolling in the other direction should be attempted.

When the basic rolling sequence has been successfully achieved, many variations can be included to offer additional challenges.

1. Rolling with hands clasped overhead
2. Rolling with one arm extended over the head and the other arm held to the side of the body
3. Rolling straight under a string line that extends about 15 feet
4. Rolling with the eyes closed and directing the body toward a sound made by the teacher
5. Making the body as round as possible and rolling down the mat like a ball

Obviously rolling can eventually lead to execution of tumbling stunts, but these should be attempted only when it is apparent that the participant is ready for elementary gymnastics.

---

*Adapted from Arnheim, D. D., and Sinclair, W. A.: The clumsy child, St. Louis, 1975, The C. V. Mosby Co.

Crawling. Crawling is a natural extension of rolling. The child moves along the floor in a face-down position by various movements of the arms and legs. Each crawling task must be executed in the proper form before the next higher level skill is attempted.

1. On the stomach, with arms at sides and feet together, each child weaves back and forth, attempting to propel the body forward. Instruction is given to maintain the arms at the sides, keep the legs straight, and move the body as a single unit. Most likely, little forward progress will be made by the child. However, when the body can be wiggled equally well on both sides and can progress forward a foot or more, the child is ready for the next progression.
2. Crawling is next attempted by moving the arm and leg on one side of the body in unison and then moving the limbs on the opposite side, as a commando would crawl. The head should be either in a straight line with the eyes looking straight ahead or turned toward the side on which the limbs are flexed.
3. Movement is then introduced in which the opposite arm and leg are flexed and the other limbs extended.

When the child can execute a cross-lateral movement with synchrony, variations are added, such as:

1. Crawling sideways in each direction
2. Crawling backwards with feet first
3. Crawling under and over an obstacle
4. Crawling up and down an incline
5. Crawling forward on a narrow board

Creeping. In creeping the child takes a hands-and-knees position. A well-skilled creeper maintains the trunk in line with the head and the shoulders. Keeping the body in good segmental alignment, the creeper should be able to move easily forward, backward, or even sideways. In general, like crawling, creeping is developed from less specific bilateral movements to unilateral and then cross-lateral movements. After the most sophisticated of creeping skills has been attained, then variations are introduced.

1. Maintaining good head and back alignment, the child moves forward by using the hands and the legs together in a homologous movement technique that is commonly described as a rabbit hop.
2. The child next progresses to a unilateral pattern by moving first the arm and leg on one side and then both limbs on the other side.
3. Cross-lateral creeping is performed by extending one arm forward and placing the hand on the mat; the opposite knee follows. This movement alternates with movement of the other arm and knee.

Some variations of creeping that might be performed are:

1. The child executes the cross-lateral creeping technique moving backward instead of forward.
2. Rather than moving one limb at a time, the child moves the opposite arm and leg forward simultaneously.
3. Instead of moving forward the child moves backward, moving the opposite leg and arm simultaneously. The child moves sideways left and then right in the four-point position. The child drags the legs like a seal.

Ladder climbing. In some respects ladder climbing can be considered a direct extension of creeping because it involves the coordinated use of both legs and arms. In much the same way as crawling, creeping, and walking, climbing a ladder evolves from a unilateral skill to the most sophisticated cross-lateral skill.

1. Unilateral climbing is performed by placing the right foot on the rung, extending the right arm to grasp a rung, placing the left foot on the rung, and extending the left arm to grasp a rung.
2. Another type of unilateral climbing is performed by simultaneously moving first the right leg and arm and then the left leg and arm.
3. Cross-lateral climbing using one limb at a time begins with the right leg. Then the left arm is moved, followed by the left leg and then the right arm.
4. In cross-lateral climbing incorporating simultaneous movements, the right leg and left arm move first, followed by the left leg and right arm.

Walking and stair climbing—level II. Level II introduces transport activities executed while in the upright posture and includes activities in which some part of the body is in contact with the supporting surface at all times, such as in walking on a level surface and stair climbing. Level II is a natural extension of level I, following the basic principles of developmental direction. At level I the child requires a great deal of physical support, while at level II he has progressed to the point that balance and locomotion are possible in the bipedal position.

A wide variety of outdoor terrain should be available to the children, including differently textured surfaces, slopes, elevations, and stairs.

Walking

1. In an upright position with good posture, the children propel themselves forward with a cross-lateral technique, first swinging one arm and then the opposite leg. This is followed by an alternating of the other limbs.
2. The children walk forward while moving opposite arms and legs simultaneously.

Some variations of walking are:

1. Walking while moving the arm and leg on the same side in unison
2. Cross-lateral walking backward
3. Walking backward while moving

the arm and leg on the same side in unison

4. Walking sideways to the left and then to the right
5. Walking forward, backward, and sideways on the toes
6. Walking forward, backward, and sideways on the heels
7. Walking with feet turned out
8. Walking with feet turned in
9. Walking on different textures, for example, grass, cement, sand, soft mat, wood floor, rug, gravel, or dirt
10. Walking up and down inclines
11. Walking with the feet on different levels

Stair climbing. Ascending and descending stairs are natural extensions of creeping and walking.

1. Ascending stairs
   a. Creeping upstairs in a unilateral fashion
   b. Creeping upstairs in a cross-lateral movement
   c. Walking upstairs in a unilateral fashion
   d. Walking upstairs in a cross-lateral movement
   e. Creeping upstairs in a supine position
   f. Walking upstairs backwards
2. Descending stairs
   a. The child sits with hands flat on the same step and feet flat two or three steps lower. From this position the child moves down to the next step by first moving the seat and then both feet, continuing down the stairs like an inchworm.
   b. Following the performance of bilateral scooting just described, the child moves down the stairs in a unilateral manner.
   c. The child descends using cross-lateral movements with feet first.
   d. Standing at the top of the stairs either holding on to a banister

or free and maintaining good posture, the child steps down the stairs in a unilateral fashion always beginning with the right foot.
   e. As in d above, the child walks down the stairs, but always beginning with the left side.
   f. Maintaining good posture alignment, the child descends the stairs in a cross-lateral fashion without holding on to a railing.

Jumping, hopping, and skipping—level III. The ability to propel the body upward from a supporting surface requires much strength, balance, and confidence. Jumping, hopping, and skipping are direct extensions of walking.

Jumping
1. Jumping with both feet together, leaving the ground, and landing with the body under control
2. Jumping with both feet together, swinging the arms, bending the knees, propelling the body over a line or very low obstacle such as the edge of a Hula-Hoop, and landing with both feet together under good control
3. Jumping over a 3-inch wide space with both feet
4. Jumping over a 6-inch wide space with both feet
5. Jumping over a 9-inch wide space with both feet
6. Jumping over a 12-inch wide space with both feet
7. Jumping with both feet over a space equal to the length of the child's lower leg
8. Jumping over a 3-inch obstacle with both feet
9. Jumping over a 6-inch obstacle with both feet
10. Jumping over a 9-inch obstacle with both feet
11. Jumping with both feet over an obstacle equal to the height of the child's knee

12. Jumping from a 2-inch step, landing with both feet together and the body under good control
13. Jumping from a 6-inch step, landing with both feet together and the body under good control
14. Jumping from two steps or a box approximately 18 inches in height, landing on both feet
15. Jumping from three steps or an equally high box, landing on both feet
16. Jumping with a two-foot takeoff over a space, landing in a balanced position on either the left or the right foot

Hopping
1. Hopping once on the left foot
2. Hopping once on the right foot
3. Hopping twice on the left foot
4. Hopping twice on the right foot
5. Hopping three times on the left foot
6. Hopping three times on the right foot
7. Hopping forward on the left foot ten times
8. Hopping forward on the right foot ten times
9. Hopping backwards on the left foot three times
10. Hopping backwards on the right foot three times
11. Hopping backwards on the left foot ten times
12. Hopping backwards on the right foot ten times
13. Hopping sideways to the left on the left foot three times
14. Hopping sideways to the right on the left foot three times
15. Hopping sideways to the right on the right foot three times
16. Hopping sideways to the left on the right foot three times
17. Hopping once on the left foot and twice on the right
18. Hopping twice on the left foot and once on the right

19. Hopping blindfolded or with the eyes closed

Skipping. Skipping is a cross-extension movement of hopping, that is, a movement consisting of alternating hops on each foot to move forward.
1. Skipping forward
2. Skipping backward
3. Skipping to the right
4. Skipping to the left
5. Skipping up a ramp
6. Skipping down a ramp
7. Skipping up stairs

Running and leaping—level IV. The activities of level IV are the most difficult of the locomotor skills. They require the child to have a good foundation in the lower level skills.

Running. When the child gains confidence in the bipedal position, walking and running develop almost simultaneously; however, controlled running does not occur until after child has reached the toddler stage. Running is an extension of walking with the difference that there is no time when both feet are in contact with the ground. In essence, there are three phases in running: pushoff, flight, and landing. The faster a person runs, the more the body is inclined forward and the more he or she runs on the balls of the feet. As the persons runs more slowly the pelvis is inclined backward and each foot is in contact with the ground for a longer time. In all running tasks the child should be encouraged to run in good alignment with arms and legs moving freely cross-laterally. Deviation from this form produces inefficient running and expenditure of more energy than is necessary.
1. Running or jogging slowly with the feet flat
2. Running slowly with the weight slightly forward on the balls of the feet
3. Running forward at medium speed with the weight on the balls of the feet

4. Running forward fast with the weight on the balls of the feet
5. Running alternately slowly and then fast
6. Running backward
7. Running slowly through a zigzag obstacle course
8. Running fast through a zigzag obstacle course
9. Running up a ramp
10. Running down a ramp
11. Running up stairs

Leaping. A leap is a synchronous movement that in most cases is an extension of running. In the leap one foot is used to push off and the other to land. The runner bends the knee of the leg that is in the back position and, with an exaggerated step of the front leg, lands on the front foot. The leaper attempts to literally sail through the air, making a landing that is as soft as possible.

1. Stepping and leaping, landing on the right foot
2. Stepping and leaping, landing on the left foot
3. Running slowly and leaping, landing on the right foot
4. Running slowly and leaping, landing on the left foot
5. Running fast and leaping, landing on the right foot
6. Running fast and leaping, landing on the left foot
7. Running fast, leaping over a knee-high hurdle, and landing on the left foot

Body and space perception

Body and space perception consists of three major interrelated factors: body knowledge, body image, and spatial awareness, as discussed in some detail earlier in this chapter. Tasks to develop body and space perception may fall into the categories of directive progressions and reflective or mimetic progressions.

Directive activities are those activities initiated by verbal or tactile directions. Reflective activities, on the other hand, are initiated without verbalization or touching but are conducted by having the child mimic the teacher's body positions or copy the attitudes of some graphic display such as a picture.

Body perception is best taught in an area that is uncluttered and has a non-distracting background such as a blank wall. A full-length mirror should be available so that both the child and the teacher can view themselves as they perform; a blindfold is also needed.

In both the directive and reflective techniques the teacher should face the class, who may be standing, sitting, or lying on their backs.

The teacher should make the directions as concise and concrete as possible, omitting words that only tend to confuse the child. Each direction should be repeated twice and should be followed by an immediate positive response such as praise when the child successfully completes the task. However, if the child fails at a certain body perception task, a few more directives should be given to determine whether the missed task was an accurate indication of the child's functional level.

Directive progressions. The teacher gives the directions listed and each child carries them out.

Level I

1. Body planes (using one or both hands)
   a. Touch the front of your body.
   b. Touch the back of your body.
   c. Touch the side of your body.
   d. Touch the top of your body.
   e. Touch the bottom of your body. (Child touches the bottoms of the feet.)
2. Body parts
   a. Touch your head.
   b. Touch your arm.
   c. Touch your leg.
   d. Touch your foot.
   e. Touch your face.

f. Touch your elbow.

g. Touch your knee.

h. Touch your nose.

i. Touch your ear.

j. Touch your mouth.

k. Touch your eye.

l. Touch your hand.

m. Touch your stomach.

3. Body movements

a. Bend your body forward.

b. Bend your body backward.

c. Bend your body sideward.

d. Twist or turn your body.

e. Bend your knees.

f. Stand on your tiptoes.

g. Bend your head forward.

h. Bend your head sideward.

i. Bend your head backward.

j. Bend your elbow.

k. Straighten your arm.

Level II

1. Body parts

a. Touch your elbow.

b. Touch your knee.

c. Touch your shoulder.

d. Touch your fingers.

e. Touch your wrist.

f. Touch your nose.

g. Touch your mouth.

2. Body movements

a. Circle your head.

b. Circle your arms.

c. Circle your leg.

d. Bend your fingers.

e. Bend your toes.

3. Laterality

a. Touch your right arm.

b. Touch your left knee.

c. Touch your right foot.

d. Touch your left eye.

e. Touch your right shoulder.

f. Touch your left elbow.

g. Touch your right side.

h. Touch your right side against the wall.

i. Kneel on your left knee.

j. Hold something in your right hand.

k. Step up on the chair with your left foot.

l. Hold up your right arm.

Level III

1. Body parts

a. Touch your thigh.

b. Touch your wrist.

c. Touch your upper arm.

d. Touch your forearm.

e. Touch your lower leg.

f. Touch your kneecap.

g. Touch your little finger.

h. Touch your big toe.

i. Touch your little toe.

j. Touch your eyebrow.

2. Body movements

a. Straighten your leg.

b. Straighten your arms.

c. Circle your foot.

d. Circle your hand.

e. Spread your fingers.

f. Spread your toes.

g. Wiggle your nose.

h. Stick out your tongue.

i. Make a sad face.

j. Make a happy face.

3. Laterality

a. Touch something to your right side.

b. Touch a ball to your left knee.

c. Touch something to your left elbow.

d. Touch something to your right ear.

e. With your right hand, touch your left foot.

f. With your left hand, touch your right ear.

g. With your right hand, touch your right ear.

h. With your left hand, touch your left shoulder.

i. With your right hand, touch your left elbow.

j. With your right hand, touch your left wrist.

k. With your left hand, touch your right eye.

l. With your right hand, touch your nose.

m. With your left hand, touch your knee.

n. With your left hand, hold on to your right ear.

o. With your left hand, grab your left ankle.

4. Directionality

a. Touch another child's right hand.

b. Touch another child's left ear.

c. Touch another child's right shoulder.

d. Touch another child's right knee.

e. Touch another child's right eyebrow.

f. Touch the left side of the chair. (Child stands facing a chair.)

g. Touch the right side of the chair.

h. With your left hand, touch the right side of the chair.

i. With your right hand, touch the left side of the chair.

j. With your right hand, touch the right side of the chair.

k. Tell me, what foot is another child standing on?

l. Tell me, what hand does another child have raised?

m. Stand with your right side against another child's left side.

n. Stand so that your left side is against another child's right side.

Some variations of directive body perception are:

1. A child gives directions to the teacher.

2. A child gives directions to self aloud.

3. A child gives directions to another child.

4. After the child's silhouette is traced on a large sheet of paper, the child colors and identifies the body parts.

5. On the directions of the teacher, the child places the body part on the corresponding part of the silhouette tracing.

6. The child verbally identifies all body parts.

Reflective progressions. Reflective body perception tasks are designed to reveal how accurately a child copies the movements or poses of another person or animal. The teacher can demonstrate in several ways, for example, by facing the class, with his or her back to them or by having both the class and himself or herself face a mirror. When the teacher faces the class, they respond as if they were viewing themselves in a mirror.

Level I. Children lie on a mat facing the teacher, who is standing at their feet.

1. Half side spread, both arms

2. Three-quarters side spread, both arms

3. One-quarter side spread, both arms

4. Half side spread, both legs

5. Three-quarters side spread, both legs

6. One-quarter side spread, both legs

7. Both arms spread overhead; half side spread, both legs

8. Half side spread, right leg

9. Half side spread, left leg

10. Half side spread, right arm

11. Half side spread, left arm

12. Half side spread, right hand and three-quarter side spread, left leg

13. Three-quarter side spread, right arm and one-quarter side spread, left leg

Some variations of level I are:

1. The child verbalizes how the arms and legs are to be moved and then the teacher and the child take that position.

2. The child watches the teacher's movement and then mimics the movement with eyes closed.

Level II. Activities are conducted in a standing position with the children facing the teacher, who stands approximately 8 feet from them. The children are instructed to follow the teacher's movements as if they were viewing themselves in a mirror. All activity tasks are conducted in silence with no verbal instructions given except prompting by the teacher to clarify how the task is executed or to provide positive reinforcement.

1. Half side spread, both arms

2. Three-quarter side spread, both arms

3. One-quarter side spread, both arms
4. Three-quarter side spread, left arm and half side spread, right arm
5. Three-quarter side spread, right arm and one-quarter side spread, left arm
6. Half side spread, right arm and three-quarter side spread, left arm
7. Half side spread, left arm and three-quarter side spread, right arm
8. Right arm extended in front of face and left arm overhead
9. Left arm extended in front of face and right arm overhead
10. Both feet spread to side
11. Both feet together
12. Right foot out to side
13. Left foot out to side
14. Right foot forward and left foot back
15. Left foot forward and right foot back

Some variations of level II are:
1. The child plays follow the leader.
2. The child mimics different animals.

Level III. In contrast to level II, level III tasks include moving both arms and legs simultaneously.

1. Half side spread, both arms and right foot out to side
2. Half side spread, both arms and left foot out to side
3. One-quarter side spread, both arms; right foot forward; and left foot back
4. One-quarter side spread, right arm; left arm extended overhead; left foot forward; and right foot back
5. Both arms extended at shoulder level and both feet spread

Some variations of level III are:
1. The child follows the teacher as they both stand in front of the mirror.
2. The teacher shows the child drawings of figures assuming various positions and the child assumes the same positions.
3. The teacher instructs the child to take the position opposite the one demonstrated.

Functional posture control

The motor development approach for young children is concerned with the most efficient use of the body in supportive tasks, such as standing, sitting, and various ways of overcoming resistance. The young child can become aware of the most efficient ways to use the body through a well-planned movement, problem-solving, and task-oriented program.

Closely associated with static and dynamic balance, posture control is concerned with the execution of body positions that involve a minimum of energy demands. Good supportive posture is the relative arrangement of the body parts and body segments that provides the greatest mechanical efficiency; poor supportive posture produces functional disharmony and mechanical inefficiency. Task progressions include activities of standing, sitting, running, and the overcoming of resistance, such as lifting, carrying, pushing, and pulling heavy objects.

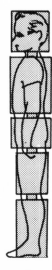

Fig. 8-12. Segmental posture alignment.

Standing. Although children are seldom at ease when they stand statically in one position, the standing posture can provide valuable information for the teacher about how well each child is segmentally aligned. Ideally, each body segment is evenly balanced over the supporting segment below (Fig. 8-12). Children can discover their own best standing posture by experimenting with the feel of contrasting positions.

To learn about the base of support, the children work in pairs with one child standing in back of the other with the hands placed on the other's shoulders. The teacher states the problem, after which the front child takes that position while the child in back pushes and pulls in an attempt to offset the partner (Fig. 8-13). Two contrasting positions are given by the teacher, and the child is asked to determine which one of the positions is the most stable. Following are examples of some contrasting positions:

The child:
1. Stands on toes or flat-footed
2. Stands flat-footed, with feet together or separated
3. Stands with knees straight or knees bent
4. Stands with feet staggered or both feet even with each other
5. Leans forward or stands straight
6. Leans backward or stands straight
7. Leans sideways or stands straight

Each child is asked to test the following good and poor standing alignments by himself or herself to see if he or she can feel the difference and decide which is better:

The child:
1. Stands with the head forward or balanced above the shoulders
2. Stands with the shoulders forward or straight
3. Stands with the back rounded or straight
4. Stands with the hips forward with the abdomen relaxed or hips straight with the abdomen held firm
5. Stands with the weight on the left foot with the left shoulder sagging or with the weight on both feet and shoulders even

Sitting and rising. Because sitting and rising from a chair are so basic to everyday life, teachers can use this element as a means of teaching proper body alignment. They should instruct the child to keep the head up and the back in good alignment when seating himself or herself in a chair. The child places one foot behind so that it touches the front of the chair and simultaneously leans the trunk forward, lowers the body to the seat, and bends the knees (Fig. 8-14). Control comes from the quadriceps muscles, which extend the knee. To rise from the

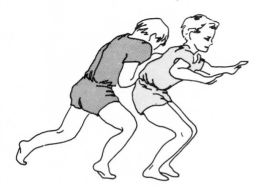

Fig. 8-13. Children learning concept of body balance and posture.

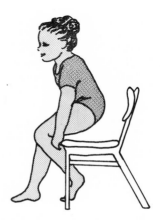

Fig. 8-14. Proper body alignment for sitting or rising.

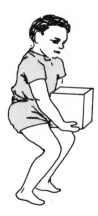

Fig. 8-15. Proper body position for lifting heavy object.

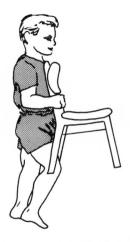

Fig. 8-16. Proper body position for carrying heavy object.

chair, the child leans forward slightly while the knee extensors straighten the legs.

Overcoming resistances. The supportive functions of lifting, carrying, pushing, and pulling are basic to a child as well as to the adult; consequently, they should be included early in a child's movement curriculum. Proper execution of these functions ensures a better application of mechanical forces, more efficiency of effort, and the prevention of muscle injury from strain.

When grasping a heavy object to lift it from a low level, the child must keep the feet flat on the floor, keep the back straight, and bend the knees (Fig. 8-15). To lift the heavy object, the child straightens the knees while keeping the head, back, and hips in good alignment. To increase the mechanical advantages of the lift, the child maintains the object close to the body.

Persons should carry objects that are heavy with both arms close to the body. To increase force and decrease the chances of muscle strain, they should keep each of their major body segments well aligned (Fig. 8-16). When carrying objects such as school books on one side of the body, they should be taught to make a special effort to keep the load close to the body and not to let the body

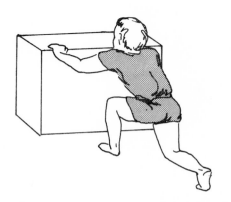

Fig. 8-17. Proper body position for pushing heavy object.

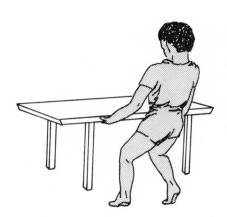

Fig. 8-18. Proper body position for pulling heavy object.

sag in the direction of the load; also frequent changes of the load from one side to the other will aid in preventing chronic postural distortions.

The physical laws applied to pushing a heavy object require the pusher to push in line with or below his or her center of gravity (Fig. 8-17). To increase pushing power, the body should be well aligned, with one foot forward and one foot back and the hips slightly bent. The primary force comes from straightening the knees.

In pulling, in contrast to pushing, force is applied upward and forward. The body is inclined away from the heavy object, with the center of gravity in line with the force of the pull. One leg is forward and the other back, with the major force of the pull coming from the extension of the legs (Fig. 8-18).

The teacher can provide children with problems that will assist them in discovering the best methods for overcoming a resistance. The child should test the differences in the following contrasting ways of overcoming resistance:

The child:

1. Lifts a moderately heavy box without bending knees, and then bending knees
2. Carries a box close to the hip and then away from the hip
3. Pushes a heavy object at shoulder height and then at knee height at the center of gravity
4. Pushes a heavy object with arms alone and then with the legs alone
5. Pulls an object higher than, lower than, and in line with the center of gravity

Balancing. Balancing skills are essential in all human movement and involve the person's ability to maintain or control a desired body position by *dynamically* moving or by maintaining a *static* position (Fig. 8-19). An individual maintains and loses balance continually in most gross motor activities; the ability to maintain balance is developed through the body's losing and then regaining the balance position.

Static balance activities. Sequences are separated into two levels. Level 1 includes a sequence of static postures without the use of equipment. Level 2 is more difficult and uses various-sized balance

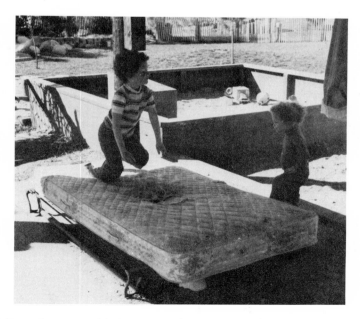

Fig. 8-19. Bouncing on an old mattress can be one way to develop an ability to balance.

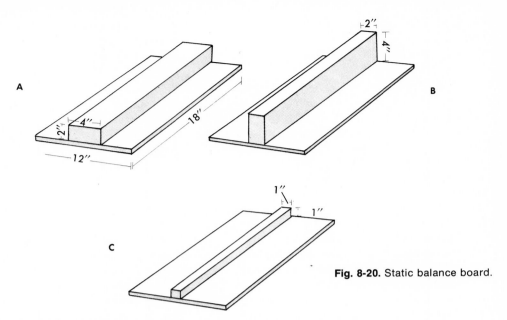

Fig. 8-20. Static balance board.

boards. In both levels, balance posture is held for a minimum of 10 seconds.

Level 1 task progressions
The child:
1. Assumes side-lying position
2. Assumes three-point position (left knee off floor and then right knee off floor) .
3. Assumes two-point position on left hand and right knee and then on right hand and left knee
4. Kneels upright on left knee, with arms crossed, and then on right knee, with arms crossed
5. Squats with arms crossed
6. Stands, feet together, with hands on waist
7. Stands, feet together, on tiptoes, with hands on waist
8. Stands, heel to toe, left foot in front and then right foot in front, with hands on waist
9. Stands on left foot and then on right foot, with arms crossed
10. Stands on left foot and then on right foot, with arms crossed, blindfolded

Level 2 task progressions. Balance board dimensions are indicated in Fig. 8-20.

The child:
1. Stands, heel to toe, with left foot forward and then with right foot forward, on the 4-inch surface
2. Stands, heel to toe, with left foot forward and then with right foot forward, on the 1-inch surface
3. Balances on right foot and then on left foot, with hands on waist, on the 4-inch surface
4. Balances on right foot and then on left foot, with hands on waist, blindfolded, on the 4-inch surface
5. Balances on right foot and then on left foot, with hands on waist, on the 2-inch surface
6. Balances on right foot and then on left foot, with hands on waist, blindfolded, on the 2-inch surface
7. Balances on right foot and then on left foot, with hands on waist, on the 1-inch surface
8. Balances on right foot and then on left foot, with hands on waist, blindfolded, on the 1-inch surface

Variations of static balance activities
The child:
1. Balances statically while assuming different poses

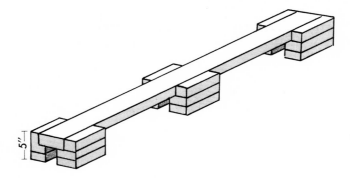

5"

Fig. 8-21. Balance beam.

2. Plays catch while balancing
3. While standing in one position, balances other objects, such as broomsticks on fingertips and beanbags on head
4. Plays "statue"—takes different positions and holds them

Dynamic balance activities. As is static balance, dynamic balance is divided into two task areas: those that are conducted on the floor or ground and those that are done on the balance beam. Success in a specific task is determined when a child can slowly and deliberately perform for a minimum of ten steps on the balance beam. A dynamic balance task is not accomplished if the performer speeds up, stops, or wavers out of control before ten steps have been completed.

Level 1 activities. All tasks must be conducted with hands on hips.

The child:
1. Walks forward in a 6-inch track
2. Walks sideward (left and then right), foot to foot, in a 6-inch track
3. Walks backward in a 6-inch track
4. Walks, heel to toe, forward on a line
5. Walks, heel to toe, sideward (left and then right) on a line

Level 2 activities. The balance beam, which is 10 feet long, is illustrated in Fig. 8-21.

The child:
1. Walks forward on the balance beam, heel to toe
2. Walks sideward on the balance beam to the left and then to the right, foot to foot
3. Walks backward and then forward on the balance beam, heel to toe
4. Walks forward on the balance beam, heel to toe, blindfolded
5. Walks sideward on the balance beam to the right and then to the left, the following foot stepping over the leading foot
6. Walks backward on the balance beam, heel to toe
7. Walks sideward on the balance beam, blindfolded, and then backward, blindfolded
8. Walks forward on the balance beam, stepping over obstacles of different heights

Variations of dynamic balance activities

The child:
1. Crawls on the balance beam
2. Bounces ball while walking on the beam
3. Catches and throws while walking on the beam
4. Performs rebound activities on the balance beam
5. Bounces on a pogo stick
6. Walks on stilts
7. Skates with either roller skates or ice skates
8. Rides a two-wheel bicycle
9. Plays hopping games like hopscotch

Rebound or airborne skills. Jumping from a surface or being projected upward provides children with a stimulating kinesthetic experience. While suspended in air, the body must make a multitude of neurophysiological adjustments in order to stabilize itself in space. Balance and gross muscle control are greatly enhanced through rebound and airborne activities.

The teacher should be aware of the number of factors essential to coordinated airborne activities: balance, bilateral gross motor control, strength of jump, and jumping pace. Balance is important to good jumping, so that the body follows the position of the head. The child should be able to change the direction of the jump easily by shifting body weight to the left or right. Smooth jumping requires the coordinated use of both sides of the body. Arms should be level with each other, and feet should be parallel to the jumping surface. The child should be able to alter the height and speed of the jump, on the teacher's command, in repetitive jumps. A child who displays stiffness and improper body control should be encouraged to participate in a wide variety of airborne jumping tasks.

Activity progressions. Flexboards, tires, or springboards are used.

The child:

1. Jumps up and down with both feet
2. Jumps up and down with the right foot and then with the left foot
3. Jumps up and down, alternating feet
4. Jumps up and down twice and then jumps with both feet to the ground
5. Jumps sideward to the right to the ground and then sideward to the left to the ground
6. Jumps backward to the ground
7. Jumps and turns to the right one-fourth turn, one-half turn, three-fourths turn, and then a full turn
8. Jumps and turns to the left one-fourth turn, one-half turn, three-fourths turn, and then a full turn

Variations of jumping activities

The child:

1. Jumps and claps hands before landing
2. Jumps and catches an object in the air
3. Jumps over an obstacle
4. Jumps and does a forward roll
5. Jumps and throws an object
6. Jumps on a trampoline, which is one of the devices used for learning postural control

Management of objects in play

Dealing with objects in space is basic to successful game playing. Children must be able to propel and/or receive objects efficiently if they are to play a wide variety of games and sports.[9] Like all motor skills, object control develops from a hierarchy of movement patterns and subskills that are built on each other to eventually emerge as a highly integrated motor act.

Throwing activities

Lead-up skills

The child:

1. While seated, pushes a 9-inch playground ball with both hands to a receiver sitting 3 feet away
2. While seated, pushes a 9-inch playground ball with both hands to a receiver sitting 6 feet away
3. While seated, pushes a 9-inch playground ball with both hands to a receiver sitting 10 feet away
4. While seated, pushes a 9-inch playground ball with the left hand to a receiver sitting 10 feet away
5. While seated, pushes a 9-inch playground ball with the right hand to a receiver sitting 10 feet away
6. While kneeling, bounces a ball straight into the hands of a receiver sitting 10 feet away
7. While kneeling, bounces a ball with the right hand into the hands of a receiver sitting 10 feet away
8. While kneeling, bounces a ball with the left hand into the hands of a receiver sitting 10 feet away

9. While standing, throws a ball with both hands from an overhead position, straight to the receiver
10. While standing, bounces a ball with the preferred hand to a receiver
11. With foot opposite the throwing arm forward, throws a small ball to a receiver

When children can efficiently execute the last directive, the teacher should then teach them the mature way of throwing an overhand ball, as follows:

12. Preparatory movement (right-handed throw is described):
    a. Pivots by rotating the body to the right and shifting the weight to the right foot
    b. Swings the throwing arm backward and upward and, from this position, is ready to execute an overhand throw
13. Final sequence of throw:
    a. Steps forward with the left foot in the direction of the throw and with the toes pointed in direction of the throw
    b. Rotates the hips, trunk, and shoulders to the left while pulling the throwing arm back to the final position before starting the forward arm movement

c. Leads the right elbow forward horizontally, extends the forearm, and snaps the wrist just before releasing the ball
d. Executes the follow-through by continuing to move the arm in the direction of the throw until the muscular energy has been dissipated (Fig. 8-22)

Throwing skills

The child:
1. Plays catch with another person
2. Throws balls or beanbags at a target
3. Throws to a pitch-back device
4. Throws, using a variation of projectiles, such as Hula-Hoops, beanbags, fluff balls, baseballs, soccer balls, and footballs
5. Plays games like dodge ball
6. Passes a football
7. Learns different ways to project, such as underhand pitch, push pass, hook pass, and shot put, and becomes aware of the differences and similarities of the various techniques

Catching activities

Lead-up skills. The ball used in learning should be partially deflated for ease of handling. Also objects other than balls, such as hoops or beanbags, can be used.

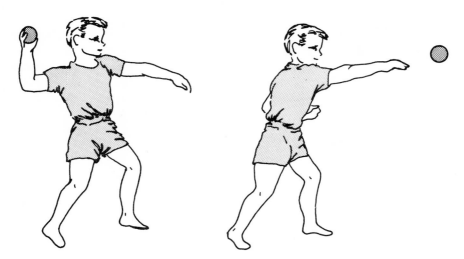

Fig. 8-22. Mature overhand throw.

The child:
1. While seated, traps a rolling 9-inch playground ball
2. While seated, stops a rolling 9-inch playground ball with both hands
3. While in a kneeling position, stops a rolling 9-inch playground ball
4. First while kneeling and then while standing, handles a bouncing 9-inch playground ball (Catching an aerial projectile requires the performer to overcome the fear of being hit in the face. The child with fear will have more success with a paper or cloth ball.)
5. Forms a scoop with the arms into which the leader throws the ball, first, from a distance of 3 feet and then from as far away as 10 feet
6. Catches the ball, first, with arms and body, then just with the arms, and eventually just with the hands
7. Uses gradually reduced sizes of balls
8. Catches objects with either hand

Catching skills

The child:
1. Plays catch
2. Catches different types of objects, such as beanbags, Hula-Hoops, fluff balls, baseballs, and footballs
3. Catches an object with a baseball glove or in a container such as a tin can, basket, or bag

Kicking activities. Kicking or striking of an object with a foot emerges after the child is able to run.

Lead-up skills

The child:
1. Pushes or nudges a stationary large playground ball
2. Kicks a stationary ball with either foot
3. Kicks a stationary ball backward with inside, outside, and then bottom of foot
4. Kicks a stationary ball to a target
5. Kicks a stationary ball and makes it airborne
6. While standing, kicks a rolled ball
7. While walking, kicks a rolled ball
8. While running, kicks a rolled ball

Kicking skills

The child:
1. Plays kickball
2. Plays games like soccer
3. Kicks a soccer ball as it drops from his or her hand
4. Kicks a football

Striking activities

Lead-up skills. The sequences described are designed to lead to such activities as handball, tennis, golf, and baseball.

The child:
1. While sitting on the floor, hits a balloon with each hand, usually in an overhand movement
2. While kneeling, hits a balloon in front of the body, at the side of the body, and overhead
3. While standing, hits a balloon with a table tennis paddle or with a rolled-up newspaper
4. With a table tennis paddle, hits a balloon in an overhand manner, with the same motion as in an overhand throw
5. With a table tennis paddle, hits a balloon from a side position
6. Holding a light plastic bat with both hands, hits a balloon
7. Holding a plastic bat with a correct batting grip, hits a large playground ball off a batting tee
8. Bats a variety of airborne balls, such as fluff balls, tennis balls, 6-inch playground balls, softballs, and baseballs
9. Using a plastic bat, hits a variety of objects on the ground
10. Using a variety of implements, such as sticks, golf clubs, croquet mallets, and hockey sticks, hits a ball from the ground

Striking skills

The child:
1. Bats off a tee for accuracy
2. Bats off a tee for distance
3. Plays base games

Table 8-1. Correcting common throwing problems

Problems	Probable causes	Possible corrections
1. Lack of force or distance	a. Releases object at wrong time b. Fails to follow through c. Fails to shift weight forward as object is released	a. Practice throwing at a target while seated in a chair. b. Practice pointing the hand directly at the target following the throw. c. Practice throwing while standing down an incline.
2. Poor accuracy	a. Does not fix attention on target b. Releases object at wrong time c. Grasps object improperly d. Cannot project object because size and/or weight is incorrect	a. Practice saying "hit" the exact moment the object reaches the target. b. Practice releasing object when hand is directly in line with the face. c. Practice grasping and throwing a variety of objects with the thumb and first finger. d. Practice with objects that can be easily projected.

Table 8-2. Correcting common catching problems

Problems	Probable causes	Possible corrections
1. Hands do not contact object.	a. Fears being hit by a hard or large object b. Closes eyes as object approaches c. Fails to keep eyes on object	a. Practice with soft objects, such as cloth, rope, or paper. When a ball is introduced partially deflate it. b. Practice with a soft object. Have child watch for a spot on the object. c. Practice watching the entire flight of the object from the time it leaves the hands of the thrower until it arrives at its destination.
2. Object bounces out of hands.	a. Makes hands and arms stiff on contact with object b. Does not position hands to meet the object properly	a. Practice making the hands loose on contact with an object. b. Practice first stopping a swinging ball (tether ball), using both hands together, and progress to catching a tossed object in a scoop fashion, always reaching out for and bringing the object to the body.

Table 8-3. Correcting common kicking problems

Problem	Probable causes	Possible corrections
1. Misses ball	a. Removes eye focus as foot contacts ball	a. Practice observing a mark on the ball until foot contact is made.
	b. Tries to kick too hard	b. Stress making good foot contact and follow-through.
2. Lacks power	a. Does not complete full leg swing	a. Practice swinging leg from the hip and kicking a stationary ball.
	b. Fails to step forward with the nonkicking foot	b. Practice stepping forward with the nonkicking foot, first with a stationary ball and then with a moving ball.
	c. Fails to follow through after the kick	c. Practice having the kicking foot follow the ball after contact.
3. Is inaccurate	a. Does not keep eyes on ball	a. Practice watching foot make contact with the ball.
	b. Does not position foot to contact ball squarely	b. Practice kicking a stationary ball with the side and top of the foot and then progress to a moving ball.

Table 8-4. Correcting common striking problems

Problems	Probable causes	Possible corrections
1. Misses or contacts object poorly	a. Failure to focus on object until it has been hit	a. Practice watching a mark placed on the object to be hit.
	b. Failure to contact object squarely	b. Practice striking first from a stationary batting "T" and then striking an object suspended on a string or rope.
2. Lacks power	a. Facing incorrectly	a. Practice keeping forward shoulder aimed at the projected object.
	b. Poor weight transfer	b. Practice striking an object while the forward foot is down an incline.
	c. Poor follow-through	c. Practice pointing the striking implement in the direction of the hit.
	d. Improper contact with the object	d. Practice watching the object and striking implement meet. Practice making contact just in front of the forward foot.

4. Plays golf
5. Plays hockey
6. Plays croquet
7. Plays table tennis
8. Plays handball
9. Plays paddle ball games
10. Plays paddle tennis

• • •

Tables 8-1 to 8-4 cover ways of correcting problems in the four areas of throwing, catching, kicking, and striking.

Rhythm control

Essential to a child's success at play and in the classroom is the ability to sense a rhythm and to respond to it with synchronized movement. All movement patterns, whether they are basic, as in locomotion, or complex, as in a gymnastic routine, require the ability to respond rhythmically. The basic body management program should include progressive sequential tasks requiring the synchronization of specific body movements. Training in rhythm can occur by the use of metronomic pacing or a drum or sticks hit together. Barsch suggested a beginning cadence of 48 beats per minute.[4] The cadence can be altered by increasing the number of beats per minute or by varying the beats from slow to fast and vice versa. The child moves in time to the beat, progressing from unilateral to bilateral to cross-lateral movements. For example, the child may be asked to blink to a cadence, first one eye, then the other eye, and finally both eyes alternately, or the child can elect to engage in large muscle rhythms, such as moving the limbs, then progress to the smaller muscles of the body.

Planning and instructing

Of the three methods of instruction common to teaching—teacher-directed, individualized, and problem-solving—the area of basic body managment is best taught by the teacher-directed and individualized methods.[16]

In order for the teacher to effectively instruct body management skills, goals and/or objectives must be established that are both long term, or terminal, and short term, including a sequence of objectives leading to the terminal performance goal. For example, a terminal objective might be to learn to walk a balance beam ten steps forward and ten steps backward. The terminal objective may have to be broken down into a sequence of lesser tasks that present a hierarchy of difficulty until the major terminal objective is attained, such as walking three steps forward and three steps backward and then four steps forward and four backward, progressively until ten steps, properly performed, have been accomplished. Each instructional objective is divided into the situation in which the task will be performed, the description of the task, and the criteria within which the task will be performed.

Tasks can be made more or less difficult in two ways: by changing the conditions under which the task is performed or by changing the criteria under which the task is judged. For example, a condition might be altered by having the child successfully walk first a 10-foot line on the floor, then a 10-foot by 2-inch by 4-inch board placed directly on the floor, and finally a 10-foot by 2-inch by 4-inch beam raised 5 inches off the floor. On the other hand, the criteria might be altered by having the child successfully walk first a 5-foot beam, then an 8-foot beam, and finally a 10-foot beam. The teacher must remember that instructional objectives must represent the performance level of the child in a specific task area, the exact conditions under which each task is to be performed, and a specific standard for the completion of each task.

CLASS ACTIVITIES

1. Design an obstacle course that will develop dynamic balance and spatial awareness.

2. Observe three children using the movement observation survey in the text.
3. Take a child through a relaxation sequence.
4. Discuss the advantages and disadvantages of developing skills in throwing and catching objects other than balls.
5. Break a complex skill down into its logical component parts to be used as a sequence of tasks.
6. Plan a sequential development program using a common piece of equipment, such as a balance beam.

REFERENCES

1. Arnheim, D. D., and Sinclair, W. A.: The effect of a motor development program on selected factors in motor ability, personality, self-awareness and vision, J. Am. Correct. Ther. Assoc. **28**(6):167-171, 1974.
2. Arnheim, D. D., and Sinclair, W. A.: The clumsy child, St. Louis, 1975, The C. V. Mosby Co.
3. Ayres, A. J.: Sensory integration and learning disorders, Los Angeles, 1973, Western Psychological Services.
4. Barsch, R. H.: The perceptual motor myth: report from workshop, Whittier Area Cooperative, Special Education Program, Feb. 11, 1969.
5. Chaney, C., and Kephart, N. C.: Motoric aids to perceptual training, Columbus, Ohio, 1968, Charles E. Merrill Publishing Co.
6. Frederick, A. B.: Tension control, J. Am. Assoc. Health Phys. Educ. Rec. **38**:42-44, 78-80, 1967.
7. Glenn, H.: The unimportance of visual and auditory perception in reading, The Commentator, Pepperdine University, School of Education **1**(1):23-27, 1976.
8. Godfrey, B. B., and Kephart, N. C.: Movement patterns and motor education, New York, 1969, Appleton-Century-Crofts.
9. Humphrey, J. H.: Improving learning ability through compensatory physical education, Springfield, Ill., 1976, Charles C Thomas, Publisher.
10. Jacobson, E.: Progressive relaxation, Chicago, 1938, University of Chicago Press.
11. Jacobson, E.: Self operation control, Philadelphia, 1964, J. B. Lippincott Co.
12. Knapp, B.: Skill in sports, London, 1963, Routledge & Kegan Paul Ltd.
13. Oxendine, J. B.: Psychology of motor learning, New York, 1968, Appleton-Century-Crofts.
14. Rarick, G. L., editor: Physical activity, New York, 1973, Academic Press, Inc.
15. Rathbone, J. L.: Relaxation, Philadelphia, 1969, Lea & Febiger.
16. Sinclair, W. A.: The effect of motor skill upon specific dyslexia, Doctoral dissertation, Albuquerque, 1970, University of New Mexico.
17. Singer, R. N.: Motor learning and human performance, New York, 1968, The Macmillan Co.
18. Smith, H. M.: Implications for movement education experiences drawn from perceptual motor research, J. Am. Assoc. Health Phys. Educ. Rec. **41**:30-33, 1970.
19. Valett, R. E.: The remediation of learning disabilities, Belmont, Calif., 1967, Fearon Publishers, Inc.

RECOMMENDED READINGS

Bateman, B. D.: Temporal learning, San Rafael, Calif., 1968, Dimensions Publishing Co.
O'Donnell, P. A.: Motor and haptic learning, San Rafael, Calif., 1969, Dimensions Publishing Co.

9

Movement education: a challenge to process and qualities

Movement education has grown into a highly viable and well-accepted way to approach the teaching of physical education. Stressing individualized and creative movement, it de-emphasizes the highly structured and formalized physical education environment. Broadly conceived, movement education encompasses many of the ideas that are current innovations of contemporary education. Three of these concepts that can be directly related to movement education are the decreased importance given to grade level, the importance of individualized teaching, and the growing emphasis placed on prescriptive teaching.

Rudolf von Laban, born in Bratislava (now in Austria), was the originator of the basic precepts of movement education. Laban's major interests were in activities associated with the theater, such as stagecraft, drama, and, most particularly, dance. In his early career, Laban became deeply interested in the creation of a dance form other than the popular classical ballet.[12] Increasingly, Laban's interest expanded to encompass almost the entire spectrum of human behavior, with special focus on architecture, mathematics, and psychology. He was a successful choreographer and teacher of dance in Germany until 1935, when the Nazi government sent him to Staffelberg as an undesirable citizen. While he was in Staffelberg, Laban's inquisitive mind began to center on how children discovered

and adjusted to the concept of space. This interest continued to grow even after he moved to England in 1938. During the World War II years in England, Laban actively engaged in both the arts and in industry. More concerned with the qualitative aspects of movement than with the quantitative aspects, he centered the major thrust of his energies on dance as an educational medium. Known in the beginning as movement exploration, Laban's educational dance later acquired its current name of movement education.

Rudolf von Laban's philosophy set forth that a person gains knowledge of the world and himself or herself through the act of moving. He considered that movement reflects the natural harmony in life and that there is a distinct relationship between all things in life. He considered that movement provided human beings with a closer contact with the creative forces inherent throughout the universe.[12] In general, Laban was vitally concerned with personal discoveries that are made by an individual while he or she is moving, how the person moves, and the qualities that are communicated by the movement.

A NEW DIMENSION IN PHYSICAL EDUCATION

The increasing popularity of movement education in the western world reflects the struggle of persons against the

191

shackles of externally imposed conformity. It expresses modern Western society's desire to be free of the many forces that dehumanize and relegate a person to predictable behavior. It also reflects the existential philosophy, which puts forth the proposition that people should "do their own thing," and the humanistic philosophy, which emphasizes the importance of the individual as compared to the group. It also represents many Americans' growing disenchantment with organized sport, which so often perpetuates the myth that winning is everything.[13]

Physical education, throughout history, has mirrored the nationalistic requirements of the country in which it was practiced. Traditionally, for example, American physical education has been taught mainly by the command method, in which the teacher is the director, demonstrator of the skill, and evaluator of the performance. Movement education, on the other hand, gradually shifts the roles of teacher and student. The teacher, using indirect methods, serves as a guide and stimulator, allowing children to make many, but not all, of their own movement decisions. Movement education's primarily indirect style is designed to foster a sense of creativity within the child, at the same time allowing for a keen awareness of the body's potential for movement and the development of a positive acceptance of self.

MOVEMENT EDUCATION TODAY

Increasingly schools are becoming more concerned with teaching children at their own particular levels in a given subject area than with emphasizing grade and age levels. Currently there is less importance being placed on marks and more on personal achievement, self-analysis, and self-evaluation. Through analysis and evaluation, the teacher and student can mutually arrive at educational goals that are appropriate for a student's personal progress. Movement education attempts to provide the child with the best conditions for individual growth. As a result, the highly structured, ordered setting of traditional physical education is being replaced by a method that is planned to be more spontaneous and self-motivating. Ideally the child who is fortunate enough to be in a good movement education program will be given the opportunity to develop to his or her full physical potential in a less inhibited atmosphere, promoting creative and inventive experiences.

INSTRUCTIONAL FOUNDATIONS

Stanley writes that "the study of principles which govern the purposeful control of living movement and the acquisition of skill in exerting that control, together with the self-understanding which attends such learning, is the purpose of movement education."[11] In other words, movement education is a means by which children learn about their bodies in all of their great variety and potential. Through experiencing rhythm and the contrast of being restricted or free and active or quiet, the child gains a sense of being unique and an individual.[10]

The framework of movement education is comprised of four basic components: the tool of movement (the body), where the body is moved (the space), how the body is moved (the quality of effort), and with whom or what the body is moved (the relationship between persons or objects) (Fig. 9-1).

The tool of movement

The body is a tool with which movement is carried out. Movement education separates the gaining of body awareness into four subareas: the body as an instrument, the body as a weight bearer, the body as an activator, and the body as a shaper.

The body as an instrument. It is important to view the body as an instrument

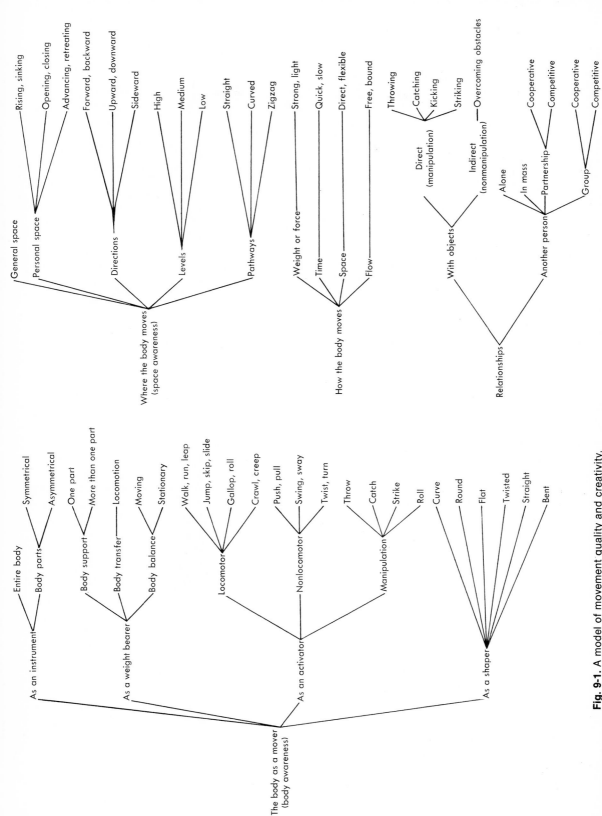

Fig. 9-1. A model of movement quality and creativity.

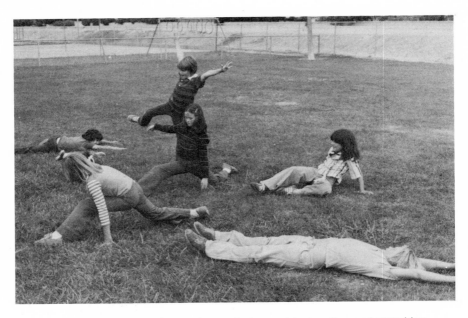

Fig. 9-2. The body can be used as an instrument by bending and stretching.

of movement much like an instrument on which one would play music. Movement education is concerned with the awareness of each body part and its relationship to a particular movement pattern. The body in its entirety, as well as its parts, can bend, curl, stretch, or twist (Fig. 9-2). The mover should become aware of those parts that can produce a turn, come closer together, or move farther apart, whether each part leads an action or follows the action or is moved symmetrically or asymmetrically.

The child moves in a symmetrical manner when the entire body or its many parts are moved proportionally on each side of the body, whereas the body moves asymmetrically when the parts are unequally moved. For example, the movement is considered symmetrical when the arms move simultaneously out to the side or to the front of the body, but if one arm moves in a different direction than the other, the movement is asymmetrical. It is obviously more difficult to move the legs symmetrically than the arms, especially if they are bearing the weight of the body. A standing long jump is a good

example of both arms and legs moving in a symmetrical manner. In general, asymmetrical movement patterns are associated with greater movement possibilities but usually offer much less stability. The transport activities of walking and running, using cross pattern movements of the arms and legs, are asymmetrical.

The body as a weight bearer. A child's awareness of the body as a weight bearer is essential before there can be efficient movement. Generally speaking, weight refers to the heaviness of an object and the amount of resistance that may be required to overcome it. Before a child can understand the concept of body weight and its effect on moving, he or she must experiment with the center of gravity, how body weight can be distributed in different ways, and the concept of balance or equilibrium as it relates to body weight. Each child should be made aware of the body's center of gravity by performing movements in low, medium, and high positions (Fig. 9-3). The child might execute movements while fully reclining, on all fours, kneeling, or standing flat-footed or on tiptoe. Each child explores

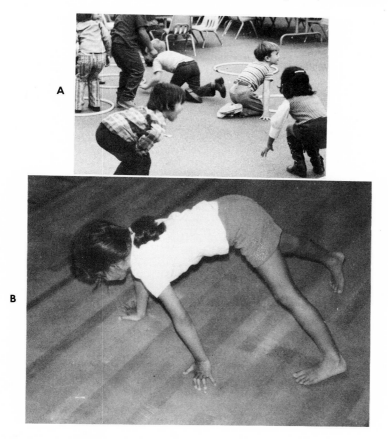

Fig. 9-3. The body is a weight bearer, with the center of gravity changing when in different positions.

his or her equilibrium by altering the center of gravity while performing various activities of locomotion on a piece of apparatus, such as a balance beam or overhead ladder. The child should test the losing and regaining of balance while exploring a variety of static and dynamic positions. Rapid changes of body position should be explored, such as moving from lying on the back to standing and moving from standing to a four-point position. The logical outcome of exploration of body weight balance change is progression from transporting the body or maintaining a stationary position to gradual involvement in simple stunts and later in highly skilled gymnastic routines.

Movement education is concerned with children experiencing three important aspects of weight bearing: the body that supports weight, the body that transfers weight, and the body that balances its weight. The child learns to become aware of the body's ability to support weight by experiencing support on different parts of the body; for example, weight may be borne on one foot, just on the seat, or on an elbow and one knee. Weight transference takes place when support shifts from one body part to another. The entire human transport system, including such movements as rolling, crawling, creeping, walking, climbing, and swinging, is operated by transferring the body weight from one part to another.

Balance is defined as the ability to maintain equilibrium while performing some transport activity or while the body is maintained in a stationary posture. One should note that the force of gravity is

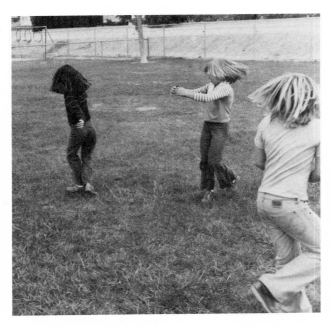

Fig. 9-4. The body is an activator; it can spin slow or very fast.

always acting on the human body, attempting to force it to the center of the earth. Gravity exerts its force vertically, and on the standing person it is directed mainly at some point in the hip region, which is known as the center of gravity.

Balancing body weight has essentially two categories: dynamic and static. Dynamic balance is a series of gaining and losing one's balance, while static or stationary balance requires the center of gravity to be directly over its base of support. Walking a balance beam or leaping over an obstacle is an example of weight transference and dynamic balance. Sitting, standing, and performing headstands are movements in which body weight is not transferred but maintained in a stationary or static balance position.

The body as an activator. Body actions may be generally separated into curls, stretches, and twists. Actions can move the body over a terrain, such as in stepping, sliding, rolling or jumping, or they can propel the body upward to be suspended for a brief moment in the air, such as in a leap in dance or a jump on a trampoline. The body may be turned quickly, slowly, partially, or completely, as in a spin (Fig. 9-4). Body actions may express gestures common to body language. Thorton[12] explains that gestures that are conducted by the arms and legs can be organized into the actions of scooping, surrounding, or scattering. The lack or absence of movement is also considered an element of the body as an activator because the state of being quiet can express a mood or accentuate a movement that has happened or is about to happen.

The body as a shaper. A human being potentially has the greatest diversity of movement of any creature on the earth. The body can assume innumerable shapes to express moods or feelings or to deal with space in a special way. For example, the body can be made into curves, rounded like a ball, flattened like a wall, elongated like a spear, twisted like a corkscrew, or widened like a doorway (Fig. 9-5). Children should be encouraged to explore the many different body shapes they can perform.

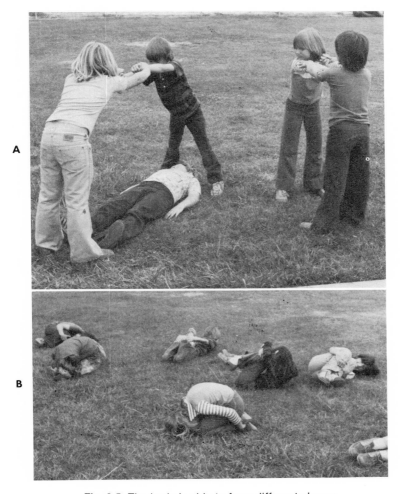

Fig. 9-5. The body is able to form different shapes.

Where the body is moved

Where the body is moved is called space, and the sensation that comes from the feeling of being in and a part of space is called spatial awareness. Space may be further defined as that expanse or receptacle in which all things are contained.[2] Space extends in all directions, having the three dimensions of height, width, and depth. From the basic premise in movement education, space may be described in two ways: general and personal. Personal space is the establishment of the body's own position orientation, while general space uses a means of orientation from outside the body. In other words, personal space is immediate to the body, while general space cannot be experienced without physically moving the body about the terrain (Fig. 9-6). In their personal space, children should experiment with contrasting movements of rising and sinking, opening and closing, and advancing and retreating.

The concept of levels should also be tested. As was mentioned in discussion of the body as a weight bearer, the child should experience the body in low, medium, and high levels. While experiencing these different levels, children should become aware of the differences in body stability that each presents. Each

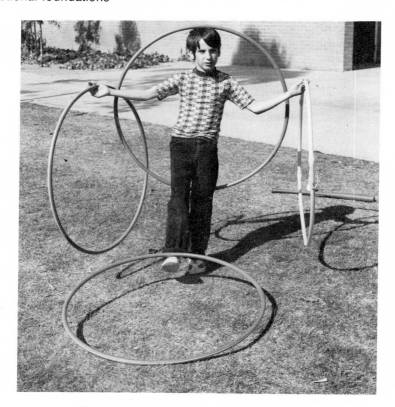

Fig. 9-6. Solving a problem in personal space.

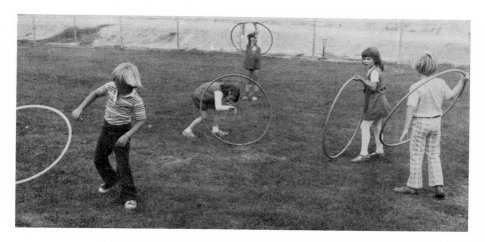

Fig. 9-7. Exploring general space with a Hula-Hoop.

child should be challenged to perform as many different movements as possible in each level, in both personal and general space.

Space awareness and self-image. The physical aspect of the self-concept, or how one views oneself, is awareness, or body image. It is more accurately defined by personality theorists as the perceptions, attitudes, and values that a person holds of himself or herself.[3] Body image is the assessment of the body from a spatial point of view. It may be described as the ability to answer the question, "Who am I?"[3] It is the total of all external and internal impressions made on the individual about his or her body.

From the time of conception, the human organism is structuring a personal system of space awareness. The physical image is dependent on innumerable factors that produce the uniqueness of the individual. One can speculate that maturation of space awareness occurs as a continuum, unfolding from birth to death. All the senses interplay in an intricate concert to form the awareness of the body in its spatial environment. As in the other factors of motor development, the awareness of the body matures from head to foot and from midline outward.

While exploring space, children should be challenged to experience varying pathways that can be made on the floor and in the air. While moving in general space, each child should solve movement problems involving straight lines, curved lines, zigzag lines, or lines forming letters or numbers that they are challenged to create (Fig. 9-7). Besides using the body as a whole to form patterns, the child can use the hands and arms to form patterns in the air.

How the body is moved

The effort qualities in human movement are given the descriptive elements of weight, time, space, and flow. These elements singularly or in combination are used to describe how the body moves.

Element	Quality range
Weight	Strong, vigorous, or heavy to weak, light, or weightless
Time	Quick, explosive, or short to slow, continuous, or sustained
Space	Directed or straight to flexible or wavy
Flow	Free or fluid to bound, restrained, or broken

Weight. Weight is a quality of effort that is constantly managed by persons either by dealing with their bodies as entities in themselves or by managing objects (Fig. 9-8). Children should become aware of the muscular exertion and tension required in all movements, especially in the contrasting of strong and vigorous actions with light, weightless movements.

Time. The awareness of time and its many ramifications is a necessary requirement for all children. Time, or temporal awareness, has been defined as the "experience of duration,"[4] or the factor of "whenness."[3] A more precise definition is that it is "the system of those relations which any event has to any other as past, present, or future; indefinite continuous duration regarded as that in which events succeed from one to another."[1] Whatever definition one accepts, awareness of time is essential in coping with a series of temporal changes occurring within a specific act. This is true in both complex, specific motor skills and in more basic fundamental skills, such as those involved with locomotion. Time is movement between two points in space.[3] Rhythm is a tempo, a uniform recurrence of beat, or measured movement. Time, space, and rhythm are inseparable. A child's concept of time develops from a primitive subjective state to an outwardly objective universal state in adulthood.

Time may be divided into four domains: physiological, physical, milieu, and cognitive. Physiological time consists of the varied periods of internal bodily processes such as heartbeat, respiration, sleep, and wakefulness. Physical time is night and day; clock time of seconds, minutes, and hours; calendar time of days, weeks, months, years, and seasons; and historical time of eras, eons, and ages. Physical time also refers to spatial estimates of distance and the concepts of here, far, there, now, then, fast, and slow. Milieu time refers to life periods of events such as infancy, early childhood, childhood, late childhood, adolescence,

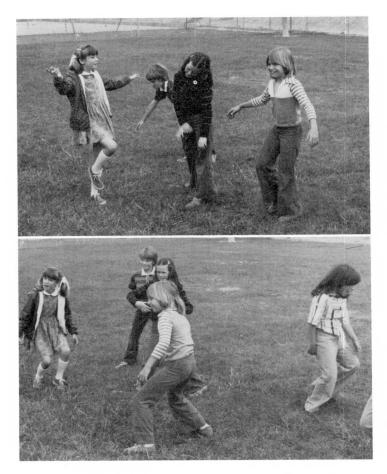

Fig. 9-8. Making the body light and heavy—an effort quality.

adulthood, and old age. Within each period are characteristic events, such as speaking the first word, walking, going to school, driving the car, going steady, marrying, or having the first child. Cognitive time is the most complex of the four domains, involving the duration required for the perceptual process to take place and consisting of reaction time, recognition time, and memory.[3]

The acquisition of time concepts is progressive, sequential, and ongoing and is completed when a person is about 16 years of age. The time schema (Table 9-1) illustrates some of the temporal skills and relationships acquired by adulthood.

Time and movement. In order for a child to move efficiently and in a coor-dinated manner, there must be an accurate awareness of time. Temporal relationships and space have a common bond. Coordinated movement requires an ability to judge the extent of neuromuscular system activation and to perceive time and distance factors associated with objects in space. Distance is a concept perceived as duration over time. If children lack accurate awareness of time, they may not have the ability to organize events or perceive subtle differences in speed. Inability to sustain a movement sequence will result in faulty motor performance.

Rhythm and time. The major portion of the information on rhythm currently known has originated from the fields of

Table 9-1. Time schema

Time concepts	Illustrative activities		
	Past	Present	Future
Objective time			
1. Terminology, definite	Yesterday, 1921, 10 years ago.	Noon, winter, to-day, this month.	Day after tomorrow, next Friday.
2. Terminology, indefinite	Many years ago when daddy was little.	Right now.	After a while, in a minute.
3. Spatial representation of time (measurement)	Time lines, calendars.	Clocks, calendars.	Calendar, time lines.
a. Fixed, equal	1 inch = 1,000 seconds, hours, or years.	Space between clock numerals = 5 minutes or 1 hour.	Same as past and present, except perhaps in science fiction.
b. Quantitative relationships	1 inch = 1 day; 7 inches = 1 week.	24 hours = 1 day.	
4. Relationships within eras	Which was invented first? What was happening in China in 1776?	What time is it in London?	Explain the twin problem in space travel.
5. Relationships among eras	Discuss speed of transportation in 1810-1820 compared to 2010-2020.	Relativity.	What can we do to prepare people for more leisure time in 1980?
Perception of time			
6. Estimation of duration	How long did it take to build a pyramid? How long is a second?	How fast did he run the 100-yard dash?	How long would it take to walk around the block?
7. Rhythm and sequence	Were those two rhythms the same or different? Digit repetition.	Dance to this beat. Reading, spelling.	Complete a rhythmic sequence.
Subjective time			
8. Awareness, control, and use of time	Recognition of apparent variations in lengths of elapsed time; e.g., each year seems shorter than the year before. Explain "Don't cry over spilled milk."	Punctuality.	Estimating and allotting time for completion of task. Long-term planning and goals.

From Bateman, B. D.: Temporal learning, San Rafael, Calif., 1968, Dimensions Publishing Co.

psychology, physiology, physical education, and art. Time does not exclusively involve rhythm, but rhythm must involve time for its orderly application. Rhythm may be described as that label given by humans to those experiences resulting from the mind's effort to make sense out of the space-time-force phenomenon.[8] In essence, all human beings are rhythmical organisms. Every cell, organ, and organ system functions in a rhythmical pattern. Rhythm may be defined as the controlling of force or the measure of energy that gives form to movement.[7] The four aspects of rhythm can be designated as cosmic, biological, performance, and perceived.[3] Cosmic rhythm refers to rhythm of the universe and nature, such as earth rotation, seasons, and day or night. Biological rhythm involves the physiological patterns functioning within each person, such as heartbeat, respiration, and digestion. Performance rhythm refers to those patterns of movement characteristic of each individual. Perceived rhythm consists of the awareness of cadences and ordered patterns that are both external (from the environment) and internal (from within the body).[3]

Rhythm is a necessary factor in the maintaining of growth and fine motor movements. In essence, efficiency in all motor responses implies a regular, patterned sequencing of muscular contractions (Fig. 9-9). Rhythmical movement also suggests a certain quality of motion. A person moving rhythmically is able to easily and gracefully cope with the internal and external variables of space, time, and force. The rhythmic child is able to move smoothly and with regularity equally well in small and in large spaces, to move fast or slow, to engage in short or sustained movement patterns, and to move lightly or heavily.

Space. Space is an effort quality that is direct and straight or flexible or wavy. For example, the child may utilize space by moving only in a straight line, such as in threading a needle or walking heel-toe along a line, or by moving in wavy patterns, taking in all of the available space in a room.

Flow. Flow may be described as the act of moving continuously and smoothly. Free flowing movement is on-going and uninhibited; bound movement is restrained and inhibited and without continuity. Continuity of movement refers to changes in speed, direction, and pattern.

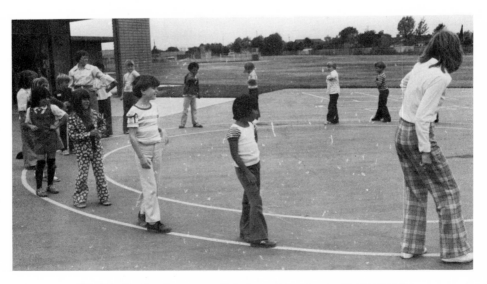

Fig. 9-9. Rhythm is an essential element in movement education.

A complex skill contains the elements of rhythm, order, and direction. A movement pattern that flows is one in which the body part moves without interruption. Discrimination of movement continuity or flow from discontinuous movement develops when the child is able to apply the concepts of slow versus fast, rhythmical versus arrhythmical, controlled versus uncontrolled, straight versus angular, angular versus zigzag, and abruptly stopping versus following through. In essence, "flow is the effort quality element which binds together a variety of actions so smoothly that the separate phases of preparation for action, and recovery from action, are indistinguish-

able from each other."[6] To acquire this quality children must learn to smoothly lead one movement into another and then, in contrast, perform a bound movement in a slow, restrained manner.

Combining effort qualities. Laban has combined the effort qualities of weight, time, space, and flow into effort actions that he calls thrust, press, slash, dab, float, flick, glide, and wring. These are defined as:

1. *Thrusting action* consists of a sudden hitting or pushing force that requires great vigor, suddenness, and directness, such as in punching a heavy boxing bag.
2. *Pressing action* is a steady force that

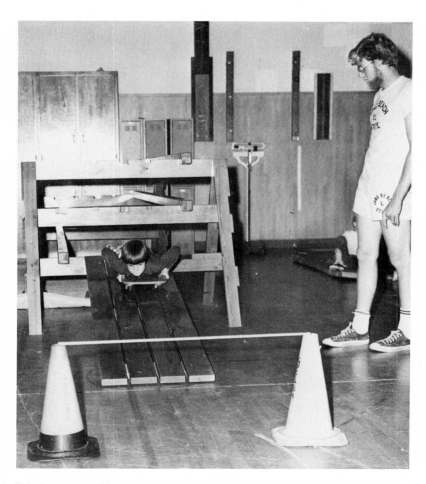

Fig. 9-10. Relating to an object means adapting one's self to that object rather than vice versa.

has strength and is sustained and direct, such as in pushing a heavy table.

3. *Slashing action* is related to a thrust, but instead of being direct, it is flexible, such as in sword fighting.

4. *Dabbing action* is an effort action of a series of taps or pats requiring the qualities of lightness, quickness, and directness.

5. *Floating action* refers to a gentle weightlesslike movement that is light, sustained, and flexible, such as in gliding in an airplane.

6. *Flicking action* requires light, quick, and flexible effort actions combined to create a movement like that of flipping an insect from one's clothing.

7. *Gliding action* is sweeping or sliding smoothly over a slick surface and displaying the qualities of weightlessness, continuity, and directness, such as in ice skating.

8. *Wringing action* refers to twisting and is vigorous, sustained, and flexible, such as in squeezing water from wet clothes.

With whom or what the body is moved

Children's movements are often related to objects in the environment or to other persons. Object relationships are direct or indirect. Direct object usage may be concerned with handling projectiles, such as in throwing, catching, kicking, or striking. In indirect object control the child adapts his or her body movements to the object rather than vice versa (Fig. 9-10). This is especially apparent when the child is performing on large apparatus such as the balance beam, rope, climbing bar, or ladder. It is important that children become aware of how they personally relate to objects and, conversely, how objects relate to them. Ways of controlling specific objects should be tested as well as the various qualities of

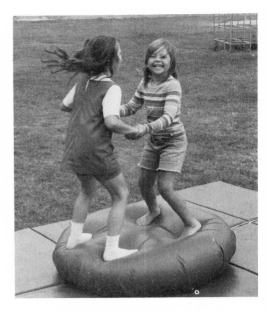

Fig. 9-11. Partner relationships can be cooperative or competitive.

each object, such as weight, size, shape, and texture, and the number of ways the objects can be used.

An important experience for the child is to move along without any association with another person. To do so the child must be totally by himself or herself. The child should then contrast this experience by moving alone but as part of a group and contrast that by moving in relationship to a partner. Moving alone in general space without the presence of another person means that the mover must relate only to himself or herself. Moving alone in a group, however, means that the mover will have some interrelationship with others even if only glances. Partner relationship requires cooperation or competition between two or more individuals (Fig. 9-11). A cooperative partnership implies that participants move together toward a common end, such as lifting a heavy load, pulling a rope, or executing a rhythmical pattern in dance. Competition, however, is a relationship that pits the movement of a person or persons against others with defeat of the opposing person or persons as the goal.

ESTABLISHING A MOVEMENT EDUCATION CURRICULUM

Although movement education stresses individuality rather than group conformity and stereotyped behavior, it still requires personal discipline on the part of the performer. Movement education seeks to give the child a sense of the joy of movement for movement's sake instead of teaching isolated skills that, according to the serious proponents of movement education, only serve to restrict the child to a prescribed set of rules and regulations.[5] In essence, movement education stresses how a mover moves rather than to what end he or she moves. In other words the process and quality of the movement become more important than the outcome of the movement.

The curriculum of movement education should offer children experiences that develop their awareness of the physical laws governing all human movement and especially that help them in gaining awareness of the wide range of movements available to them and, conversely, of the movement restrictions that are imposed by body structure and the forces of nature. The curriculum should also provide opportunities for gaining awareness of the basic elements of movement quality, such as weight or force, flow, and space and the interrelationship of these elements that is inherent in efficient movement. Every effort should be put forth to provide the child with experiences with a variety of small and large apparatus.

Movement education can be an important extension of the classroom; for example, animal actions can be portrayed, drawings can be acted out in some expressive movement, emotions can be expressed, famous personalities can be portrayed, and history lessons can be put into

the form of creative dance using the basic principles of movement education.

TEACHING IN MOVEMENT EDUCATION

As stated earlier, in contrast to the direct and structured method of teaching so common to traditional physical education, the teacher of movement education is a guider and initiator, encouraging self-direction by the child. In movement education the teacher or a designated child selects a movement challenge and asks a movement question but avoids indicating how the movement is to be performed and offers an assessment by recognizing the child's response in a complimentary manner.

Using a movement education vocabulary

A movement education vocabulary uses two expressions to describe curricular guidelines: the movement *theme* and the movement *phrase* or *sentence*.

A movement theme refers to an instructional unit in which there is a central idea that can be carried out in a specified number of lessons; for example, the general theme of body awareness might include lessons that challenge the child to move in different directions, to move at different levels, to move in the air, or to move in different patterns. Themes should be developed according to a hierarchy of difficulty with progress from the simple to the more complex. In each theme the child is allowed to freely explore, self-test, and refine skills based on his or her individual needs and abilities.

Once a movement theme has been decided upon, as well as the lessons that come under each theme, the teacher should make up movement challenges in the form of phrases or sentences, sequences of two or more words representing a meaningful unit.

The teacher then challenges the child

Movement Education Lesson Plan (Sample)

Unit: *II - Where the body moves*   Date: *Oct. 23*
Theme: *Moving in personal and general space*
Equipment and space needed: *hula hoop for each child, gymnasium, whistle*
Concept: *limitation of personal space as compared to general space*
Safety considerations: *avoid running into another child*
Preparatory activities (time *5 min.*): *have children perform as many*
movements as possible in personal and general space

Free Floor Activities (time *10 min*)

1. Major challenge: *Without touching another child, move across floor.*
   a. sub challenge: *Now, move in a different direction.*
   b. sub challenge: *Move quickly across the floor.*
   c. sub challenge: *Move slowly across the floor.*

2. Major challenge: *How close can you get to another person without touching*
   a. sub challenge: *While close together, move in a circle - don't touch.*
   b. sub challenge: *Move in a circle as fast as possible - don't touch.*
   c. sub challenge: *When you hear the whistle - change directions.*

3. Major challenge: *Show me another way to move in general space.*
   a. sub challenge: *Move that way with another child.*
   b. sub challenge: *Move quickly in that new way.*
   c. sub challenge: *Move slowly in that new way.*

Apparatus Activities (time *10 min*)

1. Major challenge: *Without touching the sides, put your body inside the hoop.*
   a. sub challenge: *Put two body parts in and two outside the hoop.*
   b. sub challenge: *Can you put different parts outside the hoop?*
   c. sub challenge: *Can you put different parts inside the hoop?*

2. Major challenge: *What different low level movements can you do inside the hoop?*
   a. sub challenge: *Can you do a low level movement while balancing on one foot?*
   b. sub challenge: *Can you do a low level movement while balancing on one foot and a hand?*
   c. sub challenge: *Can you do another low level movement while balancing on one foot?*

3. Major challenge: *How far outside the hoop can you reach with your hand?*
   a. sub challenge: *Reach as far as you can with your foot.*
   b. sub challenge: *Reach as far as you can with your hand.*
   c. sub challenge: *Reach as far as you can with your elbow.*

Suggestions for future lessons: *Moving in different*
pathways.

Fig. 9-12. A movement education lesson plan.

with a movement problem to solve. Instruction is provided by the teacher in the form of concise and clearly stated problems. The teacher allows the child to move in his or her own way without verbal guidance or cues. This allows the participant to gain insights while building movement patterns, one after another, that will eventually form a skill.

Problems can be presented to the child by a verbal phrase, by an auditory signal such as a whistle or bell, or by visual signals such as flash cards. Usually verbal challenges elicit the best response from the child. Challenges that start with words such as "can you," "how can you," "what can you," "show me," "show a," "how," and "be" provide the child with clear directions. Some examples are as follows: *Can you* find a better way to climb up the ladder? *How can you* move along the balance beam using both your arms and legs? *What can you* do to move faster over the hurdle? *Show me* how many ways you can move across the floor. *How* far can you jump backwards? *Be* as many different animals as you can.

Planning the movement education lesson plan

Each lesson should be planned before it is given; however, it should be unstructured enough to allow for easy change if the needs of the children or a certain situation call for an alteration (Fig. 9-12). The teacher should always remember that the child should feel the joy of moving and engaging in self-discovery. Each plan should include the unit, the theme, needed equipment and space, safety considerations, warm-up activities, challenges that are conducted as free floor activities, and challenges that utilize small- or large-apparatus activities.

The unit should represent one of the four curricular areas, such as effort qualities or becoming aware of relationships. The theme usually is a general idea under the unit that expresses the fact that the

problem solving will be confined to a certain area, such as becoming aware of weight or becoming aware of moving alone in a group. The equipment and space needs must be indicated on the lesson plan. It is highly desirable that each child have his or her own mat and piece of equipment in order that there be no waiting for turns or standing in line. Safety factors must always be considered in every activity. Although the movement education approach is extremely safe, activities requiring great speed or the use of large apparatus must be considered capable of producing injury. Every theme should be preceded by warm-up activities that physiologically prepare the child for movement, such as by increasing circulation, and that also motivate the child to do his or her best. Each lesson should provide activity challenges both in free floor space, in which the child solves problems in both personal and general space, and on small and large apparatus.

Challenges are divided into major challenges and subchallenges. A major challenge expresses a problem to the child that reflects the basic theme, while subchallenges establish additional problems that have stemmed from the major challenge; for example, under the unit on relationships a major challenge might be "In the space indicated, how fast can you move without touching anyone?" A subchallenge to this might be "Move as fast as you can and move in a different direction without touching anyone."

MOVEMENT EDUCATION WITH OTHER APPROACHES

Movement education is an approach in physical education that may be used by itself or in conjunction with other approaches. Some teachers prefer to interchange methods depending on the types of activities that are to be experienced; for example, movement education may be chosen for the teaching of basic movement activities, creative dance, or elementary gymnastics, but the traditional direct skills approach might be the teacher's choice for games, sports, folk dances, perceptual-motor training, or physical fitness activities. Some teachers prefer to introduce the basic skills needed for a certain activity through the movement problem approach and, from this base, gradually structure the teaching when rules, regulations, and specific skills are required. Within a single lesson, a teacher might elect to use several methods, depending on the emotional maturity and skill level of the students. Children with very poor self-control often will be unable to benefit from a program using nondirected movement education and must be restricted to the more structured approach until such time as they can tolerate more freedom. Although movement education can be an effective approach to learning sports, dance, and gymnastics, we prefer it as a major approach for the developmentally younger child.

The following are some samples of movement education challenges:

The tool of movement

1. Stand with your front toward me.
2. Show me your right arm.
3. Show me the top of your head.
4. Touch your elbows.
5. Move your elbows.
6. Show me a different way to move your arms.
7. Make yourself into a ball.
8. Make yourself into a square.
9. Make yourself into a corkscrew.
10. How many ways can you make a triangle?
11. Can you make yourself look like a table?
12. Can you make yourself look like an elephant?
13. Can you go away from "home" and return on a signal?
14. Can you go away from "home" and return using another movement?
15. Cross the room by taking as many steps as possible.
16. Move across the room; then move in a different direction when the whistle blows.
17. Can you balance on one leg?
18. Balance on another part of your body.
19. Can you move while you are balancing?
20. Pick your own "home" space anywhere on the floor. Pick out another spot, move to it, do a stunt or make a statue shape, and then return to your "home" spot.
21. Go away from "home," trace a figure-of-eight on the floor, and return to "home."
22. Move so that one foot is always off the ground.
23. Run, leap, and roll; then run, collapse, and roll.
24. Twist and lift your body, twist and smile, and then lift your arms and grin.
25. Hop, turn around, and then shake.
26. Reach, jump high, and sit down; then reach and twist.
27. Curl, roll, and jump; then twirl and make a statue.

Where the body is moved

1. Change direction and the way you move when I clap my hands.
2. How low can you make yourself?
3. Can you get any lower?
4. How high can you get?
5. Raise your body from a low level to a high one.
6. Raise only one part of your body.
7. Raise it another way.
8. Raise one part of your body, and let another part fall.
9. Walk tall.
10. Find a space and sit down.
11. How far can you reach without touching your neighbor?
12. How little space can you take up?

13. How much space can you take up?
14. Walk in one direction around the circle.
15. Slowly go to another spot without touching anyone.
16. Quickly go to another spot without touching anyone.
17. Move around the room using another movement and not touching anyone.
18. Move in another direction.
19. Move in every direction you can think of.
20. Move from the sides of the room to the center and back.
21. Run, change directions, and then collapse.

How the body is moved

1. Walk very softly.
2. Show me a different way to move softly.
3. Make your feet heavy.
4. Show me how strong your hands can be.
5. How strong can your body be?
6. Show me another way to have a strong body.
7. How fast can you make your body go while staying in one place?
8. Can you swing your arms slowly?
9. Move to the right as slowly as possible.
10. How fast can you get back to "home?"
11. Make your shoulders do something fast.
12. Make them do something at a different speed.
13. Move your body smoothly.
14. Make your body quiver.
15. Jerk one part of your body.
16. Move one part of your body smoothly.
17. Show me a smooth walk.
18. Show me a smooth run.
19. Walk or run smoothly another way.
20. Move from one side of the room to the other without stopping.

With whom or what the body is moved

1. Change places with a neighbor while walking.
2. Move across the room with a partner.
3. Move together in a different way.
4. Move in a circle so that one partner goes first.
5. Can you stand up while holding hands with a partner?
6. Show me another way to stand up while touching your partner and not using your hands.
7. Can you climb in and out of your Hula-Hoop?
8. Put one part of your body in the hoop and one part outside.
9. How high can you throw the hoop?
10. How high can you throw the ring?
11. Throw the ring another way.
12. Catch the ring before it hits the ground.
13. How many different ways can you go over the bar?
14. How many different ways can you go under the chair?
15. How many different ways can you go around the ball?
16. How many different ways can you go through the hoop?
17. Balance three beanbags any way.
18. Bounce the ball as many ways as you can using one hand and then the other.
19. How many ways can you catch the ball?

CLASS ACTIVITIES

1. Teach a ball skill using the movement education approach.
2. Teach a creative dance using the movement education approach.
3. Demonstrate as many different qualities of movement as you know.
4. Teach a popular activity using the indirect movement approach; then teach the same activity using the direct-teaching approach.
5. Using a movement education lesson plan, develop a complete lesson incorporating apparatus or equipment.

REFERENCES

1. Auxter, D.: Developmental physical training for better motor functioning, experimental edition, Slippery Rock, Penn., 1969, Western Pennsylvania Special Education Regional Resource Center.
2. Barnhart, C. L., editor: The American college dictionary, New York, 1961, Random House, Inc.
3. Barsch, R. H.: Enriching perception and cognition, vol. 2, Seattle, 1968, Special Child Publishing, Inc.
4. Bateman, B. D.: Temporal learning, San Rafael, Calif., 1968, Dimensions Publishing Co.
5. Broer, M.: Efficiency in human movement, Philadelphia, 1966, W. B. Saunders Co.
6. Gilliom, B. C.: Basic movement education for children, Reading, Mass., 1970, Addison-Wesley Publishing Co., Inc.
7. H'Doubler, M. N.: Movement and rhythmic structure, Madison, Wis., 1946, Kramer Business Service.
8. Kirchner, G.: Introduction to movement education, Dubuque, Iowa, 1970, William C. Brown Co., Publishers.
9. Larson, L. A., editor: Encyclopedia of sport sciences and medicine, New York, 1971, The Macmillan Co.
10. North, M.: Movement education, New York, 1973, E. P. Dutton & Co., Inc.
11. Stanley, S.: Physical education: a movement orientation, New York, 1969, McGraw-Hill Book Co.
12. Thorton, S.: Laban's theory of movement: a new perspective, Boston, 1971, Plays, Inc.
13. Tutko, T., and Bruns, W.: Winning is everything and other American myths, New York, 1976, The Macmillan Co.

RECOMMENDED READINGS

Fait, H. F.: Physical education for the elementary school child, ed. 3, Philadelphia, 1975, W. B. Saunders Co.

Frostig, M.: Movement education theory and practice, Chicago, 1970, Follett Publishing Co.

Latchaw, M., and Egstrom, G.: Human movement, Englewood Cliffs, N.J., 1969, Prentice-Hall, Inc.

10

Physical fitness and movement efficiency

Elementary schools should be concerned with helping children to use their bodies efficiently. If children have movement efficiency, they can use space to their best advantage and control the physical forces of equilibrium, inertia, and gravity to their fullest capacity. In this chapter we will discuss the major areas of movement efficiency, physical fitness, flexibility, strength, stamina, balance and postural fitness, coordination, appraising fitness, and conducting a program of fitness, along with how physical fitness can be incorporated into all aspects of elementary physical education.

MOVEMENT EFFICIENCY

In this chapter the expression *movement efficiency* has a physiological connotation, referring to work output and the amount of energy expended. Physiologists accept the fact that the human's ability to take in and utilize oxygen through the cardiorespiratory system is currently the most valid measure of movement efficiency.

The human organism spends a lifetime building and refining a movement repertoire. Movement efficiency in childhood has a direct effect on personal health and well-being in later life. A high degree of physical fitness allows the child to fully engage in abundant play and to fully express the joy of moving (Fig. 10-1).

Efficiency in movement has been more specifically labeled as *motor fitness*, or the ability to perform a specific motor task.[9] It is one factor in the larger area commonly called *total fitness*. Total fitness includes organic health, physical abilities to meet emergencies, emotional and psychological stability, the ability to solve problems and make concrete decisions, attitudes and values that stimulate a zest for living, and finally, a moral and spiritual foundation that provides an ethical basis for behavior in our current culture.[1] *Physical fitness* is the term commonly given to the attributes of flexibil-

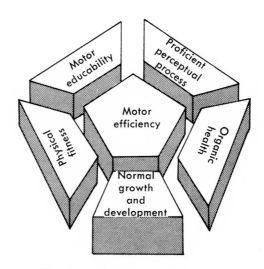

Fig. 10-1. Schema of motor efficiency.

ity, strength, muscle endurance, and cardiorespiratory endurance.

In organic health the organs and organ systems of the body are functioning properly. Also the organs have an inherent capacity to respond when stimulated by activity.

Growth and development is particularly important when imposed exercise demands exceed a child's limitations. (See Chapter 7.) Size, posture, and bone and muscle maturity play an extremely important role in how well a child performs a specific movement task.

Proficiency in the perceptual process, as discussed in Chapter 8, allows the child to interpret, store, and respond to internal and external stimuli. Without the ability to interpret or retrieve information, the child will often find many movement tasks difficult to perform.

PHYSICAL FITNESS

Physical fitness in general is that aspect of a child's physical capacity that allows for efficient motor performance and requires specific physical attributes necessary for successful performance. These attributes consist of joint flexibility; muscular strength; stamina, both muscular and cardiorespiratory; balance; and coordination.

Historical implications

Concern for motor fitness and, more specifically, physical fitness is as old as mankind. Historically it has meant the ability to survive in a hostile environment. Down through the ages strong, agile persons with great stamina and strength could more easily fend off invaders and protect themselves and their families. History has shown that a physically fit populace is in a better position to withstand the rigors of abnormal daily stress, the devastations of war, and the ravages of nature than less fit populations.

As automation increasingly provides us with opportunities for sedentary lives, the need for exercise becomes increasingly more apparent. Each year more evidence comes to light indicating that many diseases commonly affecting adults arise from lifelong inactivity. It is an accepted premise that many diseases stemming from or aggravated by obesity, hypertension, stomach ulcers, and low-back syndromes and some cardiorespiratory conditions can be prevented, or at least decreased in terms of incidence, if a lifetime regime of reasonable exercise is maintained. Our society's low physical fitness level can be overcome by helping each child to understand the need for and the enjoyment of a well-balanced daily program of vigorous physical activity. It is essential that elementary schools do everything in their power to increase the physical fitness level of each child.

Because of the amount of time that children spend watching television and the growing trend toward spectatorism, lack of physical fitness is fast becoming a problem of epidemic proportions in the United States. A positive attempt to overcome the low level of fitness of individuals in the United States came about at the result of important studies in the early 1950s, showing that American children were inferior in physical fitness to comparable European children. President Eisenhower in 1956 established a study commission on physical fitness. This commission developed the Council on Youth Fitness to promote physical fitness in Americans. To date, the council has played an important role in bringing to the citizenry important information and in stimulating interest in all activities that develop physical fitness.

Toward better academic achievement and the cognitive domain

It is generally agreed that there is no dichotomy between the body and mind. A child's total behavior is based on the interrelationship of motor, emotional, social, and intellectual factors. This holistic point of view implies that enhancement of any one factor can positively affect some factors and, conversely, can adversely affect other factors.[17] Many studies and observations have been reported that show a positive relationship between motor traits and academic achievement,[7] but there is little current evidence that intelligence and motor ability are positively correlated. However, evidence does point to the fact that children's learning potential may be enhanced or diminished by the level of their physical fitness. In other words, children who are above average in physical attributes, such as size and physical fitness, in general also have a proportionately higher level of academic achievement in comparison with children with a low level of physical fitness.

Affective domain

It is essential that the teacher help each child to develop a positive attitude toward being fit for a lifetime. One major way of accomplishing this is for the teacher to be an example of physical fitness and to display a joy and exuberance for motor activities. It is a mistake for a teacher to coerce or embarrass a child into greater feats of physical fitness. A more positive approach is to encourage each child to self-test in a given area of physical fitness and then to set personal goals based on reasonable expectations. Through positive reinforcement, the teacher should help the child to internalize the good feelings that stem from being fit, such as being able to do an activity longer or with more skill or efficiency.

Living optimally through exercise

Health factors that are positively affected by the attainment of a high level of physical fitness are mental and emotional health, growth and development, prevention of injury, physical restoration, and the aging process.

Mental and emotional health. Exercise is a desirable medium for emotional release. Pent-up emotions causing high levels of abnormal muscular tension often can be "drained off" through vigorous physical activity. Recuperative rest and sleep are promoted by the fatigue that comes from exercise, whereas mental and emotional health benefit through the self-expression that emerges from engaging in motor activities. Children gain self-confidence and positive self-concepts when they can execute well a variety of body movement skills. Good body control often parallels good emotional control.

Growth and development. Growth, development, and movement are inextricably interwoven in a child's life. Without muscular activity, the child is deprived of the stimulus necessary for him or her to reach full maturity. This fact becomes apparent when children are bedridden or confined to limited movement. The inactive child is often small or overweight in comparison to active children of the same age. An active childhood tends to increase height and produce stronger muscles, denser bony structure, and generally sturdier bodies with more normal weights.[11,18]

Prevention of injury. Injury prevention is aided by the physical fitness attributes of strength, joint flexibility, endurance, and movement skill. All these factors come into action when physical trauma is imminent. The active and well-conditioned child is able to withstand the rigors common to childhood, particularly the extreme forces that are continually being imposed on muscles and joints.[15] Exercise increases the stability of the most often injured joints, the ankle, knee, and shoulder, and a variety of vigorous activities increases the strength of both the muscles and the ligaments that support these joints.

Physical restoration. For the most part, physical restoration is the regaining of a functional level of physical conditioning after a major medical problem. After prolonged bedrest or injury to the body, a planned program of rehabilitative exercises designed to restore full motor function may be required since muscles atrophy, or decrease in size, and joints become rigid when movement ceases. Strength, flexibility, endurance, and skill development are all components necessary for physical restoration.

Aging. In all human beings aging is relative; it progresses at different rates for different individuals and also is variable in different cells, tissues, organs, and organ systems. The most outstanding factor of aging in any individual over 30 years of age is the gradual decrease in ability to return to a balance of function when the equilibrium has been disrupted. Research indicates that exercise plays a positive role in preventing or slowing down many of the deteriorations of aging. There is little question that proper physical exercise carried out during a lifetime will significantly delay many aspects of the aging process. The specific elements of strength, flexibility, and endurance that are acquired in the elementary school years and maintained at a high level throughout life ensure a longer period of physical and mental productivity.

Flexibility

Flexibility is that aspect of motor fitness that indicates the range of movement that can be initiated in a joint. Although the term *flexibility* may be misleading, it includes joint flexion as well as extension and rotation. In other words, in a broad sense, flexibility is the ability to move the body without encumbrances or restrictions. There is no single factor that enhances or detracts from body mobility; for example, any of the following conditions to name just a few may alter joint range: (1) joint disease, (2) deviations in bony arrangement, (3) inextensibility of connective and/or muscle tissue, (4) muscle viscosity, or (5) inability to reciprocally relax opposing muscles.

At birth, in most instances, the human organism has the ability to move freely without restriction. One has only to hold an infant in one's arms or view an infant at play to realize just how unrestricted the human body can really be. Research does point out, however, that flexibility diminishes as the individual becomes older; this is attributed primarily to the type of activity habitually engaged in rather than to some disease factor. Extensibility of joint tissue is specific for the type of activity performed. This simply means that flexibility is restricted or enhanced depending on the demands of the imposed activity. Children who spend many waking hours in restricted sedentary postures conform to those positions. To counteract this, a wide variety of large-muscle activities must be engaged in daily. There are two distinct types of flexibility: *extent flexibility*, the ability to flex or stretch the torso forward, backward, or sideward in a controlled manner, and *dynamic flexibility*, the ability to execute a number of quick, stretching muscular contractions.[12]

Evaluation of flexibility. The teacher must consider flexibility to be unique for each child; however, there is a range that may be considered normal.[8] Large deviations from this norm may require a remedial exercise program. For example, the Kraus-Weber[16] test for minimum muscular fitness includes a test to determine the length of the back and hamstring muscles; the child stands with feet together and knees locked and attempts to slowly touch the floor with the fingertips, holding that position for 3 seconds. Perhaps an even better means of evaluating a child's joint mobility is for the teacher to observe how supply and gracefully a child moves in a great many different large- and small-muscle activities. Can the child bend, twist, and stretch with ease, or are movements mechanical, awkward, and inefficient?

Increasing flexibility. Normally active children seldom have serious problems with flexibility. However, if a child habitually assumes restrictive postures, then special means must be used to increase the body's range of movement. The teacher must be alert to detect children who appear to be encumbered by poor flexibility, encouraging activities that lengthen the musculature to its fullest extent. In some cases, specific stretching exercises may have to be performed by the child to increase flexibility. If this is the case then the exercises should be executed in a prescribed manner—either by the controlled ballistic method or by the static, or passive, stretch method. Never should the teacher promote the uncontrolled ballistic type of exercise stretch in which the child literally bounces and hangs on unprotected joints. In the controlled ballistic, or rebound, stretch, the child is taught to concentrate on the muscles that are pulling the body into the stretch situation. For example, in stretching the hamstring muscles behind the thigh, the child concentrates on the pull of the abdominal muscles and the contraction of the quadriceps in front of the thigh.

Instead of the controlled ballistic stretch, the teacher might elect to have the child perform static, or passive, stretches, which are safer and decrease the possibility of muscle strain. In contrast to the ballistic stretch, passive stretch is slow and deliberate, with the child assuming the stretch position and gradually increasing the stretch for 30 seconds or longer. In general, ballistic stretches are repeated from six to ten times while passive stretching is seldom executed more than twice.

Strength

Strength is that factor of physical fitness that allows the child to overcome a resistance through muscular exertion. In growth and development, gain in strength parallels the general gain in weight, height, and circumference of the limbs. There is a decided increase in strength between the ages of 3 and 6 years and again in the prepubescent period for both boys and girls. Girls have their greatest strength gains between 9 and 10 years of age, whereas boys gain most between ages 10 and 12 years. However, from birth throughout life, boys are substantially stronger than girls.[11,18]

Strength elements. There are three separate strength attributes. The first attribute is *explosive strength,* or the ability to mobilize and expend a maximum amount of muscular energy in the execution of an activity requiring sudden movement. Explosive muscular strength is used in activities that employ speed and quick changes of direction, such as shuttle running, or activities in which the propelling of an object a great distance is important, such as baseball. The second attribute is *static strength,* or isometric strength, which is the ability to employ maximum muscular exertion, such as pushing, pulling, or lifting, to overcome heavy resistance. In comparison to explosive strength, little, if any, muscle shortening occurs in static strength activities. The third strength attribute is *dynamic strength,* or the ability of a muscle to exert repeated contractions over a sustained period of time. Another expression for dynamic strength is muscular endurance, which will be discussed in more detail under stamina.

Strength refers to the level at which a muscle can function in order to overcome stress imposed by a resistance. A child who is highly active and strong in comparison to his or her peer group is able to more completely use the muscle fibers.[3] This efficient use of muscle fibers comes as the result of employing more fully the neural and biochemical properties available in the body. In most cases the stronger individual has a greater mechanical advantage in the use of his or her muscles and is more able to find success in a variety of physical activities:[6] Of all the physical fitness attributes, strength must be considered most important to engaging in a wide variety of physical education activities.

Overload principle. When muscles work progressively harder, or are overloaded, the result is increased strength. There are several ways in which the teacher can help children to improve their strength levels, namely by increasing the intensity, duration, or rate of performance of the activity. The intensity of an activity can be increased by providing progressively more load or resistance to the muscles, for example, lifting progressively heavier and heavier weights. Duration, on the other hand, refers to length of time a muscle contraction can be maintained while the resistance is kept constant, such as in holding a specific weight out to the side of the body for increasingly longer periods of time. A certain degree of strength can also be attained by gradually increasing the rate or number of times a constant load can be moved within a specified time period. It should be pointed out that strength exercises requiring muscle contraction (isotonic exercise) should be performed six to ten times and repeated, after rest, two or three times for best results. In contrast to isotonic strength exercise, static or isometric exercise develops strength by contracting a muscle without moving the joint or part. Each isometric exercise should be held for between 6 and 10 seconds. *It should be noted that it may be dangerous for children to use isometric exercises extensively.* Continued maximal isometric and isotonic muscular contraction may produce a fracture caused by tendons actually tearing away from their attached site. Teachers of children must be aware that strength activities that allow movement are much more desirable than static activities and that maximal resistance is not necessary for strength to be developed.

Stamina

Stamina is the capacity to engage in a sustained physical activity without undue fatigue and with quick recovery after the performance is finished. One should note that in order to play activities for long periods of time the child must have two very important physical abilities, namely, muscle endurance and efficiency in the functions of both the heart and lungs.

Muscular endurance. Muscular endurance refers to the ability of a particular muscle or group of muscles to be repeatedly contracted over a long period of time. Generally speaking strength and muscular endurance are interrelated.[5] Strength and muscular endurance make possible a continuum from a single muscle contraction to repeated contractions. In essence, any sustained activity requires the ability to contract muscles repeatedly over a given period of time.

Cardiorespiratory endurance. The efficiency and capacity of the heart and lungs to deliver oxygen to exercising muscles determine a child's cardiovascular endurance. If children's hearts, lungs, and vascular systems are efficient, they will have the ability to engage in prolonged strenuous activities without becoming overly tired and will be able to recover quickly from muscle fatigue. For oxygen to be effectively distributed to all the body's tissues, especially the muscles, requires that energy-producing food substances be properly utilized.[4] The greater the amount of oxygen that can be assimilated during vigorous physical activity, the longer the delay of fatigue.

Physiologically, the cardiorespiratory systems of elementary school children are as competent to deliver oxygen to their muscles as those of adults of comparable fitness; therefore, vigorous activities that place high-level demands on the heart and lungs should not be excluded from the physical education curriculum.[14] In fact, we believe it is essential that more demands be placed on the cardiorespiratory system of the child. Most physical education activities should be provided with an additional factor, a *fitness factor*. For example, a low-intensity activity such as kickball could be given a fitness factor of fast base running for 2 minutes, or a slow game of one-bounce volleyball might be given a fitness factor of running the out-of-bounds lines between each game.

Children's progress in cardiorespiratory fitness can be determined in terms of lower resting pulse rates and faster recovery times. This, however, is difficult to ascertain in young children through pulse testing. The accurate taking of pulse rates has been positively demonstrated among children in the upper elementary levels but younger children find it very difficult. Progress in cardiorespiratory fitness can be subjectively determined by how quickly a child's breathing returns to normal or how vigorously an activity is engaged in for an extended period of time.

Balance and postural fitness

Balance and posture have been discussed throughout this text because they are inseparable and are an integral part of all areas of physical education. Position sense and the awareness of body alignment are essential to efficient movement and physical fitness. Posture may be defined as the relative arrangement of the various segments of the body. In good posture each body segment is well balanced in relation to other body segments. In other words, the head, trunk, pelvis, and lower limbs should be in such a relationship to one another that the least amount of strain and energy expenditure possible is created. With faulty posture, the mechanical performance of the body becomes inefficient because there are imbalances in those muscles that properly align the various body segments.

As the child matures, stationary and moving postural positions become automatic. Body alignment becomes a matter of unconscious self-regulation. Postural awareness becomes a coordination of visual cues, responses from the inner ear, and information given by tendon, joint, and muscle receptors. Misinformation or malfunction of any of these sense organs can cause faulty body alignment and result in a generally inefficient use of the body. Therefore, one must consider all aspects of physical fitness as affecting postural fitness.

Strength, with special emphasis on muscle balance, flexibility, and coordination, is essential to developing and maintaining good posture. The increase of strength on one side of the body without an equal strengthening of the opposite side can produce habitual postural distortions.

Optimum joint flexibility is also needed for good posture; however, too much flexibility without appropriate strength can be just as serious as inflexibility. As stated earlier, children are usually very flexible, becoming less so as they become older.

Postural fitness requires proper habitual use of the body. Teachers of elementary school children must be constantly on the alert for signs of faulty body alignment as well as improper body usage. It must be remembered that postural problems are best remedied when children are young and their bodies are plastic and highly moldable.

Coordination

Coordination is the ability to perform a movement skill; it is specific for the particular skill performed and must not be considered as a general trait. Many children who have good coordination and achieve success in a wide variety of activities have many individual skills. In other words, the well-coordinated child has many specific motor abilities that provide success in numerous activities. The most important motor abilities are based on the interrelation of strength, flexibility, endurance, equilibrium, speed, and agility. Children who display poor coordination may be considered physically clumsy or awkward.[2] Such children may have many subtle physical and emotional problems that make it impossible for them to play and learn activities effectively. All teachers of physical education should realize that the most unhappy people in the classroom are the children who are chosen last or who, if chosen at all, are always relegated to the least desirable positions in a game. Early recognition and remediation of the clumsy child are essential.

Using different parts of the body in an ordered sequence of movement to achieve a desired goal requires a high degree of neuromuscular coordination. Some skilled acts require predominantly eye-foot-hand coordination, such as in punting a football; other skills require mainly eye-hand coordination, such as in the precision task of hitting the ball in a center jump in basketball; and still others require eye-foot coordination, such as in kicking a soccer ball.

Coordination develops in children along maturational lines, with improvement consistent from birth to adolescence. Even during the rapid growth period of pubescence, coordination steadily improves. Very young children acquire movement experiences and coordination through exploration of the environment and through engaging in "pretending" type activities, in which the child pretends to be something or someone else. During the primary years in school, children explore all kinds of movement with special emphasis placed on the development of body management coordination. Children, having fully experienced the free and exploratory movement of the primary years, become increasingly concerned with more precise movement as they reach the middle elementary school years. Coordination in the late elementary school period centers on team competition and interacting actively and effectively in a peer group.

ASSESSING PHYSICAL FITNESS

One of the most important problems that elementary children have throughout the nation is that of poor physical fitness. Every elementary physical education program should include physical fitness testing as part of its regular program offering.

A teacher should ideally assess each student's level of physical fitness three times during a school year. The first test, which is given as early as possible in the first semester, determines the base or starting fitness level of each child; the second test, which is given 3 or 4 months after the start of the fitness program, determines whether or not the program is effective and if exercise changes should be made; and the third test, which should be given at the end of the school year, ascertains what improvements have been made. Once the teacher has determined the fitness level of each child, a program of activities can be designed and initiated.

There are many tests that purport to measure specific factors inherent in physical fitness. Many of these test batteries measure the fitness elements of strength, muscular endurance, cardiorespiratory endurance, and the primary element of agility. To represent this area of physical fitness appraisal, we have included selected test items and norms from portions of the Oregon Motor Fitness Test (Tables 10-1 and 10-2) and the American Association for Health, Physical Education, and Recreation (AAHPER) Fitness Test (Appendix B).

Physical fitness test items

FLEXED-ARM HANG (Fig. 10-2)

Factors measured: Strength and muscle endurance of hand grip and elbow flexors.

Age and sex: Boys and girls, 9 through 14 years of age.

Equipment: Adjustable horizontal bar or stall bar, stool to adjust subject to proper height, and stopwatch.

Regulations: The child grasps bar with over-

Table 10-1. Motor fitness standards, Oregon Motor Fitness Test: rating norms for boys (grades 4 to 6)

Test items	Grade	Superior	Good	Fair	Poor	Inferior
Standing long jump (in inches)	4	69-up	62-68	52-61	42-51	12-41
Push-up	4	25-up	18-24	7-17	1-6	0
Sit-up	4	64-up	47-63	22-46	1-21	0
Standing long jump (in inches)	5	73-up	62-72	56-65	46-55	16-45
Push-up	5	22-up	16-21	7-15	1-6	0
Sit-up	5	70-up	52-69	22-51	2-21	0-1
Standing long jump (in inches)	6	77-up	70-76	59-69	49-58	18-48
Push-up	6	24-up	18-23	9-17	4-8	0-3
Sit-up	6	75-up	55-74	25-54	1-24	0

Adapted from The Operations Council, Oregon Board of Education, Salem, Oregon.

Table 10-2. Motor fitness standards, Oregon Motor Fitness Test: rating norms for girls (grades 4 to 6)

Test items	Grade	Superior	Good	Fair	Poor	Inferior
Hanging in arm-flexed position (in seconds)	4	30-up	20-29	5-19	1-4	0
Standing long jump (in inches)	4	65-up	58-64	49-57	39-48	9-38
Crossed-arm curl-up	4	66-up	50-65	26-49	2-25	0-1
Hanging in arm-flexed position (in seconds)	5	31-up	22-30	10-21	2-9	0-1
Standing long jump (in inches)	5	75-up	68-74	57-67	46-56	0-45
Crossed-arm curl-up	5	68-up	52-67	28-51	4-27	0-3
Hanging in arm-flexed position (in seconds)	6	37-up	27-36	12-26	1-11	0
Standing long jump (in inches)	6	73-up	66-72	55-65	44-54	0-43
Crossed-arm curl-up	6	71-up	55-70	31-54	1-30	0

Adapted from The Operations Council, Oregon Board of Education, Salem, Oregon.

hand grip slightly outside the width of the shoulders and places the chin over the bar. Support is removed and the chin is maintained above the bar and elbows are flexed as long as possible.

Scoring: The stopwatch is started when the child is in a stable position and stopped when the chin touches the bar or falls below the bar. The length of time to nearest second is recorded.

Administrative hints: Pick a bar height that ac-commodates the majority of students. Each child gets one turn.

FLOOR PUSH-UP (Fig. 10-3)

Factors measured: Strength and muscle endurance of elbow extensors, shoulder, and chest.

Age and sex: Boys, ages 9 to 12 years.

Equipment: Flat, hard surface.

Regulations: The boy assumes a face-lying position with feet together, resting on toes,

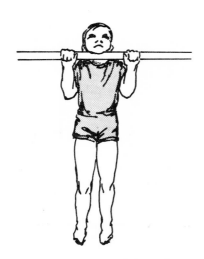

Fig. 10-2. Flexed-arm hang.

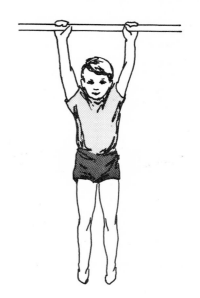

Fig. 10-4. Pull-up.

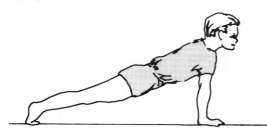

Fig. 10-3. Push-up.

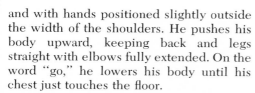

Fig. 10-5. Knee-touch sit-up.

and with hands positioned slightly outside the width of the shoulders. He pushes his body upward, keeping back and legs straight with elbows fully extended. On the word "go," he lowers his body until his chest just touches the floor.

Scoring: One point is allowed for each time the boy fully extends his elbows. Movement must be continuous with the back and legs kept straight.

PULL-UP (Fig. 10-4)

Factors measured: Strength and muscle endurance of hand grip, elbow flexors, and shoulder girdle.

Age and sex: Boys, ages 9 to 14 years.

Equipment: Horizontal bar or stall bar.

Regulations: The bar should be at a height at which the boy's legs can be fully extended. Using an overhand grip, the boy grasps the bar slightly outside the width of his shoulders. With his elbows fully extended in the hanging position he pulls himself up until his chin is over the bar. This movement is continuously executed as many times as possible.

Scoring: One point is given each time the chin comes over the bar. No points are allowed if the body snaps or swings or if the legs are not kept fully extended.

Administrative hints: The boy can be kept from swinging by the counter's placing his or her arm at a point directly behind the boy's legs.

KNEE-TOUCH SIT-UP (Fig. 10-5)

Factors measured: Strength and muscle endurance of trunk flexion.

Age and sex: Boys, ages 9 to 12 years.

Equipment: Flat surface and a thin pad or rug to lie on.

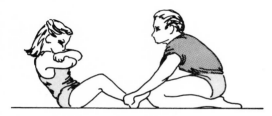

Fig. 10-6. Crossed-arm curl-up.

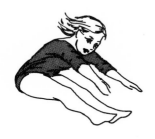

Fig. 10-7. Standing long jump.

Regulations: The boy lies on back, with hands clasped behind head, legs straight, and feet approximately 12 inches apart. His legs are held firmly in place by the counter. On the word "go," the boy touches his chin to his chest, curls his trunk upward, rotating to the right, and touches his left elbow to his right knee. He then lowers his trunk to the floor and repeats the sequence except that he rotates to the left and touches his right elbow to his left knee. The boy may bend his knees slightly when executing this sit-up. NOTE: If this activity is used for the AAHPER Fitness Test (Appendix B), as many as possible are performed in 60 seconds with the elbows touching the knees simultaneously.

Scoring: One point is given each time an elbow touches a knee. Points are not given when movement is not continuous, the boy arches his back, or he bounces off the floor.

CROSSED-ARM CURL-UP (Fig. 10-6)

Factors measured: Strength and muscle endurance of trunk flexion.

Age and sex: Girls, ages 9 to 12 years.

Equipment: Flat surface and a thin pad or rug to lie on.

Regulations: The girl lies on her back in a hook-lying position, with knees bent to about right angles, feet flat on floor, and arms folded across her chest. A partner holds the girl's feet in position. On the word "go," she curls her chin to her chest, rolls shoulders forward and curls trunk upward, coming to an erect sitting position.

Scoring: One point is given each time the girl comes to an erect sitting posture. Points are not given when movement fails to be continuous, girl arches back, or she bounces off floor.

STANDING LONG JUMP (Fig. 10-7)

Factor measured: Explosive strength of leg, thigh, and low back.

Age and sex: Boys and girls, ages 5 to 14 years.

Equipment: Flat floor surface, mat, or grassy area and tape measure.

Regulations: The child stands with feet comfortably separated and toes behind a take-off line. On the command "jump," he or she leaps with both feet simultaneously as far forward as possible, landing on both feet. The greatest distance is achieved by extending both knees at the same time and swinging both arms forward.

Scoring: The best out of three trials is scored. Measurement is taken from the closest heel to the starting point. If the child is unable to maintain balance after the jump and falls back on the hands, measurement must be taken from that point.

SHUTTLE RUN

Factors measured: Agility and explosive strength.

Age and sex: Boys and girls, ages 5 to 14 years.

Equipment: Flat surface 40 feet long, two blocks of wood 2 inches by 2 inches by 4 inches, and stopwatch. Children should wear sneakers or run barefoot.

Regulations: Two lines are placed parallel to each other, 30 feet apart. Both blocks of wood are placed behind one line. At the word "go," the child runs to the blocks, picks one of them up, races back to the starting line, and places the block behind that line; then he or she races back to the second block of wood, picks it up, returns with it behind the starting line, and places it with the first block.

Scoring: The best time is recorded for two trials.

40- AND 50-YARD DASH

Factors measured: Explosive strength and speed.

Age and sex: 40-yard dash for boys and girls, ages 5 to 9 years; 50-yard dash for boys and girls, ages 10 to 14 years.

Equipment: Outdoor grassy or dirt area and two stopwatches or one with a split-second hand.

Regulations: The runner stands behind a starting line; the timer stands at the finish line. On the command "get ready, get set, go," the stopwatch is started and the runner dashes the 40 or 50 yards.

Scoring: The time required to complete the run is recorded in seconds and tenths of seconds.

Administrative hints: To make the start more accurate, on the word "go," the timer can drop his or her hand in which is held a white handkerchief or rag.

SOFTBALL THROW FOR DISTANCE* (Fig. 10-8)

Factor measured: Explosive strength.

Age and sex: Boys and girls, ages 5 to 14 years.

Equipment: Playing field 100 yards long, tape measure, 12-inch softball, and metal or wooden spotting stakes.

Regulations: The participant throws as far as possible from a restraining area that is indicated by two parallel lines, 6 feet apart.

---

*Because of the controversy concerning use of the softball throw for distance, we recommend that it be used with caution.

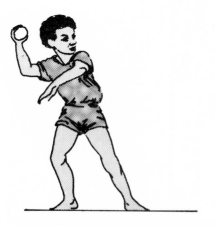

Fig. 10-8. Softball throw for distance.

The best distance of an overhand throw is marked with a stake.

Scoring: The greatest distance out of three throws is recorded.

400- AND 600-YARD RUN-WALK

Factor measured: Cardiorespiratory endurance.

Age and sex: 400-yard run-walk for boys and girls, ages 5 to 9 years; 600-yard run-walk for boys and girls, ages 10 to 14 years.

Equipment: Marked running area and stopwatch.

Regulations: On the command, "get ready, get set, go," the child runs or walks the prescribed distance. Time is called out as each child passes the finish line.

Scoring: A record is kept of the minutes and seconds required to finish the course.

CONDUCTING A PROGRAM OF PHYSICAL FITNESS

To have physical fitness is to be both physically fit and able to use the body in a coordinated manner. Ideally, the elementary school child should be able easily to meet the physical demands of daily life without undue fatigue and be able to successfully participate daily in a wide variety of large-muscle activities.

The intermediate child, who ranges from 9 to 12 years of age, should be provided with more specialized physical fitness activities than the primary child. Although in both levels there should be stress on the capacity for movement and energy expenditures, the intermediate period is the time when a lifelong desire for physical fitness can be established. The teacher concerned with a balanced activity program should make sure that developmental exercises are included in the daily regime. Every physical education activity should have an element of physical fitness built in, even games of low organization and activities that normally demand little energy output.

The sound elementary school fitness program includes three major areas: a screening test for determining each child's status, a general developmental program, and special remedial program for those individuals identified as being physically underdeveloped.

After administering a screening test, the teacher has some idea about each child's performance capacity; however, no typical state or national physical performance test can be considered as absolute in determining a child's work capacity. An absolute test would require specialized equipment not commonly available to the elementary school program. Therefore, the screening tests described in this chapter are only indicators of a child's physical performance. Children who fall below the twenty-fifth percentile should be considered for a special remedial exercise program conducted as an adjunct to the regular physical activity program.

The following exercises and activities are presented according to the level of intensity and the body area most affected. Each exercise is assigned an intensity level of low, medium, or high that corresponds to the estimated amount of energy expended or the amount of effort that must be put out for the accomplishment of the activity.

Exercises for conditioning arm and shoulder girdle

WALL PUSH-AWAY (Fig. 10-9)

Level: Low.

Purpose: Arm and shoulder strength and muscle endurance. This is a lead-up exercise to regular floor push-ups.

Equipment: Flat wall area.

Starting position: The child stands facing the wall, with the arms extended to the front at shoulder height and the feet a comfortable distance apart positioned about 2 feet from the wall.

Action: The child places the hands on the wall a shoulder width apart and directs the body to the wall until the chest touches. After the child touches the wall, the arms are extended and the body is pushed away from the wall.

Count: The action is repeated until the child can execute ten repetitions easily, at which time the child is ready to progress to the knee push-ups.

KNEE PUSH-UP (Fig. 10-10)

Level: Medium.

Purpose: Arm and shoulder strength and muscle endurance.

Equipment: Firm flat surface.

Starting position: The child extends the arms and places the hands on the floor just outside the width of the shoulders. The body is kept straight from the head to the knees.

Action: While resting on the knees and hands, the child lowers the body until the chest touches the floor and then returns to the extended arm position.

Count: One knee push-up is counted each time the child returns the body to the extended-arm position. When knee push-ups can be easily executed ten times, the child should progress to regular push-ups.

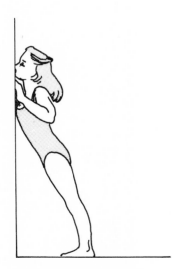

Fig. 10-9. Wall push-away.

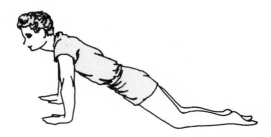

Fig. 10-10. Knee push-up.

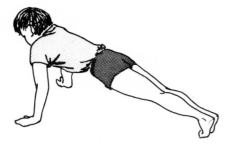

Fig. 10-11. Push-up.

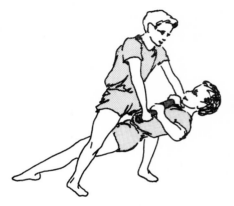

Fig. 10-12. Floor pull-up.

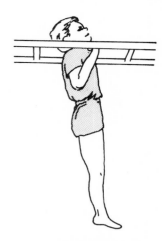

Fig. 10-13. Pull-up.

hands grasps the broomstick held by a partner who straddles the performer.

Action: While keeping the body straight, the child pulls the body upward until the chest touches the broomstick held by the partner and then slowly lets the body return to the beginning position.

Count: One floor pull-up is counted each time the child returns to the straight-arm position.

PULL-UP (Fig. 10-13)

Level: High.

Purpose: Arm, shoulder girdle, and upper body strength and muscle endurance.

Equipment: Horizontal bar, ladder, or any piece of pipe that can be grasped easily and is high enough that the child can hang fully extended.

Action: Using the overhand grip, the child grasps the bar at shoulder width. From a fully extended arm position the child pulls the body upward until the chin can be placed over the bar and then returns in a controlled manner to the starting position.

Count: One pull-up is counted each time the child pulls the chin over the bar.

Variation: A child not having enough strength to pull the chin over the bar may be conditioned by first jumping to a desired height and then slowly lowering the body until the arms are in a straight-hanging position.

LADDER TRAVEL

Level: Medium.

Purpose: Arm and shoulder girdle strength and muscle endurance.

PUSH-UP (Fig. 10-11)

Level: High.

Purpose: Arm and shoulder strength and muscle endurance.

Equipment: Firm flat surface.

Starting position: The child extends the arms and places the hands on the floor just outside the width of the shoulders. The body is kept straight from head to heels.

Action: While resting on the hands and toes, the child lowers the body until the chest touches the floor and then returns to the extended-arm position.

Count: One push-up is counted each time the child returns the body to the extended-arm position.

FLOOR PULL-UP (Fig. 10-12)

Level: Low to medium.

Purpose: Arm, shoulder girdle, and upper body strength and muscle endurance. This is a lead-up exercise to the regular pull-up.

Equipment: Broomstick and a partner.

Starting position: The child lies on the back, extends the arms upward, and with the

Equipment: Horizontal ladder.

Starting position: The position depends on the method employed, but the child is usually positioned at one end of the ladder.

Action: The goal is for the child to reach the other end of the ladder using a variety of methods, such as grasping overhand each ladder rung, skipping one or two rungs, traveling hand to hand on one side of the ladder, and alternating traveling using hands on both sides of the ladder.

ROPE OR POLE CLIMB

Level: High.

Purpose: Arm, shoulder girdle, and upper body strength and muscle endurance.

Equipment: Climbing rope 20 feet long and protection mat underneath rope.

Action: The extent to which the child exercises the arms and shoulders depends on how much the legs and feet are used in the climb. The easiest method is the leg and foot break, in which the rope passes between the legs, around one leg, and over the instep of the foot. The other foot holds the rope in place over the instep. As the arms pull the body upward, the rope slides over the instep, and the pressure of the other foot provides a braking action until the arms can recover for a new pull. A more difficult method is shinning up the rope. While the arms pull the body upward, the legs and feet, which are wrapped around the rope, push downward in assistance. One of the most difficult rope-climbing techniques is with just the arms and without the aid of the legs.

Additional activities for conditioning arms and shoulder girdle include the crab walk, wheelbarrow, and caterpillar walk. (See Part Four activities.)

Exercises for conditioning abdominal muscles

ABDOMINAL CURL
(HEAD AND SHOULDER ROLL) (Fig. 10-14)

Level: Low.

Purpose: Upper abdominal muscle strength and endurance. This is a lead-up exercise to the sit-up.

Equipment: Exercise mat.

Starting position: The child lies on the back,

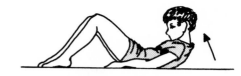

Fig. 10-14. Abdominal curl (head and shoulder roll).

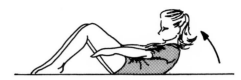

Fig. 10-15. Abdominal curl with arms extended.

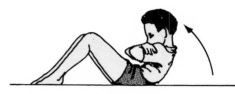

Fig. 10-16. Abdominal curl with arms folded across chest.

with the knees bent and arms at the side of the body.

Action: The child lifts the head up until the chin touches the chest and then rolls both shoulders forward and returns to the starting position.

ABDOMINAL CURL WITH ARMS EXTENDED
(Fig. 10-15)

Level: Low to medium.

Purpose: Upper abdominal muscle strength and endurance. This is a lead-up exercise to the sit-up.

Equipment: Exercise mat.

Starting position: The child lies on the back, with the knees bent and the arms extended forward.

Action: The child lifts the head up until the chin touches the chest and then rolls the shoulders forward, lifting the upper back off the mat, until a sitting position is achieved.

ABDOMINAL CURL WITH ARMS FOLDED
ACROSS CHEST (Fig. 10-16)

Level: Medium.

Purpose: Upper abdominal muscle strength and endurance. This is a lead-up exercise to the sit-up.

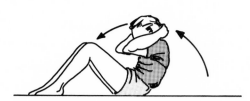

Fig. 10-17. Regular sit-up.

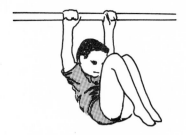

Fig. 10-18. Hanging hip curl.

Equipment: Exercise mat.
Starting position: The child lies on the back, with the knees bent and the arms folded across the chest.
Action: The child lifts the head up until the chin touches the chest, the shoulders are rolled forward, and the back is lifted from the mat to a full sitting position.

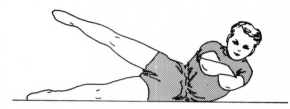

Fig. 10-19. Side abdominal curl.

ABDOMINAL CURL (SIT-UP) WITH HANDS CLASPED BEHIND NECK (Fig. 10-17)

Level: High.
Purpose: Upper abdominal muscle strength and endurance.
Equipment: Exercise mat.
Starting position: The child lies on the back, with the knees bent and the hands clasped behind the neck.
Action: The child lifts the head until the chin touches the chest, rolls the shoulders forward, points elbows toward the bent knees, rolls the trunk to a full sit-up position, touches the elbows to the knees, and returns to the starting position by uncurling.
Count: One sit-up is counted each time the child comes to a full sit-up position.
Administrative hints: Proper execution of the abdominal curl is imperative. Arching the low back and snapping the head forward to provide impetus to the curl must be avoided to prevent injury.
Variations: A number of variations can be done that increase the difficulty and/or effectiveness of the abdominal curl:
1. The child performs a curl-up, alternately touching the right elbow to the left knee and the left elbow to the right knee.
2. The child performs a curl-up and single-knee raise, alternately touching the right elbow to the raised left knee and the left elbow to the raised right knee.

3. A curl-up is performed on an inclined board.
4. A two-knee raise is performed on an inclined board, with the child bringing the knees to the chest, and returning to a fully extended position.

HANGING HIP CURL (Fig. 10-18)

Level: Medium to high.
Purpose: Lower abdominal muscle strength and endurance.
Equipment: Horizontal bar.
Starting position: With the hands the child grasps the horizontal bar keeping the feet together.
Action: Keeping the arms straight, the child raises both bent knees and curls the lower trunk upward as far as possible, uncurling very slowly.
Count: Each consecutive hip curl is counted as one.
Variations: When able to perform at least ten hip curls, the child can derive increased benefits by alternating the curls, first to the left and then to the right. Added intensity can be provided later by having the child curl upward with the knees in an extended position.

SIDE ABDOMINAL CURL (Fig. 10-19)

Level: High.
Purpose: Lateral abdominal muscle strength.

Equipment: Exercise mat.

Starting position: The child takes a side-lying position, with the legs straight and together and with the arms folded across the chest.

Action: The child raises the top leg and at the same time curls the trunk sideward toward the raised leg.

Count: Each consecutive side sit-up is counted as one.

Exercises for conditioning back

STRAIGHT BACK RAISE (Fig. 10-20)

Level: Low.

Purpose: Back extensor strength.

Equipment: None.

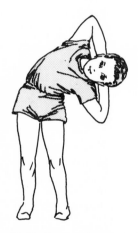

Fig. 10-20. Straight back raise.

Starting position: The child stands with legs comfortably spread and hands clasped behind the neck.

Action: Keeping the back straight and the elbows even with the ears, the child slowly bends from the waist to a right-angle position and returns slowly to a standing position.

Count: One straight back raise is counted each time the pupil returns to the straight-standing position.

UPPER BACK LIFT (Fig. 10-21)

Level: Medium to high.

Purpose: Upper back muscle strength.

Equipment: Exercise mat and a pillow or rolled up towel.

Starting position: The child lies face down, with the feet together and the hands clasped behind the head. A pillow or rolled up towel is placed under the pelvis.

Action: Keeping the back straight and the toes touching the floor, the child raises the chest about 2 inches off the mat.

Count: The child holds the back lift position for about 10 seconds and then slowly returns to a relaxed position. The exercise is repeated three times.

Precaution: At no time should the child attempt to arch the back.

LOWER BACK LIFT (Fig. 10-22)

Level: Medium to high.

Purpose: Lower back strength.

Equipment: Exercise mat and pillow or rolled up towel.

Starting position: The child lies face down,

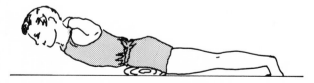

Fig. 10-21. Upper back lift.

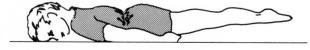

Fig. 10-22. Lower back lift.

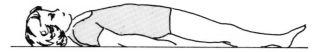

Fig. 10-23. Front-lying hip raise.

with the feet together, legs straight, arms at side, and weight of body resting on the forehead. A pillow or rolled up towel is placed under the pelvis.

Action: With the toes pointed backward and the legs straight, the child lifts the legs about 4 inches off the mat.

Count: The child holds the back lift for 10 seconds and then returns the legs to the mat. The exercise is repeated three times.

Precaution: The lower back should *not* be arched.

FRONT-LYING HIP RAISE (Fig. 10-23)

Level: Progressions for low to high intensity.
Purpose: Neck and back muscle strength.
Equipment: Exercise mat.
Starting position: The child lies on the back, with the knees bent, the feet flat on the floor, and the arms at the side.
Action: The child lifts the hips, holds them in the raised position, and lowers them slowly to the floor.
Count: The child holds the hips in a raised position for 10 seconds and then lowers them to the mat. The exercise is repeated three times.
Precaution: The child should avoid arching the back to the extent that weight is borne on the neck.

Additional activities for conditioning the trunk and back include the measuring worm, partner get-up, backward roll, human ball, and scooter. (See Part Four activities.)

Exercises for conditioning legs and pelvic girdle

JUMP AND REACH (Fig. 10-24)

Level: Low to medium.
Purpose: Leg strength and muscle endurance.
Equipment: Flat surface.
Starting position: The child stands with the arms at the side and the feet comfortably placed apart.

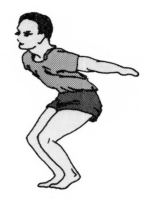

Fig. 10-24. Jump and reach.

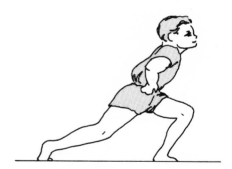

Fig. 10-25. Front lunge.

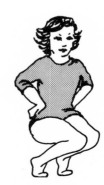

Fig. 10-26. Half squat.

Action: Keeping the back straight, the child bends the knees to right angles; swings the arms back, forward, and then upward; extends the knees forcibly and springs up until the feet leave the floor; and then returns to the standing position.

Count: One jump and reach is counted each time the child returns to a standing position. Ten consecutive jumps should be attempted.

FRONT LUNGE (Fig. 10-25)

Level: Low.

Purpose: Leg strength and muscle endurance.

Equipment: Flat surface.

Starting position: The child stands straight with hands on hips.

Action: The child lunges with the left foot forward, shifting the weight forward and keeping the trunk straight, and then returns to the starting position and lunges with the right foot. The movement should be quick.

Count: Each lunge executed is counted as one.

HOP

Level: Low to medium.

Purpose: Lower leg strength and muscle endurance.

Equipment: Flat surface.

Starting position: The child stands straight with the arms at the sides.

Action: The child hops on each foot a prescribed number of times.

Count: Each jump is counted as one.

HALF SQUAT (Fig. 10-26)

Level: High.

Purpose: Leg strength and muscle endurance.

Equipment: Flat surface.

Starting position: The child stands straight with feet spread comfortably and hands on hips.

Action: Keeping back straight, the child squats and then returns to the standing position.

Count: One half squat is counted each time the child returns to the standing position.

General strength and agility exercises

SIDE-STRADDLE HOP (Fig. 10-27)

Level: Medium.

Purpose: Arm and leg conditioning, leg strength, and muscle endurance.

Equipment: None.

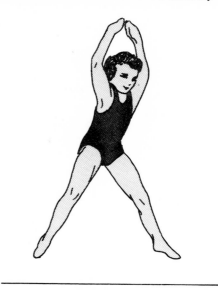

Fig. 10-27. Side-straddle hop.

Starting position: The child stands erect, with the arms at the side and the feet together.

Action: The child jumps, spreading the legs to the side; at the same time the arms are brought overhead.

Count: One side-straddle hop is counted each time the child returns to the erect standing position.

STOP AND GO

Level: Low.

Purpose: Ability to move and stop readily when a signal is given.

Equipment: Whistle.

Starting position: The children are informally scattered.

Action: They run as fast as they can when the whistle is blown once and stop as fast as possible when it is blown twice.

Count: There should be 10 to 20 stops and starts.

HEEL TOUCH (Fig. 10-28)

Level: Low to medium.

Purpose: Coordination and leg strength.

Equipment: Whistle.

Starting position: The child stands erect, with the hands at the side.

Action: At the sound of the whistle, the child jumps up and touches both heels with the fingers.

Count: Each jump is counted as one.

Variations: The child can touch different parts

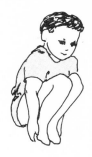

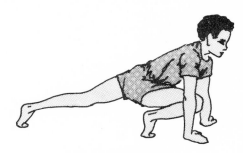

Fig. 10-30. Treadmill.

Fig. 10-28. Heel touch.

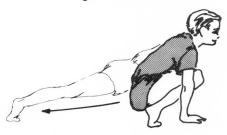

Fig. 10-29. Squat-thrust.

of the legs. Heel touch may be a lead-up activity to a stick or short-rope jump. Holding the ends of a 16-inch rope with both hands, the child jumps over the rope without loosening either grip.

SQUAT-THRUST (Fig. 10-29)

Level: Medium to high.
Purpose: Agility and general trunk and leg strength.
Equipment: Exercise mat.
Starting position: The child stands straight, with the arms at the side and the feet together.
Action: The child bends the knees and places the hands on the floor in a squat position, thrusts the feet and legs backward, assuming a push-up position, and then returns to a squat position and stands erect.
Count: One squat-thrust is counted each time the child resumes the standing position.
Variation: Push-ups may be added to the basic squat-thrust exercise.

TREADMILL (Fig. 10-30)

Level: Medium to high.
Purpose: General strength and muscle endurance of trunk and legs.

Equipment: None.
Starting position: The child assumes the push-up position with one leg forward.
Action: The child keeps the hands in place while alternately bringing one leg forward and extending the other leg in a running fashion.
Count: One treadmill exercise is counted each time the child brings the right leg forward.

ZIGZAG RUN

Level: Low.
Purpose: Agility.
Equipment: Any objects, such as chairs, that can be positioned to provide an obstacle course.
Starting position: The child stands erect at a starting line.
Action: At the word "go," the child runs as fast as possible in a zigzag course around the obstacles.
Count: The time required to complete the course is recorded.

Exercises for cardiorespiratory endurance development

MARCH

Level: Low to medium.
Purpose: Cardiorespiratory endurance and leg muscle endurance.
Equipment: Rhythmic device such as a metronome.
Starting position: The children stand in pairs, side by side. Each stands straight, with the arms at the side.
Action: At a moderately paced rhythmic beat (70 beats per minute), the children march

shoulder to shoulder with their partners. At each beat, they lift one foot approximately 5 inches off the floor, first the left foot and then the right foot.

Progressions: The teacher can provide increased cardiorespiratory stress by speeding up the tempo, by having the children lift their legs higher, and by increasing the length of time of the march. The teacher might keep a record of how many steps the children perform per minute.

RUN IN PLACE

Level: Medium to high.

Purpose: Cardiorespiratory endurance, leg strength, and muscle endurance.

Equipment: None.

Starting position: The child stands erect, with the arms flexed at the side.

Action: At the signal "go," the child alternately lifts the left knee and then the right knee to a right-angle position, swinging the arms forcibly in opposition. The cadence can be varied to increase the exercise intensity.

Progressions: The teacher can provide a progression from medium to high cardiorespiratory stress by changing the tempo from 80 to 90 to 100 steps per minute. The teacher can also vary the duration of the exercise.

JOG AND RUN

Level: Low to high.

Purpose: Cardiorespiratory endurance, leg strength, and muscle endurance.

Equipment: Outdoor or indoor running area.

Starting position: The child stands erect with the feet staggered, one foot ahead of the other.

Action: At the signal "go," the child walks, jogs, or runs a prescribed distance or length of time.

Progressions: Very low level: 150 yards in 1 minute (5 minutes, 750 yards).

Low level: 200 yards in 1 minute (5 minutes, 1000 yards)

Medium level: 250 yards in 1 minute (5 minutes, 1250 yards).

High level: 300 yards in 1 minute (5 minutes, 1500 yards).

Conditioning hints: The teacher can use this chart to roughly determine the cardiorespiratory level of each child as well as to devise a training program. He or she can initiate training progressions by increasing

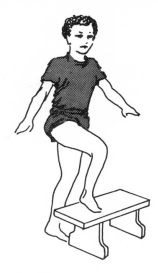

Fig. 10-31. Bench step.

the distance covered and by increasing the movement time.

BENCH STEP (Fig. 10-31)

Level: High.

Purpose: Cardiorespiratory endurance, leg strength, and muscle endurance.

Equipment: Bench 10 to 16 inches high.

Starting position: The child faces the bench, standing in an erect position with the feet together and the arms at the side.

Action: At a signal, the child steps up on the bench, stands erect with both feet together, and then steps back down and returns to the starting position. Tempo and length of time are variable; 30 steps per minute for 5 minutes is considered a high-intensity exercise.

Count: One bench step is counted each time the child steps down.

INTERVAL SPRINT

Level: High.

Purpose: Cardiorespiratory endurance, leg strength, and muscle endurance.

Equipment: Running space and a whistle.

Starting position: The child stands erect with one foot forward.

Action: The purpose of interval training is to increase the work capacity of the heart and lungs. This is accomplished by a series of sprints intermingled with recovery periods. The teacher can vary the program in any way feasible. Following is one type of interval program:

Day 1: all-out sprint 2 seconds, walk 25 seconds (5 repetitions).
Day 2: all-out sprint 3 seconds, walk 20 seconds (6 repetitions).
Day 3: all-out sprint 4 seconds, walk 20 seconds (6 repetitions).
Day 4: all-out sprint 5 seconds, walk 15 seconds (7 repetitions).
Day 5: all-out sprint 5 seconds, walk 15 seconds (8 repetitions).
Day 6: all-out sprint 6 seconds, walk 15 seconds (8 repetitions).
Day 7: all-out sprint 7 seconds, walk 10 seconds (8 repetitions).
Day 8: all-out sprint 8 seconds, walk 10 seconds (9 repetitions).
Day 9: all-out sprint 9 seconds, walk 10 seconds (9 repetitions).
Day 10: all-out sprint 10 seconds, walk 10 seconds (10 repetitions).

Exercises and special fitness programs

There is no better feeling than that of feeling physically fit. Children usually love to exercise if they are motivated by vibrant teachers. The program of physical fitness can be formal, with specific conditioning exercises, or informal, with the conditioning built into all the physical education activities. Ideally, it should be both formal and informal. One excellent method of imparting fitness is through an obstacle course that employs the circuit training method. Circuit training is a technique of conditioning that can develop all the attributes of physical fitness. This approach is designed to provide children with opportunities and personal incentives, causing them to be self-motivating. Circuit training is one of the most appropriate conditioning methods available for use at the elementary school level. Little equipment is required, and an entire class can be conditioned in a very short period of time with a great deal of fun, but at the same time each child is performing on an individual basis.[17]

Establishing each child's exercise load. On the first day of the circuit program, the teacher establishes the number of desired exercise stations. Normally there will be from six to eight stations. After determining the type of exercise to be initiated at each station, the teacher has the children go through the entire circuit, executing as many repetitions of each exercise as possible. The number of repetitions is recorded by the teacher. Each child's maximum number of repetitions is then reduced by one third. The next day, each child is given a particular number of exercise repetitions for each station and instructed to go through the circuit three times, completing all of the exercise stations within a specified target time (usually between 15 and 30 minutes).

Class organization. If there are 30 children in the class and six stations have been selected, five children can be placed at each station. In the beginning, if a target time of 30 minutes has been selected, each child would have 10 minutes to complete one circuit trip. A possible time distribution at each station could be 1 minute for completion of an individual exercise dosage plus 40 seconds for each child to record his or her progress and move to the next station.

Increasing the work load. The teacher can increase the work load by increasing the number of exercise repetitions, by decreasing the time in which to execute the repetitions, by increasing the difficulty of the exercise, by decreasing the rest time between stations, and by adding to the number of circuit trips that the children perform.

Exercise organization. Each station should have exercises that are designed to provide required strength, muscle endurance, cardiorespiratory endurance, and coordination. No muscle group should be exercised twice in a row.

Motivation. One advantage of the circuit program is that it helps to build a positive self-concept. One child's result is not compared to another's, but each child is encouraged to improve individually. Teachers who want to motivate and increase the aspiration levels of their classes should establish a predetermined performance level for a circuit, with accomplishment levels set at low, medium, and high. Each level may be distinguished by a color, such as red, green, or gold, or by an animal symbol, such as a bear, tiger, or lion.

Fitness obstacle course

The obstacle course is one of the best devices to improve the child's fitness level. Like the circuit program, the obstacle course is separated into stations at which the performer executes a specific movement or series of movements. Unlike the circuit, the obstacle course is usually executed one time only and usually against a time factor.

The course can be made up of permanent fixtures established outdoors, or it can be made from available portable equipment and set up indoors.

INFORMALIZING PHYSICAL FITNESS

In general, increasing physical fitness requires a structuring of selected activities and a plan for overloading each activity in order that development will take place. Structuring does not necessarily mean that a teacher has to be a drill sergeant leading a group of soldiers in calisthenics. The command style of teaching is traditional for fitness activities but is often the most undesirable style, especially if the teacher wants each child to be self-motivated in this area. This is not to say that doing exercises in a prescribed manner is not important or that calisthenics conducted by the teacher are not expedient for a short time allotment. However, this method often does not instill in many children a desire to improve their level of fitness. It is desirable that children become acquainted with their own

levels of fitness and become self-motivated to increasing these levels. This requires that the child become directly involved with the decision-making as to how, when, and what extent physical fitness will be improved. Once selected fitness activities have been properly taught by the teacher, more informal methods should be tried, especially with children who are self-motivated and responsible. One method that has the elements of both structure and self-motivation is the *Parcourse*. The Parcourse is an 18-station outdoor fitness trail along which participants jog between stations. At each station the participant performs a specific exercise that is geared to his or her individual developmental level. The Parcourse is described in detail in Chapter 16.

Another method of both informalizing and individualizing physical fitness is through the contract method. After being tested, a child sits down with the teacher and, through discussion, establishes a program that involves both home and school activities. The contracted program can involve many elements, such as what activities will be performed, the goal for each child, and when the activities will be accomplished. It is highly important that the teacher encourage the child to include common home activities that can be performed every day, such as bicycle riding, walking, or swimming, and selected exercises. Once an individual fitness program has been agreed upon, the teacher encourages the child to make a fitness chart that shows weekly progress.

TEACHING EXERCISES
Warm-up

Any program of physical conditioning should always be preceded by a program of warm-up and flexibility exercises. The warm-up includes body movements, such as jogging or running in place, designed to increase the circulation of blood to the deeper muscle tissue. It is generally accepted that a proper warm-up assists the efficiency of contracting muscles and at the same time prevents injuries that arise from overstraining the musculotendinous unit.[15] Flexibility exercises, particularly those of the static stretch type, normally follow the warm-up regime. Stretching exercises performed at this time provide an additional factor of safety and increased function. The flexible joint is less likely to become injured when stressed by a high-level conditioning program.

Conditioning exercises

Generally each exercise has three elements: a *starting position,* the *exercise proper,* and the *finished aspect* of the exercise. To teach children exercises, the instructor must first organize the class into the most practical and expedient formations. Exercise formations can be roughly categorized into informal and formal. In the informal formation, the teacher instructs the class to take any spot on the floor, keeping an arm's length away from any other person. The formal type of class formation is generally conducted from squads or predetermined floor markings. To expedite formal exercise, schools often paint spots, numbers, or letters on the floor spaced to provide adequate room for exercises. In the squad method, children line up, one behind the other, usually in groups of about six. They face the front and move double arm's length to the right, make a right face again and move double arm's length to the right, and then make a half left face.

In teaching each exercise, the instructor calls out the name of the exercise, demonstrates it for the class, has the class execute the exercise, and finally, evaluates how the class performed, pointing out errors that must be corrected. Each exercise should be performed to a cadence of four beats. The instructor and the class count, putting the number of the exercise at the beginning (1, 2, 3, 4; 2, 2, 3, 4; 3, 2, 3, 4; and so on) or at the end (1, 2, 3, 1; 1, 2, 3, 2; 1, 2, 3, 3; and so on) of each sequence.

Hints for proper exercise execution

Following is a list of suggestions for the instructor in conducting the conditioning program:
1. Conduct a proper warm-up before engaging in vigorous activities.
2. Avoid the forceful locking of the elbow and knee.
3. Be sure that each child knows why an exercise is given.
4. Avoid forceful deep knee bends.
5. Avoid straight leg raising from the back-lying position.

Understanding signs of overexertion

Any teacher working with children who are engaged in physical activities that produce stress must be aware of the signs of overexertion. Children who respond adversely to reasonable physical activity given by the teacher must be referred to a physician. The following signs may indicate that the program is too intense or that a child is in need of medical assistance:
1. Excessive breathlessness apparent long after exercise is completed
2. Blue lips or nail beds that are not characteristic of a reaction to cold weather
3. Cold, clammy skin
4. Profound fatigue and poor recovery rate
5. Shakiness that is most apparent in hands more than 10 minutes after exercise
6. Muscle soreness lasting more than a day
7. Systemic complaints and problems, such as headache, dizziness, fainting, sleeplessness, heart pounding, and stomach upset

CLASS ACTIVITIES

1. Administer the AAHPER test for physical fitness (see Appendix B) to a child or children.
2. Plan a semester's exercise program of physical fitness for a sixth grade class.
3. Include a fitness overload factor into the common lead-up sports activities found in third and fourth grades.
4. Observe a class of elementary school children and determine who is posturally fit and unfit.
5. Test the flexibility of children by having them attempt to touch their toes while seated. Measure the distance that some children can reach beyond or short of their toes.
6. Teach a child to take his or her pulse rate before and after activity.

REFERENCES

1. American Association for Health, Physical Education and Recreation: Fitness series no. 1, Washington, D.C., 1958, The Association.
2. Arnheim, D. D., and Sinclair, W. A.: The clumsy child, St. Louis, 1975, The C. V. Mosby Co.
3. Clarke, H. H., editor: Toward a better understanding of muscular strength. Physical Fitness Research Digest, series 3, no. 1, Washington, D.C., Jan. 1973, President's Council of Physical Fitness.
4. Clarke, H. H., editor: Circulatory-respiratory endurance. Physical Fitness Research Digest, series 3, no. 3, Washington, D.C., July 1973, President's Council on Physical Fitness.
5. Clarke, H. H., editor: Development of muscular strength and endurance. Physical Fitness Research Digest, series 4, no. 1, Washington, D.C., Jan. 1974, President's Council on Physical Fitness.
6. Clarke, H. H., editor: Strength development and motor-sports improvement. Physical Fitness Research Digest, series 4, no. 4, Washington, D.C., Oct. 1974, President's Council on Physical Fitness.
7. Clarke, H. H., editor: Athletes: their academic achievement and personal-social status. Physical Fitness Research Digest, series 5, no. 3, Washington, D.C., July 1975, President's Council on Physical Fitness.
8. Clarke, H. H., editor: Joint and body range of movement. Physical Fitness Research Digest, series 5, no. 4, Washington, D.C., Oct. 1975, President's Council of Physical Fitness.
9. Cratty, B. J.: Movement behavior and motor learning, ed. 3, Philadelphia, 1973, Lea & Febiger.
10. Espenshade, A. S.: The contributions of physical activity to growth, Res. Q. Am. Assoc. Health Phys. Educ. **31:**351-364, 1960.
11. Espenshade, A. S., and Eckert, H.: Motor development, Columbus, Ohio, 1967, Charles E. Merrill, Publishing Co.
12. Flieshman, E. A.: Examiner's manual for the basic fitness tests, Englewood Cliffs, N.J., 1964, Prentice-Hall, Inc.
13. Ismail, A. H., and Bruber, J. J.: Integrated development, Columbus, Ohio, 1967, Charles E. Merrill, Publishing Co.
14. Karpovich, P. V., and Sinnings, W. E.: Physiology of muscular activity, Philadelphia, 1971, W. B. Saunders Co.
15. Klafs, C. E., and Arnheim, D. D.: Modern principles of athletic training, St. Louis, 1977, The C. V. Mosby Co.
16. Kraus, H., and Hirschland, R. P.: Minimum muscular fitness tests in school children, Res. Q. Am. Assoc. Health Phys. Educ. **25**(2):178, 1954.
17. Morgan, R. E. and Admanson, G. T.: Circuit training, London, 1958, G. Bell & Sons Ltd.
18. Rarick, G. L., editor: Physical activity, human growth and development, New York, 1973, Academic Press, Inc.

RECOMMENDED READINGS

Annarino, A. A.: Developmental conditioning for women and men, ed. 2, St. Louis, 1976, The C. V. Mosby Co.
Hockey, R. V.: Physical fitness, the pathway to healthful living, ed. 3, St. Louis, 1977, The C. V. Mosby Co.
Morehouse, L. E., and Gross, L.: Maximum performance, New York, 1977, Simon & Schuster, Inc.

11

Integrated learning and classroom activities

What is integration? It can be thought of as a *blending of mind and body to successfully bring together all one's faculties in actions that lead toward the achievement of a goal.* For integration to be effective, it must be thoroughly planned with specific goals in mind. Through integrating classroom subjects with movement activities and involving the greatest possible number of sensory responses, the teacher can better design the learning experience.[2]

Many teachers fail to realize the potential of movement activities as complementary factors to the learning of cognitive skills. One must, however, understand that little can be learned in any subject without some movement response. Getman[1] has stated that all primary learning demands movement; speech, reading, writing, acting, and art all require some type of physical movement or muscle control. However, he also has cautioned that not all movement necessarily produces learning. This places responsibility on the teacher that cognitive activities be well planned and based on specific objectives. It is up to the teacher to make learning through movement meaningful and to directly relate the movement to the cognitive task.

For those teachers working with children who have learning disabilities, integration has increased value. Children who are designated as slow learners often find it much easier to learn cognitive skills by identifying them with some type

of motor activity. Although the learning period is sometimes extended for the slow learner, the challenge of activity and repetition, occurring in a fun situation, are often the experiences needed to ensure interest and success on the part of the child.

CLASSROOM MOTOR SKILLS

It is generally agreed that learning behavior is developed and expressed through motor responses. The language skills of reading, writing, and arithmetic depend to a great degree on the child's perceptual abilities, involving vision, audition, touch, and kinesthesis. Integration of these perceptual functions provides the basis for a child's cognitive and physical development. Physical education can provide many activities that may assist the child in the classroom. As in all education, some children learn easily through the auditory mode, whereas others are more visually oriented, and still others learn best by becoming physically involved with the material to be learned. It also should be noted that children with deficits in auditory and/or visual perceptual modes use the haptic sense, a combination of the kinesthetic and tactile senses, as their primary learning avenue.

One of the greatest advantages of integrating movement skills with classroom learning is the motivational factor. When children actively participate in any learn-

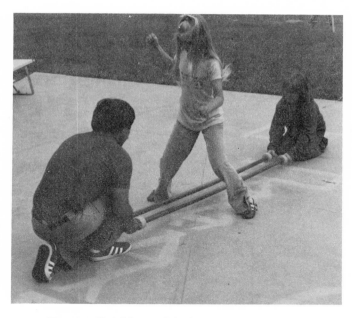

Fig. 11-1. Tinickling activity from the south Pacific.

ing activity, cognition is more quickly achieved and more likely to be lasting. As mentioned earlier in the text, there is a need for more research relating physical activity to classroom achievement. However, those who have experienced and planned integrated movement lessons are usually quite pleased with the results, because children enjoy learning classroom subjects taught through well-planned games and dance.

If the school has a physical education specialist, then there exists an excellent opportunity to initiate the team-teaching approach to learning. Through this team approach, the classroom teacher often obtains a better understanding of the aims and objectives of the physical educator and the physical education teacher has a better opportunity to understand the goals of the specific subject matter being taught in the classroom. When appropriate, the classroom teacher and the physical education specialist can work together in presenting activities that complement each other in a particular area of study. For example, if a unit on a foreign country is being taught in the classroom, the physical education specialist can present dances or games that are appropriate to that particular part of the world (Fig. 11-1). Participating in games and activities from countries around the globe brings about an understanding of world cultures second only to that derived from travel and personal experience. In this case, with integrated teaching, children can begin to understand that people of other countries have more similarities than differences.

Physical education plays an important role in the total educational scheme, whether taught by a specialist or in a self-contained classroom and whether developed through the traditional games approach or through experiences in movement problem-solving tasks. Orchestrating physical activity with academic concepts provides a challenge to the intellect as well as the body and is a definite child motivator.

Auditory skills

To successfully learn, children must have the ability to hear, discriminate or interpret, and respond in a meaningful way to sound. Children having difficulty in auditory-motor association may have difficulty in responding to instructions given by the teacher or may fail to find success in activities common to the primary grades.

To assist children in their auditory skills, a basic motor training program should be instituted that gives opportunities in motorically responding to sound.

Identification of sounds. The primary child should be able to name many different sounds. A lesson in naming sounds might include taking a walk around the school; while the children are listening for different sounds, the teacher might ask what sounds are different in different locations. In the classroom, a game may be played in which the children try to identify common sounds in the classroom, such as those of a chair moving, a pencil sharpener working, a window opening, or a door closing. Each child should be able to distinguish between sounds that are soft and loud, those that are slow and fast, and those that are first and last.

Localization of sound. Children can learn to localize sounds by closing their eyes and listening. There are numerous activity possibilities in helping a child localize sounds. The teacher might make various sounds around the room and each time have the children point, with their eyes closed, to the spot where the sound originated.

Following of a sequence of directions. Essential to a child's success in life is the ability to accurately follow directions. To follow directions, a child must listen and remember a sequence of movements in their correct order. The teacher can give the class problems in following directions, progressing from the simple to the more complex. A simple direction might be, "Everyone stand up, and then everyone sit down," whereas a complex sequence would be, "Stand up, open the window, close the door, and then pick up these five pencils on the desk and sharpen them."

Imitation of rhythm and sound. Imitation of rhythm and specific sounds requires the ability to remember a sequence and to distinguish between subtle sounds. Moving the various body parts to a cadence and clapping, tapping, or striking the various percussion instruments common to the elementary schools, such as blocks, cymbals, or sticks, are activities that enhance rhythmical responses. Children also like to add a rhythmical beat to names such as is used in rhythms of the Orff-Schülwerk technique.[4]

Imitation of sounds assists children in accurately hearing and responding. Making animal noises, such as those of a dog barking, a crow crowing, and a kitten mewing, is exciting to the young child. To enhance what is heard, the child can imitate the physical characteristics of the animal as well.

The ability to listen and to distinguish sounds is very important to a child's motor development. Such skills as imitation of rhythm, following of directions, game skills, and classroom motor activities require that the child hear and respond correctly.

Auditory activities

1. The children identify sounds heard outdoors.
2. They identify sounds heard indoors.
3. With eyes closed, they identify sounds the teacher makes, such as pieces of sandpaper being rubbed together, glasses being hit together, a ball bouncing, bells ringing, and whistles being blown.
4. With eyes closed, they point to the source of a sound, such as a hand clap, finger snap, tongue flick, or ball bounce.
5. Using elementary musical instruments, such as drums, sticks, bells, and triangles, children reproduce rhythm in marching activities.

Form-perception skills

Form-perception skills are the ability to distinguish basic geometric forms. The ability to distinguish such forms as circles, squares, and triangles leads directly to development of the cognitive areas of reading, writing, and arithmetic.

Form-perception activities

1. Cut out forms from different materials such as sandpaper and cardboard.
2. Draw, paint, or create forms with different materials, such as clay, sandpaper, paper, water, and cornmeal.
3. Make forms from materials such as felt, foam rubber, velvet, and wood.
4. Trace around a form with eyes open and then with them closed.
5. Paste forms on a board.
6. Draw forms.
7. Reproduce forms with the body.
8. Walk or run around forms.

Blackboard and chalk skills

A planned program for development of blackboard skills can aid children in many of the motor areas required in the classroom, namely, eye-hand control, laterality, directionality, and simultaneous use of the various perceptual modes.

Blackboard activities

1. Draw geometric forms.
2. Pick a particular geometric form out of a group of forms (figure-ground discrimination) (Fig. 11-2).
3. Draw a continuous line within a narrow track crossing the midline of the body.
4. Connect consecutive numbers with a line.
5. Perform audiovisual-motor tasks as suggested by Klasen.[3]
6. Draw patterns with each hand independently.
7. Draw line patterns left to right, with both hands together.

• • •

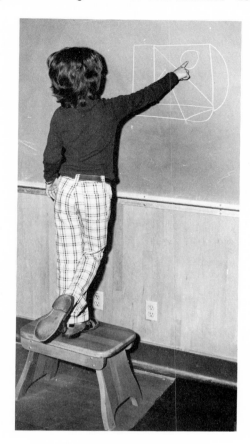

Fig. 11-2. Identifying geometrical forms.

The following activities describe some ways in which cognitive learning can be enhanced by integration with motor skills.

Mathematics

There are many ways in which numbers are used in sport activities. Too often teachers fail to realize the advantage they have in teaching mathematical concepts through games. Many games require writing numbers on targets for throwing activities such as a beanbag toss. Almost all games require some type of scoring, which involves adding or subtracting numbers to determine the winner. The stopwatch used in running events uses numbers, and all children are interested in the amount of time it takes for them to run the 50-yard dash. Linear measurement is of utmost importance in field events because everyone wants to know how far they leap or how high they jump. Measuring time and distance to compare children's abilities usually requires a great deal of accuracy since, in many cases, tenths of a second or fractions of an inch determine the winner. An easy way to teach percentages is to have students figure out their own for various games they play, like the professional and college teams do. These could be reported in the school newspaper.

The following activities deal with number concepts in a variety of settings.

Learning to tell time. Teachers can aid children in learning to tell time by letting them stand on numbers marked on the playground in the shape of a clock. (Temporary numbers can be taped on any playground circle if a permanent number circle is not available.) One additional student is placed in the center to act as the "hands" of the clock and give the answer. If the question is "Can you show us

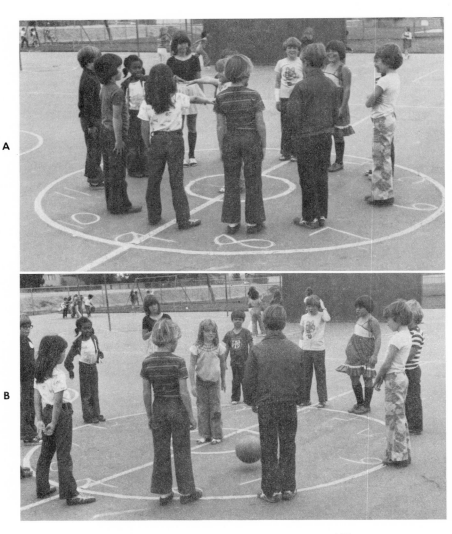

Fig. 11-3. Learning to tell time using motor skills.

three o'clock?", the child in the center joins hands with the person standing on the three and the person standing on the twelve (Fig. 11-3, *A*). The game can be varied by using an object such as a beanbag or ball to throw or bounce to the child on the correct number (Fig. 11-3, *B*). If a beanbag is used, an underhand throw would be made to the child standing on the three first, and upon return of the beanbag to the center child, the toss would then be made to the child on the twelve. The successful selection of the proper numbers incorporated with throwing and catching skills helps make learning to tell time more fun.

Making a pocket grid. Playgrounds should have numeral or alphabet grids painted on their surfaces as indicated in Chapter 3. However, for more flexibility and utility, we recommend that teachers construct a pocket grid. The advantage of a pocket grid rests with the potential for changing the numerals, letters, groups of letters, or pictures to provide a variety of activities with ease. Using the pocket grid, the teacher can change the sequence or position of numbers or other items simply by placing the material into a different pocket. When times tables are being studied, numbers depicting the products of any tables may be inserted. The activities that can be played on the pocket grid are limited only by the teacher's creativity and ingenuity.

To construct the grid, obtain a clear plastic sheet approximately 5 feet by 6 feet and at least 6 mils thick. Any number of pockets can be made, but the most practical number is 12. Divide the sheet into 12 equal parts, and outline each section with colored plastic tape. Purchase enough clear Contact paper to make 12 double pockets (about 4 yards). From the Contact paper, cut 12 rectangles 9 inches by 12 inches and 12 rectangles 7 inches by 8 inches. Remove the backing from one rectangle of each size at a time. Place the smaller rectangle on the larger one, sticky sides together, making sure they are even at the top and there is 2 inches extra on three sides. The excess sticky area will hold the pocket to the sheet. Turn the pocket over and place it on the plastic sheet in the center of one of the 12 sections. Complete the rest of the pockets and affix them to the plastic. Paper items can now be inserted for use (Fig. 11-4). Make certain that the children hop on the smooth side of the plastic so the pockets are not torn off. If the surface is slippery, the plastic sheet may be taped down.

Numeral grid. The numeral grid can be used in conjunction with addition, subtraction, multiplication, and division lessons. At the beginning level, children can play the game by jumping consecutively until they reach the highest number. Not jumping in correct sequence or stepping on the lines would constitute an error and the next child would then have a turn. This activity can become more cognitive by having a child jump into two squares and add, subtract, or multiply them, giving the correct answer. The grid can also be used as a partner game. Team 1 calls

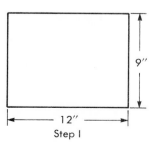

Step I

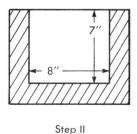

Step II

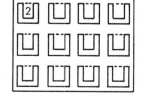

Step III

Fig. 11-4. Steps in making the pocket grid.

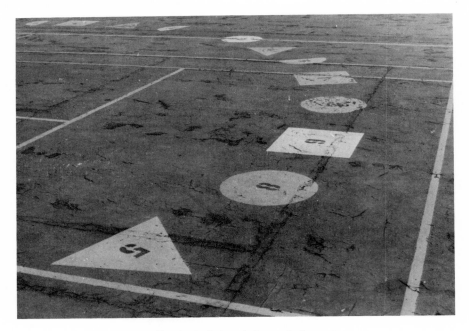

Fig. 11-5. Colored shape-circles.

out the type of computation. A member of team 2 jumps into two squares and another member of team 2 writes the answer or calls it out. A point is given for the correct answer. Other combinations can be worked out, but they must fit into the limitations of the grid. This game has great challenge when used as a problem-solving device by children.

Colored shape-circles. For this activity multicolored shapes with numerals on them should be painted in a large circle (Fig. 11-5). (Paper cutouts, taped down, may be used if permanent painting is not possible.) Children are asked to move around the circle using various means of locomotion, such as skipping, hopping, or running, and when told to stop are asked to land on a shape. Those who do not land on a shape are "out," as in musical chairs. Another way to use the shape-circle is by introducing a ball into the activity. Children can rotate around the circle, each bouncing a ball and stopping on signal on a designated shape. The children would then execute the number of bounces in-

dicated in the figure. A more difficult variation would be to have the student bounce the ball three times on a triangle, twice on a circle, four times on a square, and so on. Identification of colors and geometric shapes can be an aid in developing figure-ground relationships. Variations of the shape-circle game can help develop auditory sequencing, auditory memory, and mathematical associations.

Number hopscotch. Hopscotch has many variations (see Chapter 15). Children can begin to participate by hopping through the squares in consecutive order. Hopscotch can be played by having all children acquire a lagger (a rock, chain, or barrette) and throw it in the first square. Each participant must hop over the squares containing laggers rather than in them. After hopping in each consecutive square, the child hops back to the start, picking up his or her lagger on the return trip. The lagger is then tossed into the next section, and the game continues until one person has gone through all of the squares. An error is made in one of five

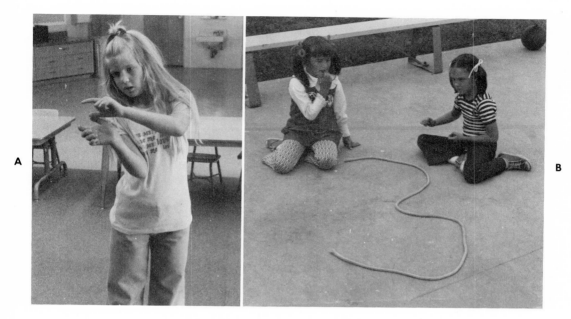

Fig. 11-6. Children making numbers.

ways: (1) if the child does not land in the proper square, (2) when a child steps on a line, (3) when consecutive order is not followed, (4) if a child hops in a square that contains a lagger, and (5) if the lagger is tossed into the wrong square.

Twelve-square jumpscotch. In this game (see Chapter 15) the children jump on consecutive numbers, attempting to turn in the air so that they can make the next jump without taking additional steps. The children add the numbers as they continue to jump; they may stay in the game until an error is made in addition or a line is stepped on.

Making numbers. A fun, total body involvement activity is for children to twist their bodies into numbers. It can be done by an individual or groups of two or three. The teacher can introduce a problem by saying, "Can you make the shape of number three by using your whole body?" Problems that can be posed are having children make the number that indicates their age, small numbers, large numbers, and even or odd numbers or having them

sit, stand or assume any creative position that the teacher can suggest and the children can solve. For a change of pace, the teacher may limit the problem by asking that only arms or fingers be used (Fig. 11-6, A). Another variation is to incorporate equipment, such as hoops, ropes, or balls, that can be arranged to display a number either with or without the child being a part of it (Fig. 11-6, B).

Counting activities. Many games involve counting consecutive numbers. The hide-and-seek or jumping rope involves counting. While bouncing on a trampoline, children can be asked to count forward to ten and then backward to one, or they can be asked to count by twos, fives, or tens. Jumping on a trampoline, or even on the sides of an old tire if a trampoline is unavailable, is invigorating and gives needed repetition for mathematic memorization if numbers are repeated while the child jumps. Sequential memory tasks, such as asking a child to jump three times, do two knee drops, do a seat drop, and then stop, incorporate counting with gross motor control and memory. The classroom teacher can bring excitement to the lesson and have fun creating new and different games using mathematical concepts in a planned program of motor activities.

Numbers relay. With the children in squad formation, a group of numbers on cardboard squares are placed randomly on the floor approximately 10 yards in front of the squad lines. On a given signal, the first child runs to the numbers, locates the number one square, picks it up, returns to the squad, and goes to the end of the line after tagging the first child in the line. The tagged child then runs to locate and pick up the number two square and returns to the line again, tagging the first child in line. This continues throughout the squad. The winning squad is the one that completes the correct sequence of collecting numbers the quickest. If the squares are placed one on top of the other when each child reaches the end of the line, an easy check can be made for errors. A set of numbers must be made for each squad playing. This game can be varied by counting by twos, fives, tens, and so on.

Language arts

Activities involving motor skills can make written and oral lessons much more exciting than normal paper-pencil tasks.

Alphabet grid. The alphabet grid can relate directly to learning and spelling lessons presented in the classroom. Students can follow the letters consecutively to help learn the alphabet or create their own games by spelling words. Similar to the numeral grid, this activity can be either teacher or child directed. Spelling the word wrong or jumping on the lines would constitute an error, and the next child would enter the game. When using a pocket grid, blends can be substituted for single letters and the child can be asked to jump on the group that is at the beginning or end of a word. This can be varied by having the child jump on a blend and then give a word that begins or ends with it.

Another activity that involves oral expression is to draw a trail of consecutive numbers with pictures or objects on each square that relate to a particular story that has been either read in class or assigned for the children to read. Selecting a number from the roll of a die, the child would hop on the square of that number and tell something about the story in relation to the object or picture in the square. An adaptation of this game would be to put single words in the square and ask the child to relate something about the story based on the particular word that was stopped on.

Making letters. This creative movement game is played in exactly the same way as Making numbers (see p. 243), except that letters are used instead. Some of the problems that might be posed are, "Using your body, make the first letter of your name," "Spell your whole name," "Show me your initials."

Jump rope rhymes. Jumping rope can be much more fun when a specific rhyme is chanted. The great variety of rhymes allows children to select favorites and become involved with the challenge of not missing a jump until the rhyme is completed (see Chapter 14).

Talking games. Games such as Midnight or Red Rover require oral expression. In the game New Orleans, children chant and pantomime a particular occupation or act in addition to the chasing activities in the game.

Storytelling games. There are a number of storytelling games that can be played, most of which end up in some kind of a chase or movement activity described in the action. One way to play the game is to have a child create and tell a story. Upon hearing a given word, previously selected by the child and told to the class, the other children are to run to a goal line before the storyteller is able to tag them. Those who are tagged can be put in "jail" until all but one is caught. The last remaining child starts a new game.

Social studies

Game activities can also be used in social studies. Each school should have a large map of the United States drawn on a plastic sheet or painted on the playground. Children may jump in the states and name them, continuing in the game until they miss or make errors. The game may be extended by having students name not only the state but the capital, major products, or primary industry. Lakes, rivers, and bordering bodies of water can also be included.

Dance and games. Dance activities lend themselves quite well to social studies lessons. When countries or cultures are being studied, dances can be taught that are specific to that particular region of the world or group of people. Activities of this nature often result in an exciting type of pageantry when native dress is worn and makes the unit of study much more meaningful. In addition to learning the dances from around the world, children also will have lots of fun learning new games that are related to a particular culture. By learning games that are played in foreign countries or are unique to specific groups, children often achieve a greater understanding and improved retention of knowledge about that country or group. When studying the Olympic Games and participating in a modified version of the ancient Olympiad, children are better able to trace the history of the event and understand its purpose in today's world.

Art

Illustrating activities. Some of children's more interesting illustrations are those of game or sport figures. Allowing students to illustrate sport activities of interest to them will result in a variety of art forms, such as drawings, posters, or collages (Fig. 11-7). By selecting a game or particular skill and attempting to show it through an art concept, children often recreate dramatic moments in sport. Many of these art projects can be used in a public relations program that will provide a showplace for student art and apprise the community of what is being done in the school's physical education program.

Color chase. The children form two lines facing each other. The teacher stands behind one line and holds up a square of colored paper. The children in the line who can see the color use nonlocomotor movements to try to describe the color to the opposite line. Children may attempt to describe objects, moods, or places that would indicate the color they are looking at. When the color is guessed correctly, the teacher goes behind the other line and follows the same procedure. The line using the fewest guesses is the winner. An adaptation of this game would be to have the children chase the team that is acting out the color as soon as the correct color is guessed. Those being tagged would move over to the other line and another game would begin.

Movement design. Children are asked to make designs of their choosing on pieces of paper. After making the drawings, each child is asked to create a movement activity that describes his or her design. One picture may be selected from the group and the total class may be asked to create movements describing the design. Children may be selected to show how they would move to describe the drawing.

Painting in space. Children may work in pairs with one "painting" an object by moving the arm through space. The second child is asked to name what the first one is painting by watching the movements. Once the object is guessed correctly, the game continues with first child acting out the color of the object created and the second child guessing. Places should then be switched.

• • •

Teachers should continually seek new ways of incorporating motor activities

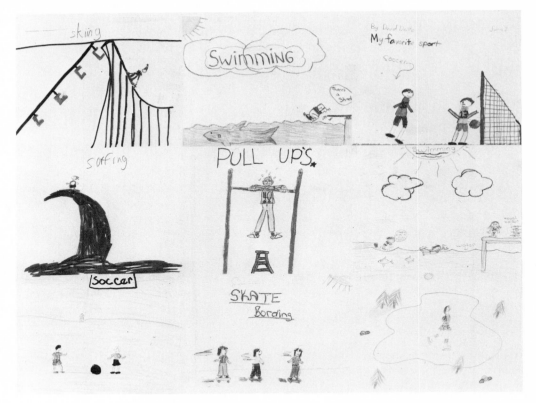

Fig. 11-7. Sample third grade art projects depicting sports activities.

with classroom learning. Multisensory learning has received increased attention in recent years. It is an untapped source of vital teaching techniques that can add immeasurably to the fun and retention of learning. One will be amazed at the many, often overlooked opportunities that could enhance the learning process in all subjects taught.

CLASSROOM GAMES

Most physical education lessons are taught in a physical education facility such as a gymnasium or playground. However, in some cases, because of inclement weather or scheduling conflicts, it is necessary to use the classroom for play space. The following activities have proved to be successful games and challenges suited to the classroom environment.

7-UP

Behavioral objective: To use strategy in deciding who to tap and self-restraint in keeping eyes closed

Developmental goal: Patience, self-control, honesty, and auditory discrimination

Space and equipment: Classroom

Number of players: 20 to 40

Procedure: Seven children are chosen to be "it" and come to the front of the room while the rest of the children in the class remain seated. The teacher or a chosen leader says, "Heads down, fingers up." Each child still seated puts his or her head down on the arms on the desk and holds up the index finger of one hand. As soon as all the children have their eyes closed and their fingers up, the chosen seven go among the players; each taps one child's finger, which the child then lowers so that a duplicate tap will not occur. The tappers go to the front of the room and the leader says, "Heads up, 7-up." Each child who was tapped stands and gets a turn at guessing who tapped him or her. A

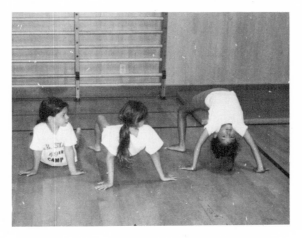

Fig. 11-8. Playing the game forty ways to get there.

child who guesses correctly becomes a tapper and the original tapper goes to his or her seat. After a child has been a tapper three times and has not been replaced, a new tapper can be chosen. Children must keep their eyes closed until they hear the signal, "heads up." It is the responsibility of the leader to disqualify peekers.

FORTY WAYS TO GET THERE

Behavioral objective: To devise original movement patterns

Developmental goal: Creativity, memory, and originality

Space and equipment: Classroom

Number of players: Entire class

Procedure: Each child is given a chance to move across the front of the room in any manner he or she wishes. Once a child has used a walk, hop, or any other movement, no one following may copy that movement. Any novel way of moving is acceptable (Fig. 11-8).

CHARADES

Behavioral objective: To interpret ideas in movements without using words

Developmental goal: Imagination, teamwork, and cooperation

Space and equipment: Classroom

Number of players: Entire class

Procedure: The children are divided into small groups. Five or six groups are selected and allowed sufficient time to work out a charade together. A captain is elected for each group. The work or object that each group chooses to act out should have syllables to make it easier to act out. All dramatizations must be in pantomime. One group acts out its charade in front of the class. The captain of the group asks the class to guess the syllable or complete word. If the word has not been guessed within a certain time, the captain tells the class and the next group takes its turn.

GOOD MORNING

Behavioral objective: To listen to a voice and correctly guess who the speaker is by his or her voice

Developmental goal: Auditory discrimination and self-control

Space and equipment: Classroom

Number of players: 5 to 40

Procedure: The children sit at their desks. One child (John, for example) stands in the front of the room with his back toward the group. The teacher silently chooses another child (Jane, for example) to play the game. Jane approaches the standing child and says, "Good morning, John." Without turning his head, John guesses the name of the speaker. If he is unsuccessful, Jane repeats her salutation. If John is still unsuccessful, he returns to his seat, and Jane becomes the guesser. If John is successful, he remains the guesser, and a new player approaches and greets him. The children should not be allowed to disguise their voices in this game.

HUMPTY-DUMPTY, STRAWBERRY PIE

Behavioral objective: To find an object and give others a chance to find it

Developmental goal: Figure-ground discrimination and self-control
Space and equipment: Classroom
Number of players: 5 to 40
Procedure: All the children except one leave the room or remain seated and cover their eyes and ears and rest their forehead on the desk. One child hides a selected object someplace within the room so that it is accessible to all but not too much in view. The children then return to the room or open their eyes and hunt for the object. As each child discovers the hiding place, he or she goes to his or her seat as quietly and inconspicuously as possible and, when seated, and not before, announces, "Humpty-Dumpty, strawberry pie!" Play continues until all have spotted the object or until the teacher calls off the hunt. The child who first discovered the object must retrieve it and then becomes the next player to hide it. In order to keep some children from being embarrassed at being last, the teacher should call off the hunt when three or four are still looking.

HENS AND CHICKENS

Behavioral objective: To listen for a sound and determine its source
Developmental goal: Auditory perception and self-control
Space and equipment: Classroom
Number of players: Entire class
Procedure: The children remain seated. One child is chosen to be the hen and goes to the cloakroom or hall. While the hen is out of the room, the teacher walks around the room and taps several children, who become chickens. All the children then place their heads on their desks, hiding their faces in their arms. The hen comes in and moves about the room saying, "cluck, cluck." All the children keep their heads down, and the chickens answer, "peep, peep." The hen listens and taps any child on the head who he or she believes is a chicken. If the hen is correct, the chicken must sit up straight; if the hen is incorrect, the chicken continues to hide his or her head. After all the chickens have been selected, the hen or the teacher selects a new hen.

FIND THE MOON ROCK

Behavioral objective: To find a hidden object through auditory discrimination

Developmental goal: Auditory perception and figure-ground discrimination
Space and equipment: Classroom
Number of players: Entire class
Procedure: The children decide on an object to be hidden. It should be a small object or pebble to represent the moon rock. The teacher chooses one player to be the astronaut and sends him or her out of the room while the class hides the moon rock. When the astronaut enters the room and approaches or moves away from the moon rock, the class may hum or clap, loudly or softly, depending on the position of the astronaut in relation to the moon rock. When the astronaut finds the moon rock, he or she chooses another astronaut.

SIMON SAYS ✓

Behavioral objective: To listen for an oral command and follow it with an action
Developmental goal: Auditory perception and honesty
Space and equipment: Classroom
Number of players: 6 to 30
Procedure: A leader is chosen to stand in front of the children, who stand or sit, but preferably stand. The leader gives commands to jump, bow, turn right, and so on. If the command is preceded by the phrase "Simon says," it is to be obeyed by all the players. If the phrase "Simon says" is omitted by the leader, the command is to be ignored. If a player fails to obey a command preceded by the phrase "Simon says" or obeys one not preceded by this phrase, he or she is eliminated. The last player to remain in the game is the winner. If the group is large, the last five or ten players may be declared the winners.

CLOTHESPIN DROP

Behavioral objective: To sight and to drop a clothespin into a bottle
Developmental goal: Eye-hand coordination
Space and equipment: Classroom or gymnasium, milk bottle, and five clothespins
Number of players: Entire class
Procedure: Each row of children in the classroom is a team. A milk bottle is placed in front of each row. The children take turns standing erect above the bottle and dropping five clothespins, one at a time, into the bottle. One point is given for each clothes-

pin that is dropped into the bottle. The row with the highest total wins.

WASTEBASKET BALL

Behavioral objective: To throw accurately at a target
Developmental goal: Eye-hand coordination
Space and equipment: Classroom, wastebasket, and ball
Number of players: Entire class
Procedure: The game may be played by teams or classroom rows. A captain is selected to keep score on the blackboard, and a child is selected to return the ball. The teacher places the basket on a chair at the front of the room and marks a line with chalk on the floor at least 5 yards from the basket. Each child takes a turn standing on this line and trying to throw the ball into the basket. Everyone is allowed three trials, with an additional trial for every ball thrown into the basket. One point is given for each ball successfully placed. After all the children have played, the captain announces the winning team or row.

CRUMPLE AND TOSS

Behavioral objective: To crumple and accurately throw a piece of newspaper
Developmental goal: Fine muscle coordination and accuracy
Space and equipment: Classroom or gymnasium, wastebasket, and newspaper
Number of players: Entire class
Procedure: The children form two lines facing wastebaskets, with the front player 6 to 10 feet from the basket. The first player in each line is given a piece of newspaper, which he or she must crumple with one hand. The player attempts to throw the crumpled paper into the basket. After the first child has thrown, he or she goes to the back of the line, and the next player moves up to the front of the line and takes a turn. The team with the largest number of papers in the basket at the end of the game wins. A half sheet of newspaper works best for crumpling and throwing. The children should crumple the paper tightly enough that it goes where they aim it. The goal of this game should not necessarily be speed, but accuracy.

NUMBERS CHANGE

Behavioral objective: To listen for numbers and to execute a movement change quickly and safely
Developmental goal: Decision making and quickness
Space and equipment: Multipurpose play area or gymnasium
Number of players: Entire class
Procedure: The children sit in a circle, with the child who is "it" in the center. The children are numbered consecutively. "It" calls out two or more numbers, such as 3, 9, and 17. The children whose numbers are called must quickly jump up and exchange seats, during which time "it" tries to take one of the seats. The player left without a seat becomes "it" and calls out other numbers.

SEAT TAG

Behavioral objective: To safely tag another child and to avoid being tagged in a limited area
Developmental goal: Agility and coordination
Space and equipment: Classroom or gymnasium
Number of players: Entire class
Procedure: One child is "it," and another is a runner who "it" chases about the room. The other children remain seated. The runner may sit down with some other pupil, and that pupil then becomes "it" and must chase the one who was "it." If "it" tags the runner, the positions are reversed, the runner becoming "it."

BEANBAG PASS

Behavioral objective: To pass an object quickly and accurately
Developmental goal: Speed and accuracy in handling an object
Space and equipment: Classroom with desks in rows and beanbags enough for each row
Number of players: Entire class
Procedure: The child in the first seat of each row is given a beanbag. On command, the beanbag is handed to the child in the seat directly behind and so on until it reaches the end of the row. When the beanbag reaches the end of the row, the last child goes quickly to the front of the row and holds the bag high. The first row accomplishing this task is the winner. To keep students from rushing to the front, the

teacher can ask that the beanbag be passed back from child to child until it is returned to the head of the line.

HOT ROCKS

Behavioral objective: To move safely and quickly

Developmental goal: Agility and object management

Space and equipment: Classroom, beanbag, record, and record player

Number of players: Entire class

Procedure: Players sit in their seats with their hands on their desks. One child is given a beanbag to carry. The teacher starts the record player and the child with the beanbag runs up and down the aisles and gives it to another player. This player gets up, runs up and down the aisles, and gives it to another child before the music stops. The one who has the beanbag when the music stops is out of the game. The last child in the game is the winner. A child must run at least the length of one aisle before giving the bag to someone else.

LAST SEAT OUT

Behavioral objective: To react quickly to a tactile signal

Developmental goal: Agility and speed

Space and equipment: Classroom with desks in rows

Number of players: Entire class

Procedure: One child from each row is selected to stand at the back of the row. On the command "go," each child at the back runs forward and touches the hand of the child sitting in the first seat of his or her row. The child who is touched stands up and the runner takes the vacant seat. The child who has just risen touches the person behind and takes that seat. This procedure continues until all the children have been touched and the child in the last seat rises and runs to the front of the row. The game is won when the last child is standing straight at the front of the row.

Paper play

FALLING LEAF

Behavioral objective: To track falling paper and catch as close to the floor as possible

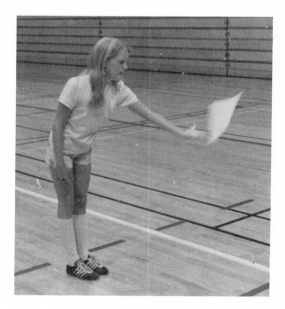

Fig. 11-9. Falling leaf.

Developmental goal: Eye tracking and hand control

Space and equipment: Classroom and onionskin paper

Number of players: Entire class

Procedure: Each child should be given a piece of onionskin paper. When holding the paper high and parallel to the floor, the child is asked to let it drop. The task is to see how close he or she can let the paper get to the floor before catching it on the edges. The paper will fall to the floor like a leaf, taking a different path each time it is dropped (Fig. 11-9).

PAPER WAVES

Behavioral objective: To keep the paper on the hand by maintaining a smooth motion

Developmental goal: Flexibility, bending, stretching, and smoothness of motion

Space and equipment: Classroom and onionskin paper

Number of players: Entire class

Procedure: Each child should place the paper flat on the palm of the hand. By keeping the hand moving, the children will be able to wave the paper through the air in different patterns (Fig. 11-10). As long as the wind resistance is kept constant the paper may be moved up and down, through the legs, and behind the back. Children should be en-

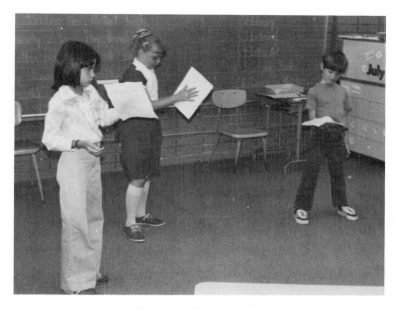

Fig. 11-10. Paper waves.

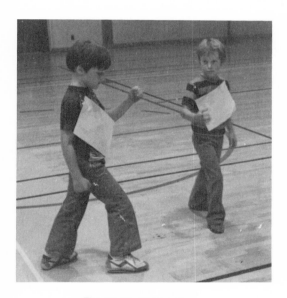

Fig. 11-11. Paper chase.

couraged to move the paper in as many different ways as possible.

PAPER CHASE

Behavioral objective: To move safely in space

Developmental goal: Agility and movement control

Space and equipment: Classroom or multipurpose area and onionskin paper

Number of players: Entire class

Procedure: The children place the paper flat on their chests and let go after beginning to move around the room. While looking to avoid colliding with other classmates, the children move in space, keeping the paper on their bodies as long as possible (Fig. 11-11). The winner is the last child moving about the room with the paper still on his or her chest. Children must move in a controlled fashion but fast enough to keep the paper pinned to their chests.

COLORED DISKS

Behavioral objective: To balance objects on the palms of the hands

Developmental goal: Flexibility and balance

Space and equipment: Classroom and two cardboard disks, 9 inches in diameter, for each person in the class

Number of players: Entire class

Procedure: Each child is given two colored disks and asked to perform a variety of balance tasks with the disks, such as balancing one in each hand (Fig. 11-12, A). The tasks can be performed by other parts of the body, such as the head, knee, or foot (Fig. 11-13). More advanced students can pass the disks between their arms and bodies, bringing the disks out to the side (Fig. 11-12, B and C), and then can bring them back the same way

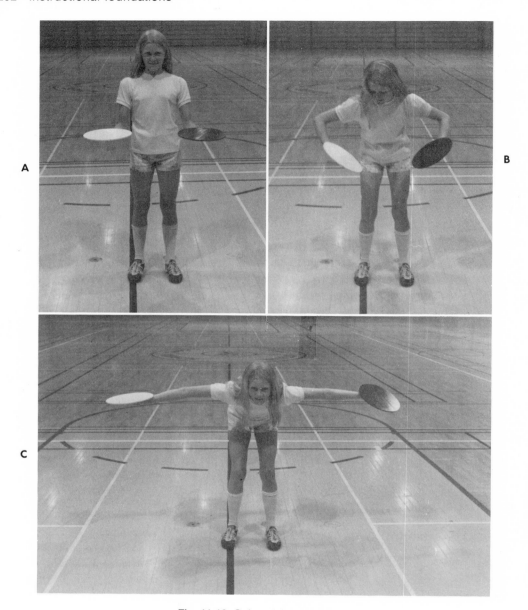

Fig. 11-12. Colored disk activities.

or perform a figure eight by passing a disk from one hand to the other, going around and through the legs.

Balloon play

A good way to develop eye-hand coordination in a limited space is to use a balloon. The slow movement of the object makes catching and striking skills much easier to accomplish.

BALLOON ACTIVITY

Behavioral objective: To listen for directions and develop accurate catching and striking skills

Developmental goal: Eye-hand coordination

Space and equipment: Classroom and balloons enough for all

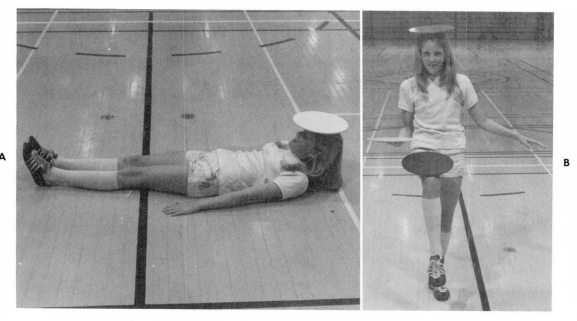

Fig. 11-13. A, Head balance; **B,** head, hand, and knee balance.

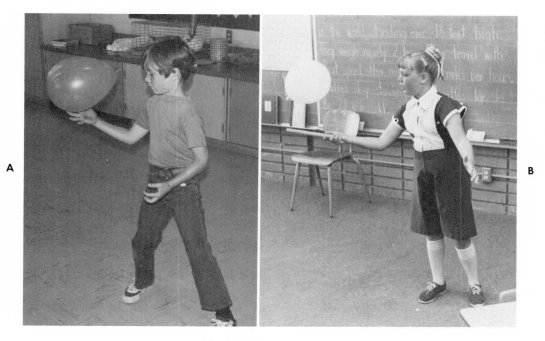

Fig. 11-14. Balloon games.

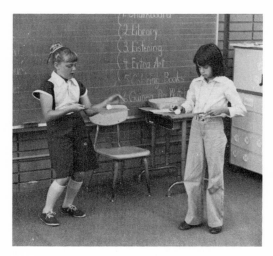

Fig. 11-15. Stretch ball.

Number of players: Entire class

Procedure: Each child is given a balloon. The teacher gives numerous directions, such as batting the balloon with the right hand and then the left hand and then alternating hands (Fig. 11-14). One can also count to see how many hits a child can make before the balloon strikes another object or falls to the ground. The same activity can be played using the foot or other parts of the body or an implement, such as a dowel stick. If space permits, simple games of balloon volleyball, using a string for a net, or target games, using a suspended hoop for a target, can be played.

Ball play

STRETCH BALL

Behavioral objective: To hit the ball as many times as possible in succession

Developmental goal: Eye-hand coordination

Space and equipment: Classroom or multipurpose room, panty hose rackets, and whiffle golf or yarn balls

Number of players: Entire class

Procedure: Each child should have a panty hose racket made out of a hanger as described in Chapter 3. By using a small yarn ball or a whiffle golf ball, children can count how many times they can consecutively hit the ball on the racket (Fig. 11-15). Better players may work in pairs and play mini-tennis by hitting the ball back and forth to each other if space allows.

Finger play

Young children like to play with their fingers. Finger games can give children a break from classroom routine and can be used with any size group. They are quiet and, because specific hand actions are required, they can be a great aid in settling down a group. Participating in finger games on a regular basis relieves classroom tensions, develops auditory skills, and provides training and enjoyment in rhythm and fine motor activities (Fig. 11-16).

As children grow older these games often develop into chanting and patting rhymes performed with a partner. Many of these chants not only feature rhythm and rhyme but cause the students to use cross-over hand patterns that help develop laterality. A further extension of fine motor training is the inclusion of string manipulation games such as cat's cradle.

THE KITE

I often sit and wish that I
  (Put hands under chin.)
Could be a kite high in the sky,
  (Lift a hand up in the air.)
And ride upon the breeze and fly
  (Make hand bob up and down.)
Whichever way I care to try.
  (Move hand back and forth.)

TWO HOUSES

Two little houses closed up tight,
  (Make two fists.)
Open up the windows and let in the light.
  (Make two small circles with thumb and index finger.)
Ten little children tall and straight,
  (Hold up fingers.)
Ready for school at half past eight.
  (Flutter fingers.)

JACK-IN-THE-BOX

Jack-in-the-box is shut up tight.
  (Make box by forming a fist with one hand with the thumb resting on top for a lid.)
Not a speck of air or light,
  (Insert index finger of the other hand inside the box for Jack.)

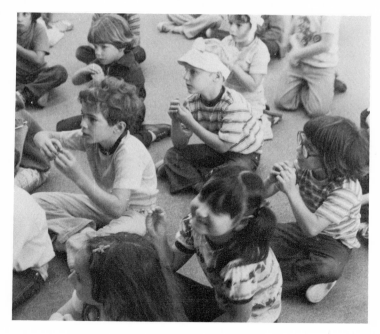

Fig. 11-16. Finger play activities.

How dark it must be,
He cannot see.
Open the lid and up he jumps.
    (Push index finger out of the box as the
    lid opens.)

AIRPLANES

Here's the little airplane,
    (Hold right hand in air, palm down.)
Zooming way up high.
    (Move hand in the air.)
Here's the bright and shining sun,
    (Make a circle with the fingers of both
    hands.)
Watching it pass by.
    (Look up and raise hands up high.)
Here's a big, black, ugly cloud,
    (Ball up the fist of the left hand.)
Dripping drops of rain.
    (Open fingers of the left hand and flutter
    them.)
Here's the thunder, booming loud,
    (Clap hands.)
Booming once again.
    (Clap hands again.)
Then here's the little airplane,
    (Move right hand in the air.)
Zooming from the sky,
    (Keep moving hand.)

Moving to its hangar where it will be so dry.
    (Cup left hand, "fly" airplane into it.)

HICKORY, DICKORY, DOCK

Hickory, dickory, dock,
    (Place right elbow in left palm. The raised
    right arm swings back and forth.)
The mouse ran up the clock.
    ("Run" fingers of the left hand up the
    right arm.)
The clock struck one,
    (Raise the index finger of the right hand.)
The mouse ran down,
    ("Run" fingers of the left hand down the
    right arm.)
Hickory, dickory, dock!
    (Hold arm upright and swing back and
    forth as in first movement.)

BEES

Here is the bee hive.
Where are the bees?
    (Cup the left hand downward with the
    fingers of the right hand hidden under it.)
Hidden away where nobody sees.
Soon they come creeping out of the hive.
One, two, three, four, five.
    (Make fingers of the right hand creep out.)
Buzz, buzz, buzz-zz-z z-zz.

(Make fingers of the right hand "fly" around.)

Tactile discrimination

THE FEELY BAG

Behavioral objectives: To identify objects or shapes and sizes by tactile discrimination

Developmental goal: Development of tactile skills

Space and equipment: Feely bag with various objects

Number of players: Entire class

Procedure: A cloth bag or a box with a cloth cover, having a hole just large enough for the hand to enter, is filled with a variety of small objects. A child reaches into it and attempts to identify an object by feel alone. The child continues to feel and identify objects until an error is made. The winner is the child who can successfully identify the most objects. A variation of the game is to place a series of like objects of different sizes into the box. Objects such as marbles, squares, or triangles are numbered consecutively from small to large. The child attempts to pick out the smallest object and progress sequentially to the largest without making an error (Fig. 11-17).

FITNESS IN THE CLASSROOM

Although the activity space may be limited to the classroom, this does not make impossible the inclusion of fitness activities. All the components of fitness suggested in Chapter 10 can be incorporated into the limitations of the classroom. Cardiovascular development, strength development, and flexibility activities are easily adapted to this area.

Cardiovascular development

Running in place. Children can be asked to stand at the sides of their desks and run in place, lifting their knees high. The teacher can control the pace by varying the tempo of the stationary run.

Jumping in place. Jumping in place is another limited space activity. On command children can jump eight times facing forward, turn a quarter turn to the right for eight jumps, and continue quarter turns until they reach the beginning position. The teacher may give directions to turn in different directions for variety.

Shadow jump rope. Children can simu-

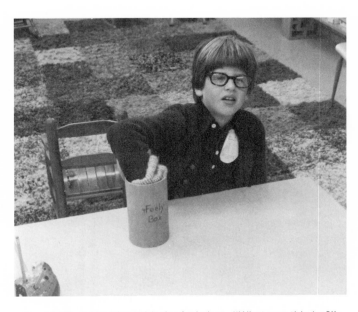

Fig. 11-17. Having fun with the feely bag. "What can this be?"

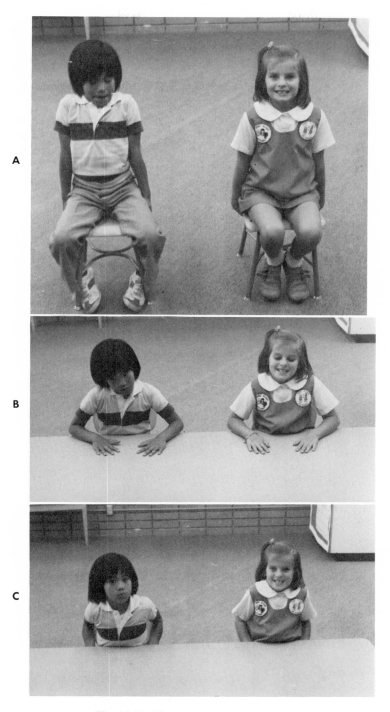

Fig. 11-18. Classroom isometric exercises.

late jump rope routines by turning their arms as if holding a rope. Different tricks can be put together to create a jump rope routine. Children can experiment and demonstrate their ingenuity through different movement patterns.

Strength development

While sitting at their desks or tables, children can develop strength through isometric activities.

Upper-body strength. Students can be asked to grasp the outside of their desks or chairs and push inward for 6 seconds and release on command (Fig. 11-18, A). By pushing down or pulling up, the children can strengthen different muscle groups (Fig. 11-18, B and C). If desks are not practical to use, the children may push their hands together or grasp other parts of the body to gain resistance as the muscles are contracted. It is recommended that a series of three, 6-second repetitions be used in each position.

Teachers should be careful not to overdo the use of isometric exercises with children since structurally they are still in the growing stage.

Leg strength. Students can hold a half knee bend for 6 seconds and repeat it at least three times. Vertical jumps for height can also be accomplished in limited space. If space permits, follow the leader can be played using the crab walk, seal walk, or other stunts requiring strength in upper- and lower-body parts.

Flexibility

Bending, stretching, and swaying in a variety of ways can develop flexibility. The teacher can ask the children to touch their toes, bend backward, or stretch to the side. For creative stretching in limited space, the teacher can ask the students to bend as many ways as possible while keeping their feet flat on the floor or to perform any other problems involving flexibility.

CLASS ACTIVITIES

1. Create a new finger play activity and present it to the class.
2. Develop a mathematics lesson using a ball.
3. Describe three ways to teach a geography lesson with a jump rope.
4. Discuss how motor skills can be incorporated into a science lesson.
5. Develop a physical fitness lesson suitable for the classroom in which the children work in pairs.
6. Write a mini-paper on the advantages of integrating cognitive learning with motor activity.
7. Develop 12 story game cards for use in the pocket grid.
8. Construct a feeley bag containing at least seven different objects.

REFERENCES

1. Getman, G.: Keynote speech, Conference of the California Association for Health, Physical Education and Recreation, Anaheim, California, 1977.
2. Kephart, N. C.: The slow learner in the classroom, Columbus, Ohio, 1960, Charles E. Merrill Publishing Co.
3. Klasen, E.: Audiovisual motor training with pattern cards, Palo Alto, Calif., 1969, Peek Publications.
4. Orff-Schülwerk: A means or an end? The School Music News (New York School Music Association) **31**:5-8, 1968.

RECOMMENDED READINGS

Block, S. D.: Me and I'm great, physical education for children three through eight, Minneapolis, 1977, Burgess Publishing Co.

Barlin, A., and Barlin, P.: The art of learning through movement, Pasadena, Calif., 1971, The Ward Ritchie Press.

Cratty, B.: Active learning: games to enhance academic abilities, Englewood Cliffs, N.J., 1971, Prentice-Hall, Inc.

Fait, H. F.: Physical education for the elementary child, ed. 3, Philadelphia, 1976, W. B. Saunders Co.

Gilbert, A. G.: Teaching the three R's through movement experiences, Minneapolis, 1977, Burgess Publishing Co.

Humphrey, J. H.: Education of children through motor activity, Springfield, Ill., 1975, Charles C Thomas, Publisher.

Latchaw, M.: Human movement: with concepts applied to children's movement activities, Englewood Cliffs, N.J., 1970, Prentice-Hall, Inc.

12

The exceptional child: from the limited to the gifted

Too often, physical educators have been guilty of lumping children into large groups without regard for individual capabilities or potential. Such groups are usually geared to the so-called normal class ability, so that the gifted or the less able children are often thwarted in their efforts to succeed. Because physical education is important to people of all ability levels and ages, provisions should be made within each school to ensure that every child has an opportunity to engage in a well-organized and well-conducted program. We believe that, ideally, all physical education should be adapted to individual needs rather than conducted on a mass basis with the child adapting to a set program; however, realistically, this may be feasible only for the education of the exceptional individual in which special provisions are made for program adaptations. There are within every school and community exceptional children with very special requirements (Fig.

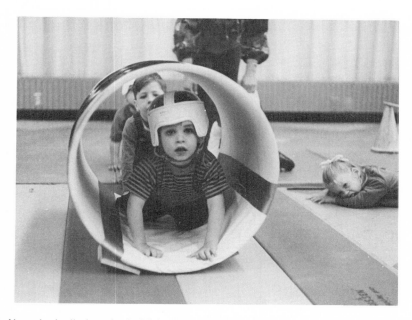

Fig. 12-1. Neurologically impaired children developing spatial awareness. (Photo courtesy Lyonel Avance and photography by Anita Delfs, Special Education Branch, Physical Education Project, Los Angeles City Schools.)

12-1). It has been estimated that over 12% of American school age children are exceptional to some degree and require a modification of school practices or special services out of the ordinary in order for them to reach their maximum potential.[1] Exceptional children are those that are physically and mentally gifted as well as those that have physical, mental, and emotional impairments or disabilities.

In the decade of the 1970s there has been a great thrust forward to provide educational services for the United States' over 6 million physically limited children, especially for those many children receiving no or minimal educational services. An important trend has been the instituting of the *mainstreaming* concept, in which handicapped children are integrated into the regular classroom program whenever feasible. Children who are mainstreamed may spend the entire day or a portion of the day with their non-handicapped peers. Those spending part of the day in the regular classroom may spend the remaining time in a special education program or may receive physical or occupational therapy.

Another highly important factor in the education of handicapped children has been PL 94-142, a federal law that mandates that, no matter the degree of disability, every child has a right to be educated to his or her fullest potential and that every state and school district must ensure the education of that child. Under PL 94-142 every handicapped child will have an individual program plan that fully promotes his or her education within the classroom and in physical education, along with additional special education and/or therapeutic services that may be required.

INDIVIDUALIZED INSTRUCTION

A number of teaching methods are currently being employed throughout the country that are designed to personalize teaching. Most of these methods have been successful with the special education and adapted physical education classes that have a limited number of students.

Modification of behavior

Out of the work of Skinner[8] and the influence of computer science have grown many current educational approaches that are designed to modify individual behavior through stimulus-response learning. Operant conditioning and positive reinforcement or variations of them are commonly employed to change behavior. Operant conditioning differs from classical conditioning in that a behavior produces the reinforcement rather than a simple involuntary reflex response as in Pavlov's salivating dog. In this approach, particular target behavior is determined by the teacher, and an intervention program is instituted to elicit that particular behavior. This is commonly known as behavior shaping. The target may be to acquire a simple behavior such as a habit of proper grooming or a more complex behavior such as overcoming a difficult reading problem or learning to perform a difficult sport skill. Positive reinforcement of a specific behavioral response might be more adult or peer attention, food, money, or permission to participate in a special activity. For children, a reward can be anything that brings pleasure, such as love or praise. Some basic rules for rewarding are as follows:

1. A new behavior that is being learned must have an immediate reward.
2. In the later stages of learning a behavior, rewards can be given less often.
3. In the early period of learning a new behavior, rewards are given for accomplishment of less complicated tasks.
4. In the later period of learning a new

behavior, rewards are given for increasingly larger accomplishments.
5. When a behavior is not rewarded, it will eventually become extinct.

Prescriptive method

Prescriptive teaching is well suited to individualized instruction in both the classroom and physical education settings. The following steps are taken in establishing and initiating an educational prescription:
1. The teacher selects an evaluation tool (test).
2. The teacher evaluates the child's achievement with the tool.
3. The achievement test is assessed.
4. From the assessment, the teacher determines an educational diagnosis.
5. From the diagnosis, a prescription of how to overcome a specific problem is determined.
6. After establishing the prescription, the teacher gives a prognosis as to when the problem will be overcome.

In most cases, the prescriptive teaching method is task oriented and utilizes operant conditioning methods; however, it is assumed that the teacher has a good diagnostic tool and that the teacher can accurately assess the test findings. This method individualizes instruction because it focuses attention on each child's personal strengths and weaknesses.

Contract method

The contract method takes the prescriptive method a step further by involving the child in the decision-making process. After assessing the child, the teacher establishes specific objectives or goals to be accomplished. Each goal is broken down into logical task steps. Conferring with the teacher, the child contracts to work on specific task areas and agrees on the reinforcement that follows the accomplishment of each task.[5] The contract method has been found to be self-motivating and extremely valuable for children with low self-esteem.[3]

Shifting of decision making

Education, in general, and physical education, in particular, have been guilty of not providing children with opportunities for making decisions. Physical education characteristically has been a field that has used the autocratic style of teaching with the major focus on the teacher as leader and the students as followers. However, the introduction of movement education has influenced some elementary schools to be more child centered (see Chapter 9).

Educators always ask how best to respond to the needs of children. There is no one best teaching method; children respond individually to various educational techniques. However, education should make it possible for each child to develop a positive self-concept and become a mature, self-reliant person with a clear understanding of his or her abilities. This concept is particularly important to exceptional children with special requirements. Before individualization can occur, a freeing process must take place that moves the student away from dependence on the teacher and toward independent thought and action.[6] The teacher can bring this about by gradually shifting decision making from himself or herself to the student.

INDIVIDUAL PROGRAMS

Four programs within physical education are specifically oriented toward the individual and modifying instruction. They are the programs for the physically gifted, physical development programs, remedial programs, and modified games and sports programs. Movement education is also mentioned because it is a teaching approach within physical education that encourages individualization.

Program for the physically gifted

Most schools and communities provide many opportunities for their physically gifted children through intramural and interscholastic sports. Intramural sports are usually offered to children in grades 4 and up. Although designed for all children within a particular school, intramural sports provide the physically well coordinated child an opportunity to learn and perform at a level higher than he or she commonly engages in as part of the regular physical activities program. A school's intramural program should consist of a variety of games and sports that encourage the development of a wide range of abilities such as locomotion, balance, agility, and eye-hand and eye-foot coordination as well as the elements of strength, endurance, and flexibility.

At the elementary school level, interscholastic sports, in which children perform against children from another school, are not widespread through the United States. However, community league, club, YMCA, and recreational department team competition is relatively common for the elementary school child. Such competition provides the athletically gifted child a chance to excel and the less-gifted child a chance to be a part of a cohesive group. Some antagonists of elementary school children's competing consider it educationally, physiologically, and psychologically harmful. This point of view has never been fully substantiated by scientific research; however, in some isolated instances physical and/or psychological harm can be directly related to sports competition at a young age (see Chapter 7). As discussed earlier, competitive sport is neither good nor bad inherently; whether it is good or bad depends on the leadership and the direction in which the child is motivated. The pro-

ponents of early athletic experience state that "engaging in athletic competition automatically instructs the participant in 'good sportsmanship.'" This is not the case; sportsmanship, like any expression of attitudes and values, must be overtly planned for and taught to the performer by the leader.

We consider it beneficial for the physically gifted child to have opportunities to excel at a sport; however, a number of dangers to the maturing child are inherent in continually engaging in one sport alone without a variety of movement experiences. Athletically gifted children, like all children, must experience a wide variety of movement activities if they are to reach their full potential. No one sport offers all that a child needs. Consequently, overemphasis of a sport must be avoided at all costs to ensure that the gifted child has a well-rounded physical, mental, and emotional development.

Physical development program

Development is that aspect of human evolving that is continuous and ongoing until full maturity is reached. Schools commonly use the term "physical development program" to refer to a program dedicated to assisting children who are physically subfit. An increasing number of school districts are providing special opportunities for children to raise their levels of physical fitness through individualized programs (see Chapter 10).

A primary goal of the physical educator is to develop within all students those physical attributes necessary for engaging in daily activities without undue fatigue and at the highest possible level of movement proficiency. Determining which children are physically underdeveloped or have poor stamina is difficult for most teachers, mainly because there are so many factors that must be considered. The diagnosis of physical and motoric deficiencies is usually determined through tests designed to measure the immediate status of the child. Selected tests should also motivate the child to improve as well as measure progress after the child has engaged in a prescriptive physical fitness program for a period of time.

Since physical development programs are individual in nature, with each child having unique requirements, the fitness program should be created cooperatively by the child and the teacher. The role of the teacher is to interpret the test findings and provide valuable information about the best way to overcome specific deficiencies. However, program decisions should be made by the child and the teacher together in a cooperative venture. Ideally, a fitness program, besides ameliorating specific problems, will be motivating enough that the child will want to maintain a high degree of fitness throughout his or her lifetime. This can be accomplished best when the decisions are personally made or agreed to by the teacher and child rather than thrust on the child from some outside source. Following are some suggested steps in decision making that the teacher may use to help the child overcome subfitness:

1. The teacher selects and administers the test.
2. The teacher discusses the test with the child.
   a. The teacher identifies weak fitness areas.
   b. The teacher suggests ways to overcome deficiencies.
3. The child and the teacher agree on ways to overcome deficiencies and the rewards to be earned.
4. The child and the teacher agree on the time to exercise each day.
5. The child keeps a personal progress record.
6. The child and the teacher agree when work load changes should be made.
7. Once the child reaches the fitness goals, the child and the teacher agree on the best ways to maintain

and perhaps increase the child's level of fitness.

Remedial program

In this text, remedial physical education (RPE) refers to that aspect of physical education concerned with working with specific physical, mental, and emotional problems through the medium of prescribed movement activities. The problems of the children who receive RPE range from minor to severe disabilities. A program of RPE may be conducted as part of a regular school curriculum or may be an integral aspect of a special school dedicated to children with specific handicaps, such as mental retardation, orthopedic handicaps, emotional disturbances, or the sensory deficits of blindness and deafness.

Primary objective. The primary objective of RPE is to assist the child in achieving the fullest potential possible in the area of mental, physical, emotional, and social development through a carefully planned and individualized program of physical education activities. The following opportunities should be afforded each child requiring special help:

1. To participate in a movement program of basic body management and perceptual-motor therapy for children with motor handicaps
2. To ameliorate postural defects and increase good body mechanisms
3. To become physically fit within limitations
4. To become aware of means of protecting himself or herself and preventing further aggravation of the disability
5. To develop desire and skill for engaging in leisure-time games and lifetime sports
6. To develop an appreciation of his or her physical and mental capabilities

Program organization. The majority of schools or school districts have children requiring modified physical education programs. At least 2% of the children in any school have medical problems so severe that they require a special class in physical education. There are a number of different ways in which a RPE program can be begun in a district. Ideally, each elementary school should have its specialists in physical education; however, in most instances this is too expensive.

One plan that has had some success is the *itinerant plan,* in which one RPE teacher is responsible for approximately three schools. Each day the itinerant teacher travels to and conducts one or two special physical education classes in the schools under his or her jurisdiction. Another plan that has found moderate acceptance is the *center plan,* in which children are bussed to a center specially designed and equipped for therapeutic physical education. Whatever plan is employed, the success of any program depends on the teachers and the backing they receive from the school administration and the community.

Identification of participants. Children may be identified as eligible for a remedial class by one of a number of sources. The classroom teacher often initiates the referral of a child who may display signs of physical, mental, or emotional problems. The regular physical educator also refers children who, because of some apparent problem in performance, are not finding success in regular physical education. Other referrals may come from physicians, nurses, and psychologists.

Advisory committee. Once children's needs for special adaptations in physical education have been identified, they are referred to an advisory committee. The advisory committee is composed of people from a number of different disciplines, the choice of which depends on the particular needs of the school and community. Commonly seen on such a committee are a physical educator, a medical representative (physician or nurse), a counselor, an administrator, a special education teacher, a parent, and perhaps a member from a community

handicap organization. The committee members support the RPE program by making themselves available for advice when special problems arise. They can be called on to assist in selecting the children who have the most need for such a program.[1]

Individualization of methods. A remedial program must be individualized in order to be successful. The teacher's approach may be similar to that in the developmental program. Children requiring specialized exercises or activities should have their programs placed on cards. Young children or those unable to record their own progress should dictate the information to a recorder. Program changes should be conducted through communication between the child and the teacher. If children understand their particular problems and are reasonable in the understanding of their abilities, they should eventually be able to develop their own programs without assistance.

Aides are extremely valuable in individualizing programs for handicapped children. Paid aides, parent aides, and student aides provide a valuable service in freeing teachers from many time-consuming chores, such as lifting children in and out of wheelchairs and putting on and removing braces, so that they have more time for individual instruction and class administration. If a teacher does not have delegated aides, the more capable children within the class can assist and thus gain personal reward and free the teacher for individual help.

Modification of activities. Extremely important to individualized instruction is the modification of physical education activities for children with special needs. In every physical education program, not just in special classes, provisions should be made to adapt games and sports. Some of the reasons for modifying activities are as follows:

1. Modifying activities gives opportunities to play games to children who otherwise would be unable to.
2. It provides possibilities for engag-

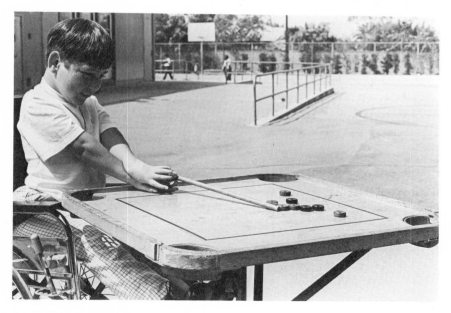

Fig. 12-2. Carom game can be enjoyed by all. (Photo courtesy Lyonel Avance, Special Education Branch, Physical Education Project, Los Angeles City Schools.)

ing in some form of active play in later life.

3. It provides a wholesome emotional release for children who may be confined.

4. It can be a therapeutic adjunct to a program of physical therapy.

5. It adds elements of fun to perhaps an otherwise monotonous existence.

Games and sports can be modified to meet personal requirements so that they are safe and at the same time developmentally sound. The innovative teacher can create many games that include competition and excitement for every performance level (Fig. 12-2). Generally, activities can be modified by changes in duration, speed, intensity, and space for performance. The teacher can modify activities as follows, when adapting them to children with special needs:

1. By decreasing the size of the playing area

2. By changing the size of the implements of the game

3. By increasing the number of players

4. By changing the rules

5. By shortening the game time

6. By reducing the number of points in a game

7. By freely substituting the players

8. By changing the positions of the players readily

Modified games and sports program

The concept in physical education of modifying games and sports is applicable to every grade and level of ability, although it is most often applied to children with special needs. It means that a teacher and the curriculum are flexible enough to accept all children as individuals and to make program modifications accordingly. The committee on Adapted Physical Education of the American Association for Health, Physical Education, and Recreation (AAHPER) defines adapted physical education as "*a diversified program of developmental activities, games, sports, and rhythms suited to the interests, capacities, and limitations of students with disabilities who may not safely or successfully engage in unrestricted participation in the vigorous ac-*

tivities of the general physical education program.'' This statement implies that physical education should be available to all children no matter what physical, mental, or emotional problems they may have.

Movement education

Movement education induces children to accept personal differences and to progress at their own rates. Through solving movement problems and analyzing themselves, children explore and discover their own motor abilities. By increasing their sensory awareness, children learn to solve complex movement problems involving the factors of space, force, and time (see Chapter 10).

SPECIAL CONCERNS

The elementary school teacher will be confronted with many children who require special considerations when engaging in physical activities. Children having special needs are often categorized as impaired, disabled, or handicapped, but these terms are not synonymous or necessarily interchangeable. An *impairment* is an identifiable organic or functional condition that may be either permanent or temporary, such as a behavioral maladjustment or the lack of a limb resulting from an amputation. On the other hand, a *disability* is a restriction in the execution of a particular skill as the result of an impairment. Finally, a *handicap* is the psychological, emotional, or social effect of an impairment or disability. A handicapped person is one who views himself or herself as being unable to overcome the obstacle of an impairment or disability.[9]

Motor disturbances

Motor disturbances can range anywhere from subtle movement difficulties to very obvious asynchronous move-

ments. There are many causes, and the assessment of them is often difficult, requiring the assistance of a professional team of neurologists, pediatricians, psychologists, and educators. Children with moderate to severe cerebral dysfunction often are under the care of a physician and a physical therapist. However, less understood but more often seen are the children who display clumsiness.

The "clumsy child syndrome" is a catch-all term for the lack of coordination of some children in the execution of certain motor tasks.[2] This deficit may be attributed to heredity, central nervous system disorder resulting from disease or injury, perceptual-motor dysfunction, sensory impairment, and emotional problem; all these factors can contribute, in part or in combination, to a child's lack of coordination. Poor coordination may be manifested by large-muscle awkwardness in running, walking, or throwing or catching a ball or in the fine eye-hand coordination activities of playing with building blocks or writing. It should be noted that every child shows clumsiness in certain movements; however, the child who repeatedly displays problems in a number of movement tasks may require special help.

Children with motor difficulties are often failures at play. They are relegated by their peer group to being chosen last and to playing in the least desirable roles or positions in a game. This chain of failure events may be compounded and cause a feeling of inferiority and a fragile ego later in life. Intervention programs should be instituted as early as possible. There is good indication that basic motor development programs provided for young children with coordination difficulties can prevent them from having many problems when they are older.

Children with movement problems should be provided with as many opportunities as possible to engage in a wide variety of movement experiences (Fig. 12-3). An individualized program should

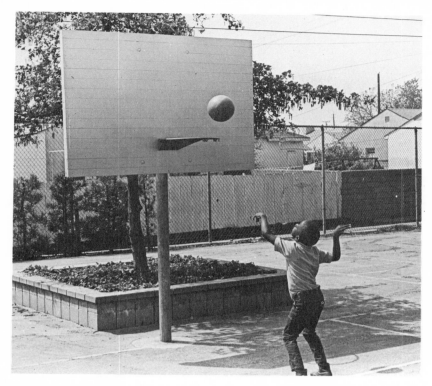

Fig. 12-3. Basketball shooting task for child with motor disturbances. (Photo courtesy Lyonel Avance, Special Education Branch, Physical Education Project, Los Angeles City Schools.)

be developed by the teacher that accentuates activities that will help to remedy a specific motor problem. Areas of remediation should be broken down into a logically sequenced set of tasks, from the simple to the more complex. For example, children with static balance difficulties might start with tasks requiring that they stand with both feet together for 10 seconds and progress to a very difficult task of balancing with one foot on a 1-inch-wide board. After successfully completing a task, the child is given the positive reinforcement of praise or a more tangible reward such as points, food, or free activity time.

Learning impairments

Children with learning impairment fall into two major categories: those with normal intelligence who have disabilities in some aspect of the learning process and those who have general intellectual retardation. Each type of child must be considered educationally unique.

Educational disability. It has been estimated that almost 20% of children in the United States who are within the normal range of intelligence are educationally disabled. These children have been variously called perceptually handicapped, neurologically impaired, minimally brain-damaged, educationally handicapped, and dyslexic. Whatever the label, this disorder is manifested primarily in the communication arts of reading and writing. Children who are educationally disabled may also be awkward and clumsy in small- or large-muscle activities, or conversely, they may be athletically gifted. Children with perceptual disorders may have difficulty in processing information in one or two perceptual channels such as vision and audition (see Chapter 11).

Mental deficiency. The American Association on Mental Deficiency (AAMD) refers to mental retardation as a subaverage general intellectual function occurring during the individual's developmental period and associated with an impairment in adaptive behavior.[1] As does a person in any segment of the population, the mentally deficient child attempts to adapt to the environment; consequently, the most descriptive evaluation of the retarded child is that of how well he or she reflects appropriate behavior in meeting the demands of the particular culture. If individuals can adequately adjust to the responsibilities of society, it is difficult to say that they are incompetent. In other words, it is very difficult to differentially diagnose the exact level at which a child is functioning since the only criterion may be poor performance in school, whereas maturation and social adjustment may be considered normal. Generally speaking, trainable mentally retarded children are unable to develop usable skills to achieve academically and are impaired in maturation and social adjustment. On the other hand, educable mentally retarded children can achieve academically, but their performances are significantly below average for their ages. In contrast to children who are classified as having learning disabilities, mentally retarded children are generally slow and have limited abilities.

Following is a list of some causes of mental deficiency in children:

Genetic irregularities
1. Inheritance that produces mental deficiency
2. Genetic disorders caused by factors such as overexposure to x rays and infections
3. Errors in metabolism
4. Rh blood factor incompatibility
Adverse events during pregnancy
1. Infections (German measles)
2. Glandular dysfunctions
3. Toxic poisoning

4. Faulty nutrition
Adverse events at birth
1. Prolonged labor
2. Too rapid birth
3. Premature birth
4. Factors that reduce the amount of oxygen transported to higher brain centers
Adverse events after birth
1. Childhood diseases such as whooping cough, chickenpox, measles, meningitis, scarlet fever, polio, and encephalitis
2. Glandular dysfunctions
3. Trauma
Adverse cultural and environmental events
1. Cultural deprivation
2. Serious emotional problems

Mentally retarded children, besides being low in intelligence, may also be limited in motor fitness, motor skills, and recreational skills. They need opportunities to experience a good physical education program. Increasing their physical ability through motor activities may provide them with opportunities for enriched leisure time and perhaps even possibilities for employment.

Basic to all movement is motor fitness. Without an efficient fitness level, the retarded child characteristically has muscle hypotonicity (low muscle tone) and is flabby and unable to engage successfully in a wide variety of movement activities. It is obvious that if the retarded child's motor fitness is increased, he or she will fatigue less, be less obese, become efficient in body mechanics, and be able to learn basic motor skills more readily.

Because retarded children mature and learn at slower rates than average children, they may be denied opportunities for learning basic movement skills, such as running, jumping, climbing, throwing, catching, kicking, and striking. Therefore, they should learn basic motor skills before they attempt more advanced activities; the learning of basic movement skills is followed by the learning of rhythms and games of low organization, which lead in turn to the learning of the more advanced activities of dance, gymnastics, and sports. Many retarded persons, depending on their level of intelligence, with patient instruction, may be able to learn complex motor activities.

Essential to a fruitful life is the ability to perform recreational skills. For many retarded persons the enjoyable experiences of life are extremely limited; therefore, the physical education program should offer instruction in recreational and leisure-time activities. Through these activities, retarded children can increase their physical capacity, social awareness, use of leisure time, and ultimately, their occupational potential. Following is a list of some techniques for teaching mentally retarded children motor skills:

1. Group the children according to interest rather than age.
2. Use small groups instead of large groups.
3. Choose games with few rules.
4. Limit competition with other children.
5. Include opportunities for immediate success in each activity.
6. Take part in the game.
7. Use exclusion from a game or a decrease in playing time as discipline.
8. Give opportunity for free play.
9. Closely supervise to recognize dangers.
10. Make explanations about activities short, concrete, to the point, and without abstraction.

Emotional disturbances

Educators are becoming increasingly aware of children who are emotionally disturbed. Characteristically, these children are inflexible in their behavior and impaired in their ability to adjust to a changing environment. More specifically, these children often find difficulty in learning, getting along with other children, engaging in motor activities, and conducting themselves appropriately under normal social conditions.

Emotional disturbance encompasses many personality and behavior traits that range from hyperactivity to hypokinesia and withdrawal. Some abnormal behavior characteristics that directly affect the learning process are hyperactivity, impulsiveness, disorganization, distractibility, figure-ground confusion, and perseveration (Table 12-1); these are generally considered impulse disorders. In general, a child with this set of behavior characteristics requires a highly structured and predictable environment. Following is a list of principles for the teacher who may be working with emotionally disturbed children with impulse disorders:

1. Remove distractions from the environment.
2. Overstimulate except in cases of hyperactivity.
3. Give concrete descriptions of rules and games.
4. Give manual guidance in learning basic skills.
5. Select tasks within each child's ability.
6. Give immediate reinforcement for an accomplished task.
7. Avoid overengaging in the same activities.
8. Encourage the child in a positive self-concept at all times.

Physical education provides many opportunities for emotionally disturbed children to develop appropriate behavior. Through a well-planned program, they can acquire basic movement and game skills as well as learn to get along with other children. Personal constraint gained from encountering frustrations with other children on the playground may carry over to the classroom.

Following is a model of a planned intervention program for children with motor impairments:

A. Primary program: efficiency in movement
B. Secondary objectives
1. General body management
2. Object control

Table 12-1. Emotional disturbances in children

Behavior disturbance	Characteristics	Intervention	Implications for physical education
Hyperactivity	Moves constantly; has high energy level; is usually aggressive; is unable to focus attention.	Decrease distractions; direct energy to one task.	Simplify rules of game; individualize instruction; pick play activities in which there are few distractions.
Impulsiveness	Exhibits unplanned, meaningless, and often inappropriate behavior.	Provide highly structured setting with no distractions; give concrete directions.	Provide activities that are distinct and maintain interest.
Disorganization	Exhibits random behavior; cannot listen; performs pointless activities; has untidy habits.	Provide highly structured setting with no outside distractions; pick short tasks with immediate reward.	Pick activities that require distinct sequencing, such as rhythms.
Distractibility	Cannot focus attention; is easily distracted by outside stimuli.	Structure the environment; decrease stimulation; use single-task approach.	Pick low-expectation activities; emphasize instruction with highly distinct aids, such as bright colors; provide individual instruction.
Figure-ground confusion	Cannot distinguish figure from background, visual and/or auditory.	Accentuate figure by decreasing background.	Play ball games against a plain, light background; give directions simply and concretely.
Catastrophic reaction	Has low frustration level; exhibits explosive behavior; has abnormal fears; overreacts to threatening situations.	Structure routine; use positive approach.	Keep games at low excitement level; prevent unexpected situations; teach rules concretely; keep distractions to a minimum.
Perseveration	Cannot shift attention; is locked into a specific behavior and automatic response.	Separate by physical means; provide distinctly different tasks.	Avoid activities that are too highly sequenced, such as bouncing a ball and marching; change activities often to create dissimilarity.

3. Body control on apparatus
4. Emotional control
C. A multisensory approach to movement: the acquisition of motor skills
D. Primary developmental areas
  1. Gross motor development

2. Fine motor development
3. Perceptual-motor development
4. Body image and spatial awareness
E. Admission evaluation in the areas of
  1. Balance

2. Gross body control
3. Eye-hand coordination
4. Dexterity
5. Simultaneous motor control
F. Specific intervention task areas in
1. Relaxation-tension recognition
2. Locomotion
3. Balance
4. Movement exploration
5. Rebounding
6. Body awareness
   a. Directive
   b. Reflective
7. Manipulation
8. Play
   a. Throwing
   b. Catching
   c. Kicking
   d. Striking
9. Posture control
10. Motor fitness
11. Classroom transfer activities
G. Gaining emotional control by
1. Behavioral modification through positive reinforcement
2. Structuring the environment
3. Gradual introduction of stress
4. Planned social behavior
5. Child counseling and family education*

Heart and respiratory problems

The elementary school teacher is often confronted with the problem of instructing children who have heart or respiratory problems. Over half a million children have heart disorders, the majority of which are attributed to rheumatic fever, which is caused by a hemolytic streptococcus infection. This infection within the bloodstream attacks the heart valves in some individuals. If the valves are af-

---

*This program model was developed by the Institute for Sensorimotor Development conducted at the California State University at Long Beach and was designed primarily for children who are considered awkward in their motor behavior, many of whom also have learning disabilities, emotional disturbances, and perceptual-motor impairments.

fected, the heart may lose its pumping efficiency. In such cases, the child becomes less able to engage in physical activity; the extent to which he is able depends on the amount of damage. Second to rheumatic heart disease in incidence is congenital malformation of the heart. Defective fetal development causes the malformation of the heart and/or blood vessels.

Graded exercise is generally considered good for children with heart or lung defects if it is given in the proper amounts based on individual capacity. It is desirable that children with heart conditions be classified by a physician as to their exercise levels. Following is a classification system based on the child's ability to engage in physical activity:

Class A: Needs no activity restriction.

Class B: May conduct normal daily activity but cannot participate in competitive activities.

Class C: Must be moderately restricted in daily activity routine and is not allowed to participate in strenuous activities.

Class D: Must be markedly restricted in all physical activities.

Class E: Must be confined to bed or chair.

Although the classifying of a child with a heart condition may assist a teacher in selecting correct activities, the best indicators are how the individual child reacts to activity. Contraindicated activities would be those that cause an accelerated pulse, shortness of breath, weakness or dizziness after exertion, undue fatigue, or a higher level of excitement.

Common to most schools throughout the country are children who have respiratory problems. The most prevalent lung condition is bronchial asthma. Asthma is obstruction of the bronchial tubes caused by muscular spasm and an excess of fluid secreted from the mucous lining. Some of the factors causing asthma attacks are irritations from air contaminants or allergy-producing substances and abnormal physical or mental stress.

Like children with heart problems, those with lung problems must be given graded activity programs based on individual requirements. Care must be taken so that an attack is not caused by overexertion or overexposure to extreme temperatures.

The teacher should adhere to the following rules in planning a program for children with heart or lung problems:

1. Avoid breath-holding activities.
2. Avoid causing breathlessness.
3. Reduce the speed of activities.
4. Reduce the number of activity repetitions.
5. Provide rest between exercise bouts.
6. Avoid high-level competition.

Most of the activities presented in this text can be specifically selected or modified to suit the needs of children with heart or lung problems. For example, if children are in class B and must avoid high-level competition, the teacher can select games for them to play, such as ball passing, nine court basketball, and steal the bacon.

Visual limitations

Children with visual limitations may be placed in special education programs or may be mainstreamed into the regular classroom. In either case, the educational curriculum must be modified to meet their unique requirements.

Two educational classifications are used for children with visual defects: blind and partially sighted. Legally, the degree of blindness is determined by a test of visual acuity. The legally blind person is one who has a visual acuity of not more than 20-200 after correction; in other words, he can see 20 feet away what a person with normal sight can see 200 feet away. A legally partially sighted person is one who has a visual acuity of less than 20-70 after correction. A person who has a visual field of 20 degrees or less (tunnel vision) also may be deemed legally blind or partially sighted.

There are four basic causes of visual limitation: refractive error, structural defect, infectious disease, and imbalance in eye muscle function. About 50% of all visual defects are caused by errors in refraction, that is, the bending of light rays as they enter the eyes that results in the focusing of images on the retina.

Children with visual impairments often have developmental lags in all areas of classroom, social, and motor responses; consequently, the expectations of these children must not exceed their particular level. This is not to say that children with visual problems cannot reach their full mental and physical potential; it does mean, however, that special efforts must be made to help them arrive at their maximum level of achievement.

Physical activity is essential in providing visually limited children opportunities for adjusting to the demands of their environment. Only through the senses of feel, movement, and hearing can these children learn about their physical world. Accurate body awareness is particularly important to blind children for acquiring knowledge of their positions in space. Before blind children can be free to move around, they must have a sense of "whereness."[4]

Through physical education the lives of blind and partially sighted children can be enhanced socially, emotionally, and physically. Many games, sports, rhythmics, and stunts are available that require use of the senses of audition, tactility, and kinesthesis. Activity adaptations can be made so that the sense that the blind child has most available is used. Through vocal guidance by a teacher or a classmate, the blind child can enjoy many ball games and stunts. Many running activities are possible for the visually limited child through the sense of feel and the guidance of a string or rope.

Lower-limb disabilities

It is not uncommon to find children with lower-limb disabilities mainstreamed into regular classrooms or placed in special classes in a regular school setting. Such children may have defects such as congenital malformation, arthritis, paralysis, and lack of a limb because of amputation. Their mobility potential may vary from limited locomotion with braces on their legs or with crutches to permanent confinement in a wheelchair. Whatever their restrictions, these children should have physical activities adapted to their particular needs. Like all children, those with lower-limb defects need social opportunities, emotional outlets, a sense of accomplishment through play, and improvement of the motor fitness factors of strength, flexibility, and stamina.

The adapted program for children with lower-limb problems may be divided into the development of basic motor skills, stunts, games and sports, rhythmic skills, and motor fitness.[7] Because of their limited mobility, children with lower-limb disabilities should be given every opportunity for experiencing basic movement activities. Success at this level will provide self-confidence and a foundation for learning high-level activities.

Stunts, games, and sports can be suited to individual capabilities. Stunts can be executed that require little leg support, if any, such as tumbling, apparatus performance, and rope climbing. Many sports can be played from a wheelchair,

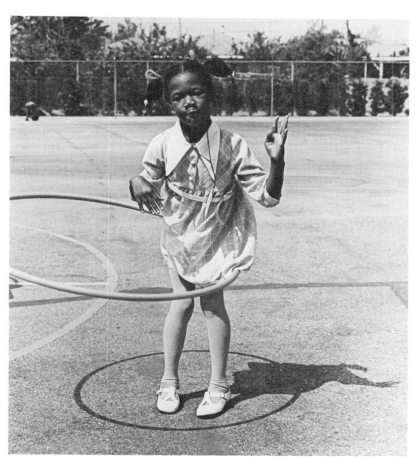

Fig. 12-4. Child with arm impairment performing a challenging task. (Photo courtesy Lyonel Avance, Special Education Branch, Physical Education Project, Los Angeles City Schools.)

such as bowling, badminton, and basketball. Other games can be modified to be played by a child in a wheelchair, such as swinging-ball games like tetherball and target games, or to be played by a child on crutches, such as soccer or relays.

Motor fitness is of extreme importance to the child with limited movement. The development of arm and shoulder strength and stamina is essential if the child is going to enjoy a full and productive life.

Upper-limb disabilities

Like children with lower-limb defects, those with upper-arm disabilities vary in their educational needs. Occasionally the teacher will have a child who, because of paralysis or congenital malformation, does not have full use of both arms (Fig. 12-4), although most frequently an affected child has single-arm involvement, such as that resulting from an amputation, with full use of the other arm. The latter children can engage in a full activities program with the major emphasis placed on posture control, balance, and motor fitness to counteract the asymmetry caused by having one affected arm.

CLASS ACTIVITIES

1. Observe children who have one or more sensory deficits at play. How is their movement similar to or different from that of a child without this deficit?
2. Compare the play behavior of children who are considered mentally retarded with that of children who are physically gifted.
3. Adapt a common lead-up activity such as kickball for a group of children who have severe lower-limb disabilities.
4. How would you modify the rules for a child who is asthmatic?

5. Develop a personalized program for a child who is exceptional. In your plan, develop a contract with the child.
6. Teach a game activity to the class while they simulate blindness by use of blindfolds.

REFERENCES

1. Arnheim, D. D., Auxter, D., and Crowe, W. C.: Principles and methods of adapted physical education and recreation, ed. 3, St. Louis, 1977, The C. V. Mosby Co.
2. Arnheim, D. D., and Sinclair, W. A.: The clumsy child, St. Louis, 1975, The C. V. Mosby Co.
3. Bannatyne, A., and Bannatyne, M.: Motivation management materials, Miami, 1970, Kismet Publishing Co.
4. Cratty, B. J., and Sams, T. A.: The body image of blind children, New York, 1968, American Foundation for the Blind.
5. Hoome, L.: How to use contingency contracting in the classroom, Champaign, Ill., 1970, Research Press.
6. Mosston, M.: Teaching physical education, Columbus, Ohio, 1966, Charles E. Merrill Publishing Co.
7. Sequenced instructional program in physical education for the handicapped, Los Angeles City Schools, Special Education Branch, Physical Education Project, Public Law 88-164, Title III, 1970.
8. Skinner, B. F.: Science and human behavior, New York, 1953, The Macmillan Co.
9. Stein, J.: A clarification of terms, J. Health Phys. Educ. **42:**63-68, 1971.

RECOMMENDED READINGS

Cratty, B. J.: Remedial motor activity for children, Philadelphia, 1975, Lea & Febiger.
Daniels, A. S., and Davies, E. A.: Adapted physical education, ed. 3, New York, 1975, Harper & Row, Publishers.
Humphrey, J. H.: Improving learning ability through compensatory physical education, Springfield, Ill., 1976, Charles C Thomas Publisher.
Sherrill, C.: Adapted physical education and recreation, Dubuque, Iowa, 1976, William C. Brown Co., Publishers.

PART FOUR

INTRODUCTION TO ACTIVITIES— FROM DISCOVERY TO COMMAND

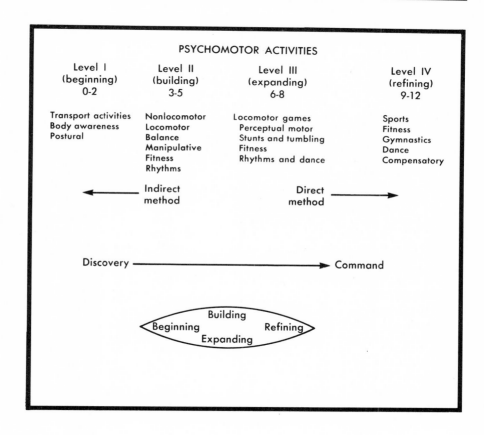

We have designed the activity section to coincide with the developmental levels presented in Part Two. Through this approach the reader will discover a logical method of selecting activities that are suited to the abilities of specific groups of children. One can further improve the activity selection process by referring to the suggested percentages of activity categories listed in Chapter 3. This procedure allows for a balanced program of body management, movement exploration, rhythms and dance, and games and sport activities, providing a variety of participation related to general developmental needs. For more sophistication, activities in levels 2, 3, and 4 are listed with behavioral objectives and developmental goals and are related to the seven-item Basic Motor Ability Test described in Chapter 2. Through the use of this test, the teacher is able to effectively prescribe a physical education program based on specific information that has been identified and computed to give a clear picture of individual and group needs.

Activities begin with an emphasis on the discovery, or indirect, method of the teaching-learning process and progress to the command, or direct, method at the higher levels, in which more sophisticated skills are learned and the child has identifiable, successful motor performance patterns. In other words, the child experiences movement activities through experimentation with what the body is capable of doing, expands to combine continued experimentation with some direct learning, and culminates with an emphasis on direct learning of sports skills along with creative innovations and the strategy of competitive activities.

It should be noted that some overlap occurs between levels, and it is quite normal for some classes to be motorically ready for activities in more than one level. It is the teacher's responsibility to identify proper levels and expand activities through creative program planning. The physical education curriculum is limited only by the enthusiasm and ingenuity of the teacher and should be individualized as necessary. When teaching specific skills, the reader is encouraged to refer back to the appropriate theory chapters for techniques and teaching methodology.

References are listed with the activity when appropriate, and a list of sources and materials is located after Part Four.

13

Level 1: Beginning

This chapter is concerned with developmental exercises and movement activities that are best suited for individuals whose levels of development range from infancy through toddling, as measured by a standardized developmental scale. We fully realize that teachers of children in preschool and elementary school would seldom work directly with children in nursery school, but these teachers may be confronted with individuals whose development in some areas of movement functioning is at level 1. This

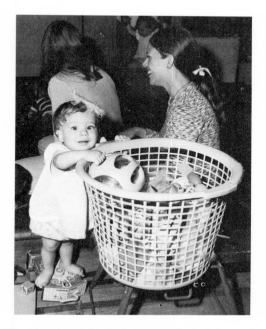

Fig. 13-1. A toddler is free to explore and to gain perceptual experiences through the medium of touch.

chapter has a three-fold purpose. It is designed to give the reader an appreciation of the fact that physical education commences at birth, that activities must be appropriate to a child's individual developmental level, and that level 1 activities may be used for remedial purposes for those children, particularly in preschool, who are performing below their expected level.

The period from birth to 2 years of age is known as the sensorimotor period. It is a time in which perception and motor responses begin to become integrated (Fig. 13-1). This chapter is organized to give the reader sample representative activities for specific developmental age levels. Two action categories are presented: *Developmental Movement Activities* and *Additional Activities and Experiences*.

FIRST MONTH AFTER BIRTH
General goals

The first month after birth is a time for the infant to adjust to living outside the mother. Activities should be concerned with producing postural adjustments, producing spontaneous reflex responses, and gaining head control.

Space and equipment

A firm surface, such as the floor or a table, that is covered with some soft material is needed.

Developmental movement activities

PICKING INFANT UP

Purpose: To stimulate the infant's postural reflexes

Procedure: The infant is picked up while lying in different positions, such as back-lying, front-lying, and left- and right-side–lying. Each time the infant is gently picked up, cradled in the adult's arms, and then returned to the starting position (repeat two or three times).

ROCKING

Purpose: To stimulate body positioning and postural reflexes

Procedure: The infant is gently and slowly rocked back and forth while held in different positions, such as on the abdomen, on the back, and on each side and while being carefully supported in a seated position (30 seconds in each position).

GRASP REFLEX

Purpose: To stimulate the grasp reflex

Procedure: Apply gentle pressure or stroke the infant's palms to cause the fingers to reflexively form a grip (repeat three to five times).

ROTATING FROM SIDE TO SIDE

Purpose: To stimulate the grasp and postural reflexes

Procedure: The infant grasps both of the adult's forefingers. Next, the infant's arms are straightened and slowly moved from side to side, causing the infant's head and upper trunk to move from side to side (repeat three to five times).

LEG STRETCH AND BEND

Purpose: To stimulate the reflex that causes each leg to straighten and bend

Procedure: Gentle pressure is applied to the soles of the infant's feet while in a back-lying position. When applied to the soles, the pressure causes the legs to alternately straighten and bend (repeat three to five times).

Additional activities and experiences

1. Show the infant brightly colored objects (18 inches from eyes).
2. Talk and smile at the infant.
3. Encourage the infant's eyes to follow a brightly colored object.
4. Rock the infant.
5. Gently stroke the infant's trunk and limbs.
6. Hum or sing to the infant.

FROM 2 TO 3 MONTHS OF AGE
General goals

By the time a month has gone by, the infant's adjustment to living outside the mother has almost been achieved. Developmental movement at this time continues to be concerned with postural control, particularly that of the head and trunk, as well as spontaneous and reflex behavior. Movement at this time should also be concerned with the development of eye and hand usage.

Space and equipment

All activities are conducted on a soft but flat surface such as a covered floor or table.

Developmental movement activities

MOVING THE INFANT'S LIMBS

Purpose: To gently stretch the major muscles of the infant's upper and lower limbs, stimulating muscle contraction (Fig. 13-2)

Procedure: While the infant is in a back-lying position, the arms or legs, either one at a time or in unison, are gently and slowly moved in a variety of directions, such as arms across the chest alternately, one arm overhead and one arm at the side alternately, or both arms overhead and to the side. The legs may be raised alternately, keeping the knees straight, or one may be rotated over the other in an alternating manner. Both feet might be brought up to touch the infant's chest or face in a rhythmical pattern while the adult sings a song or says a nursery rhyme (repeat each procedure three to five times).

SITTING UP

Purpose: To stimulate the muscles that bend the trunk forward and contract the thighs as well as the muscles of the lower abdomen

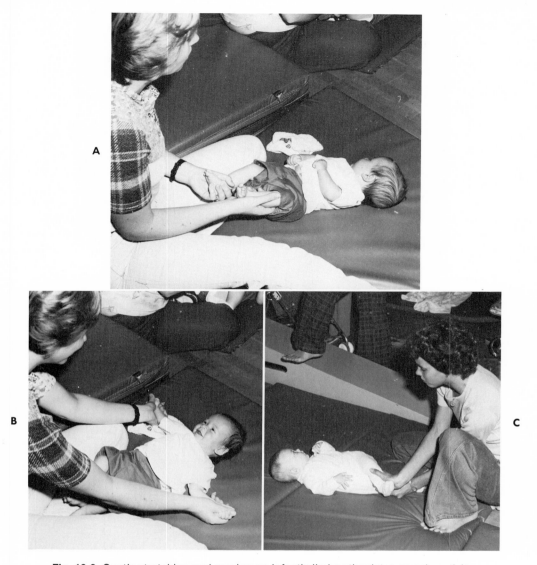

Fig. 13-2. Gently stretching and moving an infant's limbs stimulates muscle activity.

Procedure: The infant is placed in a back-lying position and the thighs are gently pressed downward at which time a sitting position is automatically assumed (repeat three to five times) (Fig. 13-3).

AUTOMATIC WALKING

Purpose: To stimulate the walking reflex which uses the muscles of the infant's legs and lower trunk
Procedure: The infant is supported firmly underneath the arms and lifted gently to a full-standing position. When pressure is

applied to the soles of the feet, because of the infant's weight on the floor, rhythmical steps will automatically be taken (repeat two or three times).

HEAD TURN AND BODY ROLL

Purpose: To stimulate the muscles of the neck and trunk
Procedure: While in a back-lying position, the infant's head is gently turned to the left and right. When the head is turned to one side the shoulders and trunk usually will rotate

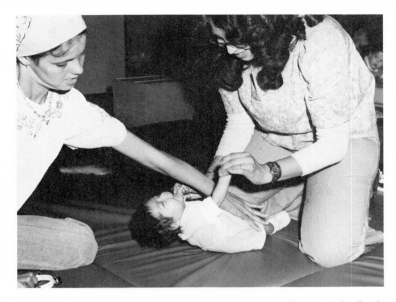

Fig. 13-3. A young infant who is placed in a back-lying position will automatically sit up when the thighs are pressed downward.

in the same direction (repeat three to five times on each side).

Additional activities and experiences

1. Change the infant's resting position.
2. Play with the infant's hands and feet and face.
3. Stroke the infant's body with hands or silky materials or both.
4. Encourage family interaction with the infant.
5. Hang brightly colored mobiles over the crib.
6. Tie a bell on the infant's ankle or wrist.

FROM 3 TO 4 MONTHS OF AGE
General goals

At 3 months the baby is able to perform voluntary activities involving the head, trunk, arms, and legs. Developmental movement at this time is designed to stimulate better postural control and encourage voluntary movement.

Space and equipment

Flat, soft surface, brightly colored toy, ball at least the size of a large beach ball; wedged-shaped pillow; two plastic rings or a ¼-inch diameter, 18-inch long wooden dowel, and a diaper, hand towel, or dishcloth are needed.

Developmental movement activities

FOLLOWING A TOY

Purpose: To track a moving object with the eyes, causing the head to be turned in the direction of the moving object

Procedure: While the infant is in a back- or front-lying position with the head in a midline position, a colorful object is introduced into his or her line of sight. By moving the object 16 to 18 inches above the infant's head, the adult can encourage movement of the eyes and head to the left and to the right (repeat three to five times on each side) (Fig. 13-4).

BODY TILT

Purpose: To stimulate postural responses

Procedure: The infant's trunk is grasped just

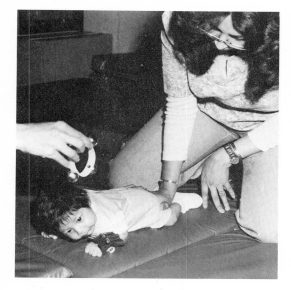

Fig. 13-4. Making a young infant visually focus on a brightly colored object while in a face-lying position stimulates the lifting of the head.

A 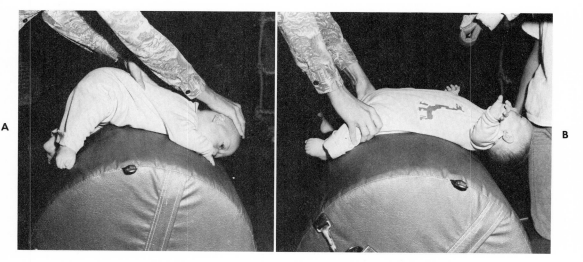 B

Fig. 13-5. A, Gently being rolled on a bolster to stimulate the balance senses. **B,** Stimulating the neck and trunk muscles.

below the arm pits. With the soles of his or her feet on a flat surface, the infant is first tilted to the left and to the right then forward and backward. The infant should maintain the head, although perhaps unsteadily, in the upright position (repeat three to five times in each direction).

ON A BALL

Purpose: To develop the sense of balance as well as muscles of the neck and trunk

Procedure: First, the infant is gently placed face down on ball at least the size of a beach ball. Supported at the hips, the infant is slowly moved back and forth and sideways in each direction on top of the ball. While face down the infant is encouraged to extend the head upward off of the ball. When at ease in the front-lying position the infant is then put in a back-lying position and again rolled in a variety of directions (repeat three to five times in each direction) (Fig. 13-5).

FLYING

Purpose: To strengthen the neck and back extensor muscles, decrease the infant's fear of heights, and adjust the infant to a relative lack of support

Procedure: The infant is placed on the adult's abdomen. The infant is held just above the hips and lifted gently above the adult's face. In this position, the infant's head will be lifted, legs extended backward, and back arched. The infant can also be moved back and forth and from side to side in this position (repeat three to five times).

LOOKING AROUND

Purpose: To stimulate neck and back extensor muscles and at the same time encourage focusing of the infant's eyes on an interesting object

Procedure: With the infant placed in a front-lying position, the lower legs are gently pressed down; this causes the head to be raised. In order to maintain this raised head position, the infant's elbows or a wedged pillow is placed under the chest. Once the infant's head is elevated correctly, a brightly colored object is placed in front of the face but just out of reach (repeat two or three times) (Fig. 13-6).

SIDE AND BACK LIFTING

Purpose: To strengthen the side and front trunk muscles (Up to this point emphasis has been placed primarily on developing back strength and control. This activity will assist in strengthening the abdominal muscles and muscles in front of the neck.)

Procedure: First, the infant is placed in a back-lying position. The adult grasps both of the infant's feet with one hand while with the other hand grasping the infant's side just below the arm pit. Gently, the infant is lifted up sideways. Both of the infant's sides should be exercised equally. Next, the infant is grasped between the hips and arm pits and gently lifted straight upward. If the infant's head sags when he or she is lifted, this exercise should be deferred until there is adequate strength in the neck (repeat each procedure three to five times on each side).

PULL TO A SIT-UP, THEN STAND-UP POSITION

Purpose: To strengthen trunk, legs, and arms and coordinate them for sitting and standing

Procedure: This is a two-fold activity. The infant is first pulled to a sitting position and then to a standing posture. In the back-lying position, the infant grasps either a dowel or

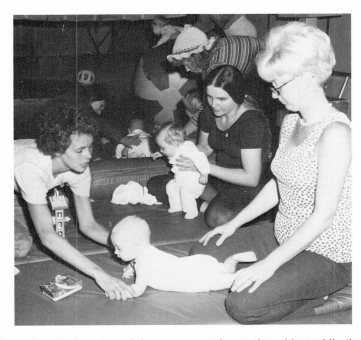

Fig. 13-6. Stimulating the focusing of the eyes on an interesting object while the head is raised.

ring held by the adult. While holding on to the object, the infant is gently pulled to a sitting position and, once sitting, is then carefully pulled upward until some weight is placed on the feet. When pressure is applied to the infant's feet, the legs will automatically extend and push down against the flat surface in a rudimentary attempt to stand (repeat two or three times).

CRAWLING IN AIR

Purpose: To stimulate those muscles that later will produce an actual crawling movement

Procedure: A diaper or cloth strip 4 or 5 inches wide is placed under the infant's chest. The ends of the strip are grasped to form a sling around the infant's trunk. The infant is then lifted 3 or 4 inches off the surface. When suspended, the infant will produce movements as if crawling or swimming (repeat three to five times).

Additional activities and experiences

1. Place a hanging ball (about 20 inches in diameter) over the crib to encourage eye-hand control.
2. Place brightly colored objects that can be touched over the crib.
3. Stimulate the infant's eyesight by moving objects in front of the face.
4. Encourage the infant to make verbal sounds.
5. Play peek-a-boo with the infant.
6. Massage the infant's skin with differently textured materials.
7. Keep the infant in places in the house and out of doors where there is activity.
8. Give the infant soft objects to manipulate.

FROM 4 THROUGH 6 MONTHS OF AGE
General goals

The major goal of developmental movement during this time is to continue to develop neck, trunk, and leg strength. Of special interest at this time is the strength of the hands and arms and their coordination with the eyes.

Space and equipment

A flat surface, a firm pillow or 8- to 10-inch diameter bolster, an 8-foot by 1-inch by 12-inch board, a toy, a 10-inch diameter suspended ball and a Jolly Jumper are needed.

Developmental movement activities

TUMMY STAND

Purpose: To stimulate those muscles that affect standing

Procedure: The infant sits on the abdomen of the adult. With his or her feet pressed against the abdomen of the adult the infant is slowly drawn upward to a standing position. As pressure is applied to the soles of the infant's feet, the legs will straighten automatically (repeat three to five times).

REACH FOR A TOY

Purpose: To combine the action of lifting the head, focusing on an object, and reaching for the object while supporting the trunk with the opposite arm

Procedure: While the infant is in a face-lying position, a toy is introduced just in front of his or her face. The infant is encouraged to focus on the toy and reach for it with one hand. The infant may have to be assisted by having the support elbow moved under the chest (repeat two or three times).

WHEELBARROW WALK

Purpose: To strengthen the arms, shoulders, and upper trunk

Procedure: The infant is placed over the edge of a firm, wedge-shaped pillow or bolster. From this position the infant is encouraged to wiggle and crawl off of the object by pushing with the legs and pulling with the arms (repeat two or three times).

OVERHEAD LIFT

Purpose: To stimulate neck and back muscles and to assist the infant in adapting to a position of less support

Procedure: The infant is grasped around the

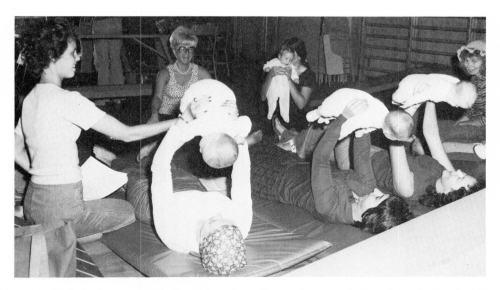

Fig. 13-7. While in the overhead lift position, these three infants are being stimulated to straighten their necks and backs.

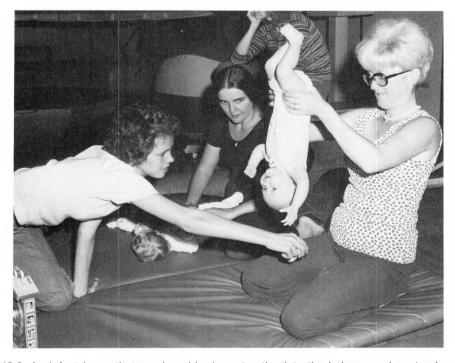

Fig. 13-8. An infant is gently turned upside down to stimulate the balance and postural senses.

trunk while in a back-lying position. The infant is then raised over the adult's head. When overhead, the infant will be stimulated to arch the back and lift the head (repeat two or three times) (Fig. 13-7).

CARRYING THE INFANT IN DIFFERENT WAYS

Purpose: To stimulate the posture senses and to develop adaptation to different body positions

Procedure: Vary the way the infant is carried, such as on the infant's back, abdomen, or side or in a back carrier (at least 30 seconds in each position).

TOPSY-TURVY

Purpose: To stimulate the balance mechanisms and adaptation to the upside-down position

Procedure: Supported just above the hips, the infant is gently turned upside-down (repeat two times and hold for 5 seconds) (Fig. 13-8).

LET'S ROLL

Purpose: To stimulate the locomotor skill of rolling and to strengthen those muscles that are involved in posture control

Procedure: Place the infant at the upper end of a ramp that has been elevated about 3 or 4 inches. Gently encourage the infant to turn the head, lift the shoulders, and roll down the ramp.

ROCKING CHAIR

Purpose: To stimulate the posture and balance mechanisms

Procedure: The infant lies face up cradled between the legs of the adult. Grasping the infant's wrists, the adult begins to rock gently back and forth, gradually increasing the length of the rock (repeat ten to 20 times).

JOLLY JUMPING

Purpose: To strengthen the leg muscles

Procedure: The infant is suspended underneath the arms or is placed in a Jolly Jumper* and gently encouraged to bounce

---

*This is a device that is suspended overhead and in which the infant sits free to push downward against the floor.

up and down by pushing against the floor (continue as long as the infant actively pushes).

HANGING BALL PLAY

Purpose: To gain leg and arm muscle control

Procedure: Suspend a 10-inch diameter, lightweight ball over the infant's crib. After elevating the infant's hips with a small pad or folded towel, the adult places the ball in such a position that pushing it with the feet is easy. After performing foot play, the infant is positioned so that hand play can be accomplished (continue until the infant loses interest).

Additional activities and experiences

1. Watch objects move.
2. Watch a stationary object while being moved.
3. Experience to different environments, such as the backyard or the park.
4. Determine where a sound is coming from.
5. Play with hands.
6. Touch one's own body.
7. Play with small objects that are different shapes.
8. Play with toys that make noise.
9. Feel different textured materials.
10. Play with cooking utensils.
11. Regard self in a mirror.
12. Play in water.
13. Play pat-a-cake.
14. Wave bye-bye.

FROM 7 THROUGH 9 MONTHS OF AGE
General goals

Some major concerns during this period are beginning locomotor activities, such as crawling and rolling, and gaining postural control of sitting and standing. This is also a time when there is a need to acquire greater control of small muscles that have to do with the skilled movements of the arms and hands.

Space and equipment

These activities require two or three obstacles, such as cardboard boxes or chairs; a regular-size ladder; a ½-inch diameter, 18-inch long dowel; a mattress or bouncy surface, such as a trampoline; a pillow; a towel; a toy; and an 8-foot by 12-inch by 1-inch ramp.

Developmental movement activities

CRAWLING OVER OBSTACLES

Purpose: To develop locomotor control and spatial awareness

Procedure: The adult sits on the floor with legs outstretched. The infant is placed on the adult's lap and encouraged to crawl over the adult's legs and chest. Once this task is accomplished, other obstacles might be used, such as pillows or rolled up towels (continue until the infant loses interest or tires).

CRAWLING UP AND DOWN A RAMP

Purpose: To strengthen the muscles involved with locomotion

Procedure: A ramp is elevated 3 or 4 inches at one end. Starting at the bottom, the infant is encouraged to crawl up and then down the ramp (repeat three or four times).

LADDER CRAWL

Purpose: To develop crawling coordination and strength in muscles concerned with locomotion

Procedure: The infant is placed at the end of a ladder laid flat on the floor. A toy is placed between two of the ladder rungs just out of reach of the infant, who is then encouraged to crawl over the rungs to the toy (repeat two or three times).

CRAWLING UNDER, THROUGH, AND AROUND

Purpose: To develop spatial awareness

Procedure: Set up an obstacle course that allows the infant to crawl under an object, such as a chair, through something, such as a tunnel made out of a box, and around objects, such as pillows or books (continue until the infant loses interest or tires) (Fig. 13-9).

HIP HANGER

Purpose: To stimulate the protective reflex mechanism of the arms and to adapt to the upside-down position

Procedure: The infant is placed in a back-lying position. Grasping the hips of the infant,

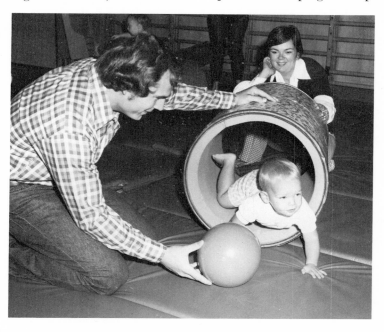

Fig. 13-9. Crawling through a tunnel helps to develop self-awareness and spatial awareness.

the adult lifts straight upward until the infant's head is off the floor by about 2 or 3 inches. When free of the floor, the infant will normally raise the arms out to the side and arch the back. The infant is then returned to the back-lying position (hold the hanging position for 5 seconds).

ROLLING THE INFANT

Purpose: To stimulate the postural and balance mechanisms

Procedure: The infant is placed on the floor and rolled first in one direction and then in the other by the adult (repeat two or three times).

TUG-OF-WAR

Purpose: To strengthen the hand grip, arms, shoulders, and upper back

Procedure: Both the adult and infant sit facing one another. Both grasp a dowel then proceed to push and pull back and forth. Movement can also be made from side to side or in a twisting fashion (repeat two or three times).

STAND UP, SIT DOWN—I

Purpose: To develop muscle strength in those muscles that are involved in standing and upright locomotion

Procedure: The adult kneels facing the infant, who is held upright by the hands. The adult bends the infant slightly at the hips and pushes backward until the infant falls gently into a sitting position. Gradually the infant is encouraged to sit voluntarily (repeat three to five times).

BOUNCY BOUNCY

Purpose: To stimulate the balance and postural mechanisms

Procedure: The infant is gently bounced while on a soft resilient surface such as a bed or trampoline in back-lying, front-lying, side-lying, sitting, and standing positions (repeat the bounce in each position five to ten times).

Additional activities and experiences

1. Climb up and down stairs.
2. Climb up a ladder with rungs between 4 and 6 inches apart.
3. Make noisy toys work.
4. Play crawl chase.
5. Walk while being supported.
6. Put small objects into a jar and then take them out.
7. Pull a pull or push toy when crawling.
8. Scoop something up with a large soup spoon.
9. Pull a drawer out.
10. Hold a glass with both hands and drink.
11. Cuddle a favorite toy.
12. Find a missing object.
13. Finger feed self.
14. Listen to different sounds.
15. Make different sounds with mouth.

FROM 10 THROUGH 12 MONTHS OF AGE
General goals

During this period the emphasis is on developing prelocomotor skills leading up to walking and postural control.

Space and equipment

For these activities a large ball, tables and chairs, two or three cardboard boxes, a balance beam or 8-foot long, 6-inch wide board, and a blanket or large beach towel are needed.

Developmental movement activities

HANDWALKING

Purpose: To encourage the development of arm and shoulder strength

Procedure: From a face-lying position, the infant is lifted by the thighs to an upside-down position. By pushing forward gently the adult can start the infant walking on the hands (continue for 5 seconds).

BIG BALL PLAY

Purpose: To develop balance and postural awareness

Procedure: The infant is positioned on a large

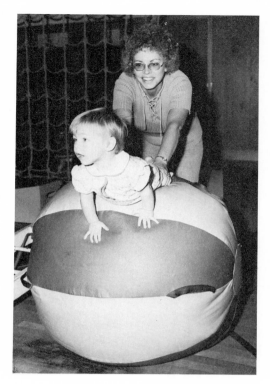

Fig. 13-10. Being moved on a big ball affords the infant opportunities for developing balance and postural awareness.

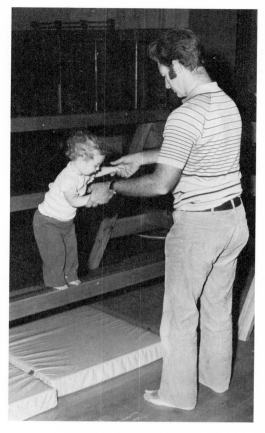

Fig. 13-11. Learning to walk a narrow beam helps in developing dynamic balance.

ball in a variety of ways. While in these positions, the infant is moved back and forth and from side to side (repeat ten to 20 times) (Fig. 13-10).

HOLD ON

Purpose: To stimulate the infant to move in an upright posture

Procedure: Set up low tables and chairs or other supports in such a way that the infant can walk while holding on to them. When the infant can accomplish the walk easily, different low objects, such as boards, bricks or sticks to step over, are placed in the way, forming an obstacle course (repeat three or four times).

STAND UP, SIT DOWN—II

Purpose: To gain leg and back strength and standing balance in preparation for walking

Procedure: Encourage the infant to sit and then stand up from a low seat such as a stair step or an 8-inch high box. At first the infant will have to hold on to a hand but will gradually

learn to perform without help (repeat three to five times).

LET'S KICK A BALL

Purpose: To develop standing balance and eye-foot coordination

Procedure: Holding on to a hand for support, the infant is walked into a large stationary ball. When the infant has learned that the ball can be moved by walking into it, kicking the ball is introduced. The infant should attempt to kick the ball with each foot (repeat as long as interest continues).

HANDSTAND WALK ON THE FLOOR

Purpose: To strengthen the arms, shoulders, and upper trunk

Procedure: The infant is grasped by the lower legs and lifted to an upside-down position placing full support on the hands. Slowly the infant is moved forward, causing the hands to move alternately (repeat four hand steps, three times).

BALANCE BEAM WALK

Purpose: To develop walking balance and confidence

Procedure: Assist the infant to walk a 6-inch wide beam or board that rests 5 inches off the floor. Support the infant under the arms. As confidence and balance are acquired, give less support (repeat three to five times) (Fig. 13-11).

HANDWALKING A BEAM

Purpose: To develop upper-body strength, balance, and coordination

Procedure: Place the infant's hands on a 6-inch wide board or beam. Lift the infant's body by the thighs into the air until the entire body weight is supported on the infant's hands. Push gently forward to cause a walking motion (repeat two to three times).

BOX CLIMBING

Purpose: To gain the ability to engage in movement problem solving

Procedure: Place the infant in a sitting position in a 12-inch deep cardboard box. Using a toy as enticement, encourage the infant to climb out of the box (repeat two to three times).

BLANKET PULL

Purpose: To develop sitting balance and trunk strength

Procedure: Seat the infant on a blanket or large beach towel. Gently pull the blanket or towel forward with the infant on it. Pull just hard enough to almost throw the infant off balance. Once forward pull is accomplished with the infant maintaining good balance, pulling can be backward or sideways (pull across the room three times).

Additional activities and experiences

1. Sit and get up without help.
2. Stack books.
3. Float a boat.
4. Get an out-of-reach toy with a stick.
5. Play in a plastic pool.
6. Roll a ball.
7. Push a ball on the floor.
8. Listen to the noise of an airplane.
9. Put a 1-inch block on another 1-inch block.
10. Pretend to drink from a cup.
11. Turn pages of a magazine.
12. Put plastic doughnuts on a spindle.
13. Try to feed self with a spoon.
14. Pretend to stir a pot.
15. Watch self eat in a mirror.
16. Find a hidden toy.

FROM 13 THROUGH 18 MONTHS OF AGE
General goals

The goals of these activities are to assist the child to develop effective locomotor and self-help skills as well as to provide the child with opportunities to explore the environment.

Space and equipment

These activities require an area of space large enough for the child to move freely without running into things and getting hurt, a Hula-Hoop, ten bricks or wooden blocks, an 8-foot by 1-inch by 6-inch board or beam, a regular-size ladder, a ¼-inch diameter, 18-inch long wooden dowel, a modified ladder with rungs 4 to 6 inches apart, and a soft pad for stunts.

Developmental movement activities

BACK AND FORTH AND SIDE TO SIDE

Purpose: To develop standing balance and postural awareness

Procedure: Facing and grasping the hands of the standing child, the adult gently begins to push rhythmically back and forth and then side to side while singing a song or nursery rhyme. Each push or pull should attempt to throw the child slightly off balance (repeat for 30 seconds).

HULA-HOOP WRESTLING

Purpose: To develop standing balance and grip strength

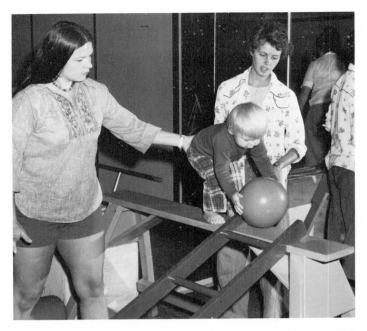

Fig. 13-12. Walking a board at a height requires balance and self-confidence.

Procedure: The child and adult face each other, griping a Hula-Hoop. The adult moves the Hula-Hoop gently back and forth, making the child step forward and backward. Next, the Hula-Hoop is moved from side to side, causing the child to move sideways. Finally, the adult slowly walks in a circle, first in one direction then in the other, still holding onto the hoop and forcing the child to follow.

BLOCK WALKING

Purpose: To develop walking balance

Procedure: Using ten bricks or 8-inch by 2-inch by 4-inch wooden blocks, make a stepping-stone–like path for the child to walk on. Each block should be placed in such a way as to ensure that the child must alternate feet in stepping (repeat three to five times).

WALKING A BOARD

Purpose: To develop dynamic balance and confidence

Procedure: A balance beam or board is placed about 5 inches above the floor. Starting at one end the child is assisted to walk forward the full length of the board. As the child's confidence and balance increase, the board is raised (Fig. 13-12).

MOVING UP A RAMP

Purpose: To gain leg strength and walking skills

Procedure: Place a board ramp on a slight incline by raising its end about 3 or 4 inches. Starting at the low end, the child is assisted in crawling or walking the board's length. When the child gains the ability to move up the ramp without help, the board is elevated 1 or 2 inches more (repeat three to five times) (Fig. 13-13).

LADDER OBSTACLE

Purpose: To develop dynamic balance and proper foot positioning in walking

Procedure: Place a regular-size ladder flat on the floor. Starting at the end of the ladder, the child is assisted in walking the full length of the ladder, stepping over each rung with alternate feet.

DOWEL HANG

Purpose: To develop grip, arm, and shoulder strength

Procedure: The child grasps a dowel in an overhand grip. Facing the child, the adult positions his or her hands over the hands of the child and, gently and slowly, lifts the child a few inches off of the floor. As confidence is

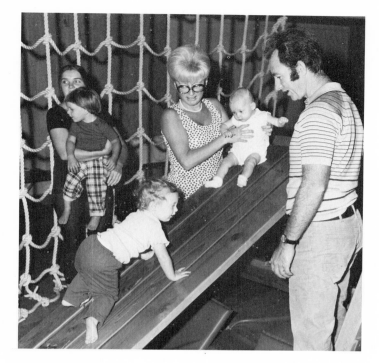

Fig. 13-13. Moving up a ramp can develop both leg and trunk strength.

acquired, the child can be raised higher and for longer periods of time. In the beginning the lift is held for 5 seconds, gradually progressing to 30 seconds.

BACK ROLL

Purpose: To strengthen and stretch trunk muscles and develop coordination

Procedure: With the child in a back-lying position, the adult lifts the child's thighs to a spot over the face. At this time, the child's head is turned to one side for protection, and the roll is completed over the shoulder opposite that to which the child's face is turned (repeat three to five times).

INTRODUCING THE FRONT SOMERSAULT

Purpose: To strengthen arms, shoulders, and trunk and to increase position sense

Procedure: The child is first placed on the hands and knees of a soft surface. The child's head is then tucked on the chest, the back is rounded, and the hips are lifted. From this position the child is gently pushed forward, executing a somersault over both shoulders (repeat three to five times).

GLIDER

Purpose: To develop back and neck strength and balance

Procedure: The adult sits on the floor with knees bent and feet flat on the floor. Standing in front of the bent knees, the child faces the adult. Grasping the hands of the child, the adult leans slowly backward to a back-lying position while pulling the child on to the lower legs. The adult's feet are then brought off the floor, and the child is lifted into the air. When suspended on the legs, the child will automatically arch the back and neck. The adult then brings the child's arms out to the side as if flying (repeat three to five times).

LADDER CLIMBING

Purpose: To develop balance and leg and arm coordination

Procedure: Place a modified ladder, which has rungs no more than 6 inches apart, on an incline of 2 or 3 feet. Encourage the child to climb the full length of the ladder using alternate feet. When the child is able to effectively execute this task, progressively

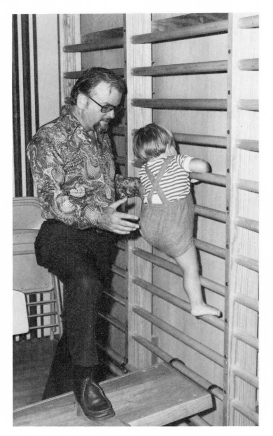

Fig. 13-14. A stall bar makes an excellent ladder for young children to climb.

increase the height of the raised end of the ladder until it is completely upright (repeat three to five times) (Fig. 13-14).

Additional activities and experiences

1. Stack more than two 1-inch blocks on top of one another.
2. Pull objects out of bags, purses, or pockets.
3. Put pegs in holes.
4. Put containers inside one another.
5. Stack objects of unequal size on top of one another.
6. Put pennies in a piggy bank slot.
7. Work a zipper.
8. Complete the pushing of a button through a buttonhole.
9. Walk and pull a toy.

10. Climb up to get something.
11. Play hide and seek.
12. Roll a ball to someone.
13. Make noise with a play musical instrument to music or a beat.
14. Play Ring-around-the-rosy.
15. Point to self in mirror.
16. Look at a picture in a book.
17. Follow direction such as stop and come.

FROM 19 THROUGH 24 MONTHS OF AGE
General goals

Activities during this period are designed to encourage the child to explore the environment, increase refinement of locomotor skills, and increase postural control, balance, and strength.

Space and equipment

Indoor and outdoor space in which to run and explore, cardboard boxes of different sizes, and boards are needed.

Developmental movement activities

TREE LIMB

Purpose: To increase upper-body strength and balance

Procedure: The child stands with the back pressed against the chest of the kneeling adult. Supported around the hips and chest, the child is leaned slowly forward. The adult then leans backward, leaving the child in an extended position at about a 45 degree angle (repeat three to five times with each extension held from 5 to 30 seconds).

KNEE HANDSTAND

Purpose: To strengthen the arms and shoulders and to develop the balance mechanisms

Procedure: The adult assumes a back-lying position with knees bent up and feet flat on the floor. The child then stands on the adult's abdomen with the hands placed on the bent knees. Gently, the child is elevated to a handstand position while supported on the adult's knees. As confidence is gained in this activity, the child maintains the handstand position while the adult's knees are gradually lowered to the floor (repeat three to five times).

ROW THE BOAT

Purpose: To strengthen the arms and trunk muscles

Procedure: The child takes a sitting position on the floor with legs straight and leans on both hands, which have been placed just in back of the hips. The child is then encouraged to pull the body backward between the hands as far as possible while dragging the legs and to continue the movement across the floor to the song "Row, Row, Row Your Boat" (repeat two or three times).

BOX JUMPING

Purpose: To develop body control in the air

Procedure: Have the child climb onto some raised area such as the bottom stair step or a box no higher than 8 to 10 inches. Support the child and encourage him or her to jump to the floor. The child's knees should be bent on landing. Gradually, remove support until the child is able to perform the task without help (repeat three to five times).

OBSTACLE COURSE

Purpose: To develop spatial awareness, balance, strength, and coordination

Procedure: Set up an obstacle course that challenges the child to balance and to walk on, over, through, and around objects. Boards should be used as ramps and balance beams and cardboard boxes as objects to go around and through. (Continue until the child loses interest or becomes fatigued.)

Additional activities and experiences

1. Attempt to lace a shoe.
2. Attempt to work a buckle.
3. Hammer a peg into a hole.
4. Turn the door knob.
5. Attempt to color between lines.
6. Use a spoon to feed self.
7. String beads.
8. Play chase.
9. Point to body parts.
10. Pretend to be an animal.
11. Pretend to do housework.
12. Listen to stories.
13. Name pictures.
14. Turn a switch on and off.
15. Play with dolls or stuffed animals.
16. Attempt to dress and undress self.
17. Attempt to turn a screw with a screwdriver.
18. Walk on tiptoes.
19. Laugh while watching television.

14

Level 2: Building

Level 2 activities are designed to offer the child enjoyment in challenges that require basic motor skills. Simple games involving nonlocomotor, locomotor, and manipulative skills and rhythms that can be learned quickly allow children to receive maximum enjoyment in physical education.

Children at this level begin to develop the skills necessary to compete successfully in activities presented in level 3. The teacher should select a variety of activities on the basis of the needs of the children as determined by the Basic Motor Ability Test. The behavioral objectives and developmental goals listed will aid the teacher in developing a well-rounded program.

NONLOCOMOTOR ACTIVITIES

Nonlocomotor activities involve movements performed around the axis of the body. They include all of the movements that can be executed while the body remains in one place. Nonlocomotor movements are performed in such positions as standing, sitting, squatting, crouching, kneeling, lying, leaning, and stooping. Nonlocomotor movements can be done in combinations, making them more fun and thought provoking. Some examples are bending-stretching, rising-falling, swinging-swaying, pushing-pulling. The most effective approach to teaching nonlocomotor skills is by indirect movement exploration or problem-solving technique.

Body awareness activities

IDENTIFICATION OF BODY PARTS

Behavioral objective: To identify body parts and learn their relationship to each other

Developmental goal: Body awareness and auditory skills

Space and equipment: Classroom or gymnasium

Number of players: Entire class

Test reference*: VI

Procedure

1. The teacher touches different body parts starting with the head and says, "This is my head, can you touch your head?" The children touch their heads saying, "This is my head" (Fig. 14-1). The teacher continues with all other body parts then repeats the same directions but asks the children to close their eyes as they do it.

2. The teacher asks the children to touch various body parts using other body parts (Fig. 14-2), such as:
   arm to leg
   foot to knee
   head to knee
   elbows to knees
   wrist to ear
   wrist to neck
   wrist to ankle
   chin to shoulder
   chin to chest
   nose to elbow
   ear to shoulder
   hands to hips

3. The teacher asks the children to touch body parts to their environment, such as:
   back to floor

---

*Test reference refers to Basic Motor Ability Test, Chapter 2.

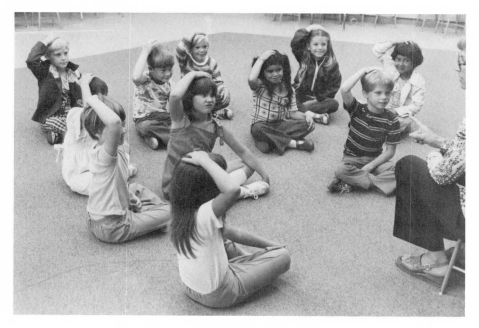

Fig. 14-1. ''Can you touch your head?''

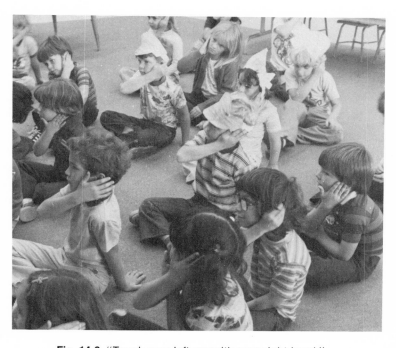

Fig. 14-2. ''Touch your left ear with your right hand.''

head to desk
nose to window
hand to wall
wrist to table
fingers to book
knees to chair
elbows to chalkboard
toes to wall

4. The teacher instructs children to move specific body parts on command, such as:
    Turn your head.
    Twist your neck.
    Bend your elbow.
    Turn your arm.
    Cover your eyes.
    Clap your hands.
    Wiggle your toes.
    Open your mouth.
    Bend your knees.
    Snap your fingers.
    Stamp your feet.
    Shrug your shoulders.

5. While the children are lying on their backs, the teacher asks them to move various parts, such as:
    Lift your head.
    Lift your legs.
    Lift your arms.
    Lift your right hand.
    Touch your elbows together.
    Touch your left heel to your right knee.

MOVEMENT OF BODY PARTS

Behavioral objective: To learn the basic movement vocabulary and explore how body parts move

Developmental goal: Flexibility, directionality, and listening skills

Space and equipment: Classroom or gymnasium

Number of players: Entire class

Test reference: III and VI

Procedure:

Rising and falling
1. Show me if you can raise different parts of your body and let them fall while you are standing. Sitting. Kneeling. Lying.
2. Can you raise your body to a standing position from a sitting or kneeling position?
3. Can you raise your head while lying on your stomach?
4. How many other parts of your body can you raise while lying on your stomach?

5. Show me how slowly you can sit from a standing position.

Swinging and swaying (Fig. 14-3)
1. Show me how many parts of your body you can swing while in a standing or kneeling position.
2. Show me how many parts of your body you can sway while kneeling or lying on your back.
3. Can you sway very slowly and then fast while you are in a standing position?
4. Show me if you can swing and sway your arms with a partner while holding hands.
5. Can you swing and sway in different ways while holding a partner's hand?

Bending and stretching
1. Can you show me how you bend your body?
2. Show me how high you can stretch.
3. Can you change from a bending position to a stretching position?
4. Can you make the top part of your body get closer to the bottom part of your body?

Pushing and pulling
1. Show me how many parts of your body you can use to push with.
2. Show me how you would pull in a tug-of-war.
3. Show me how many ways you can push and pull with a partner.

Twisting, turning, and whirling
1. Show me how many parts of your body you can twist while standing or sitting.
2. How many parts of your body can you turn while kneeling?
3. Can you twist and turn with a partner three different ways?

Jiggling
1. How many parts of your body can you shake very quickly?
2. How slowly can you shake your arm and leg?
3. Show me if you can jiggle two different parts of your body at the same time.

Relaxation
1. Can you stand like a wooden soldier with your arms, legs, and head straight, making tight fists with your hands?
2. Can you relax like a rag doll, making yourself soft and droopy and letting your body hang loosely?
3. Show me how you lie on the floor and

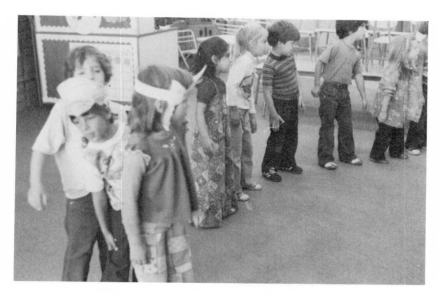

Fig. 14-3. "Show me how you swing and sway."

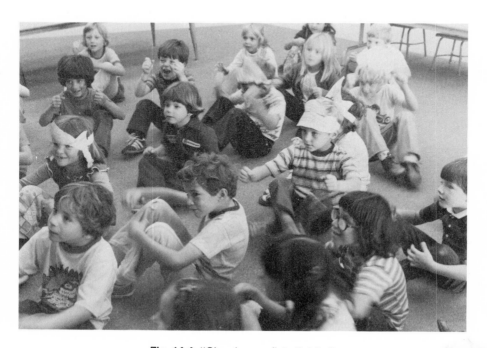

Fig. 14-4. "Clench your fists tightly."

tense your arm, then relax. Tense your leg, then relax. (Do this with all body parts, naming them as you contract the muscle.)

4. Can you stand and breathe deeply? Blow your breath out and bend at the waist with your arms and upper body hanging limp. Inhale and slowly raise up and extend your arms upward. Exhale slowly returning to the limp position.

Hands

1. Can you open and shut your hands, clenching fists tight (Fig. 14-4) and opening them wide?
2. Can you shake your hands up and down like a rag doll?
3. Show me your thumbs rotating in a circle, first to the right and then to the left.
4. Can you clasp your fingers together and "twiddle" your thumbs, right over left and then left over right?
5. Can you hold your hands with palms up and close first one hand then the other and then alternate opening and closing them?

Head

1. Show me your head moving forward and backward.
2. Can you tilt your head to the right and the left in a rhythmical fashion like a clock?
3. Can you roll your head in a circle to the right then to the left?
4. Show me how far back you can tip your head. What can you see? How many see the _____ ?
5. Can your turn your head and touch your chin to your left shoulder? Return to the original position and try to touch your right shoulder with your chin.
6. Can you lie down on your back and lift your head?
7. Show me how high you can lift your head while lying on your back. On your stomach.
8. How many different ways can you move your head?

Shoulders

1. How high can you raise your shoulders?
2. Show me how you raise one shoulder

and then the other. Do it in a rhythmical fashion.

3. Can you rotate your shoulders in a circular motion?

Torso

1. How far can you rotate your upper body to the right then to the left?
2. With your legs in straddle position and your hands on your shoulders, can you bend to the right and then to the left?
3. With your hands on your hips can you bend forward then backward?
4. With hands over your head and knees straight can you bend forward and touch your knees? Ankles? Toes?
5. Can you bend and touch your right foot with your left hand? Your left foot with your right hand?
6. How many different ways can you move your body from the waist up?

Arms

1. With your arms our in front, can you make little circles then big circles (Fig. 14-5) with your arms and then reverse?
2. With your arms to the sides, can you make arm circles in different directions?
3. How far can you swing your arms forward then backward?
4. Can you hold your arms out in front and open and close your hands quickly?
5. Show me how you use your arms to climb up a rope. Climb down a rope.

Legs

(Activities are performed from different reclining positions on the floor.)

1. Lying on your back can you move your legs in and out? Move your arms up and down at the same time.
2. Lying on your back, show me how high you can lift your right leg. Your left leg.
3. Lying on your side show me how high you can lift your leg.
4. Can you swing your leg back and forth parallel to the floor?
5. Lying on your side, can you make circles with your leg?
6. How many other ways can your move your legs?

Legs

(Activities are performed in a standing position.)

1. Can you stand on one foot and balance

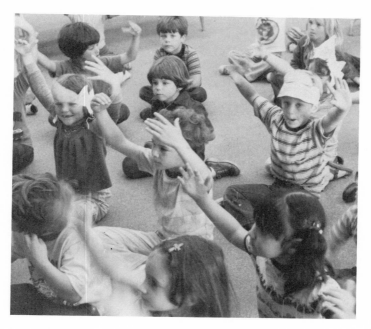

Fig. 14-5. Making big circles.

with your eyes open? With your eyes closed?

2. Can you stand with your eyes closed, keeping your balance, for 10 seconds?
3. Can you raise up on your toes and go back down in rhythm?
4. Can you stand on one foot and swing your opposite leg forward and backward? From side to side? Use slow, wide swings and fast, short swings.
5. Can you stand with one foot in front of the other, heel to toe?
6. Show me your heels together with your toes pointed outward.
7. Can you touch your toes and point your heels outward?
8. How many different ways can you stand?

Imitation

1. Can you pretend you are a wave? The ocean is very rough! Now it is calm.
2. Can you be a tree blowing in the wind? The wind is so soft.
3. Show me you are a windshield wiper. Use only your arms. Use your whole body.
4. Can you be a flower growing? Can you grow slowly?
5. Can you be a flag blowing in the wind?

The wind is very strong; now it is weaker. The wind has stopped.

NONLOCOMOTOR GAMES

ANGELS IN THE SNOW

Behavioral objective: To respond to directions for bilateral, unilateral, and cross-lateral movements

Developmental goal: Laterality and directionality

Space and equipment: Classroom

Number of participants: Entire class

Test reference: III and VI

Procedure: Ask the children to lie on the floor with their feet together and arms at their sides. Ask them to slide their arms "up" along the floor keeping them straight, until they touch their ears. Now ask them to move their legs "out" as far as possible. Instruct the children to listen carefully and do what is asked of them, such as:

Move both arms up and back.
Move both legs out and back.
Move your right arm up.
Move your left arm up.
Move your right leg out.
Move your left leg out.
Move both arms and legs at the same time.

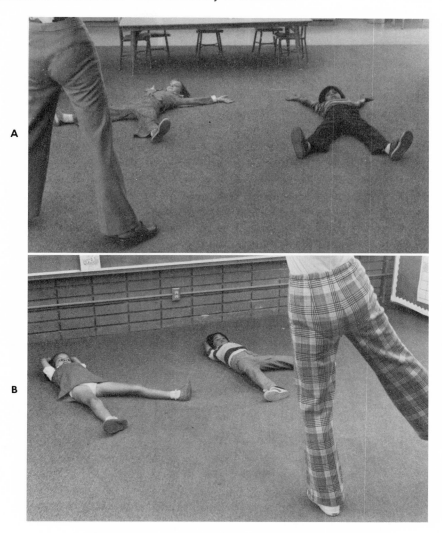

Fig. 14-6. **A,** Angels in the snow. **B,** Variation of angels in the snow.

Move your right arm and right leg.
Move your left arm and left leg.
Move your right arm and left leg.
Move your left arm and right leg.
The teacher should observe the children to check for smooth, decisive, correct movements. Children should keep body parts in contact with the floor at all times (Fig. 14-6).

WIGWAG

Behavioral objective: To respond to visual directions to move body parts
Developmental goal: Accurate perceptual translation of visual stimuli
Space and equipment: Classroom, playground, or gymnasium

Number of participants: Entire class
Test reference: VI
Procedure: This is a nonverbal activity. Children mimic whatever nonlocomotor movement the teacher is doing. Successful performance is reflecting the same movement as the teacher.

LOCOMOTOR ACTIVITIES

Locomotor activities involve body movement from one place to another. Travel through the different modes of rolling, crawling, walking, running, and skipping is experienced through individual challenges or simple game activities.

Children of level 2 ability find much enjoyment in discovering the many ways in which the body can move. Teachers should develop the program to incorporate all of the fundamental locomotor skills.

ROLLING

Procedure

1. Roll continuously in one direction: reverse direction.
2. Roll and stop on a signal.
3. Roll to a marker and stop.
4. Roll with arms overhead, at your sides, and crossed.
5. Roll up in a blanket and unroll.
6. Roll down a hill and up a hill.
7. Roll around in a circle.
8. Roll in a cardboard box, open at both ends.
9. Roll up in a ball with arms wrapped around knees. Another child rolls "the ball" in any direction; then the child returns to the original position.
10. Two or more children lie next to each other in a line with their arms overhead. All together, the children roll over and over.
11. Children lie on the floor parallel to each other like railroad ties, about 2 to 3 feet apart. The first child rolls over all children and lies down at the end of the line. The second child follows. Continue until all have participated.

CRAWLING

Procedure

1. Crawl forward.
2. Crawl down a hill; crawl up a hill.
3. Crawl around obstacles.
4. Crawl over obstacles.
5. Crawl through a low opening.
6. Crawl through a narrow opening.
7. Crawl backwards.
8. Crawl sideways.

CREEPING

Procedure

1. Creep forward on marked handprints. Backward.
2. Creep forward.
3. Creep backward.
4. Creep sideways.
5. Creep uphill and downhill.
6. Creep under, around, and through obstacles.
7. Creep on hands and feet (dog walk).
8. Creep with one arm or leg off the ground.
9. Creep with same sides of body moving forward (unilateral).
10. Creep with opposite sides of body moving forward (cross-lateral).
11. Bend forward and touch the ground, keeping knees and elbows stiff and hips elevated; walk forward.
12. Creep on knees and elbows.
13. Sit on the floor with knees bent. Leaning back on your hands, lift buttocks off the floor. Walk forward, backward or sideways (crab walk).
14. Bend forward and touch the ground with both hands. Keep knees and elbows stiff and hips elevated. Keeping feet in place, walk hands out as far as possible without touching body to the ground. Keeping hands in place, walk feet forward as close as possible to the hands. Repeat sequence (inchworm).

WALKING

Procedure

1. Walk on footprints.
2. Walk between two lines, 6 inches apart.
3. Walk on a line forward. Backward.
4. Walk uphill and downhill.
5. Walk with exaggerated movements swinging arms high and raising the legs.
6. Sidestep to the right. The left.
7. Walk up and down steps.
8. Walk on tiptoes.
9. Walk on your heels only.
10. Walk with toes pointed inward. Outward.
11. Walk in the spaces between rungs of a ladder or hoops placed flat on the ground.
12. Walk on the rungs of ladders.
13. Walk around geometric shapes.
14. Step over a rope on the ground.
15. Step over a rope raised off the ground.
16. Walk on tires or innertubes of various sizes.
17. Walk fast and slow, using big and small steps.
18. Walk around a circle marked with geometric shapes, and stop on the shape called out.

19. March to music with knees high.
20. Walk while balancing a beanbag on the head.
21. Walk while holding ankles.
22. Walk with hands on knees.
23. Walk with knees bent.
24. Walk while holding toes.

RUNNING

Procedure
1. Run forward. Backward.
2. Run uphill and downhill.
3. Run quietly. Loudly. Faster. Slower.
4. Run and change directions on a signal.

JUMPING (TWO FOOT TAKEOFF)

Procedure
1. Jump up and down like a jumping jack.
2. Jump like a rabbit.
3. Jump uphill and downhill.
4. Jump forward. Backward. Sideways.
5. Jump in and out of a hoop.
6. Jump up and touch the sky.
7. Jump in place with eyes closed.
8. Jump over a line.
9. Jump over a rope. slightly raised..
10. Jump to rhythm or music.
11. Jump, making quarter turns to the right while in the air. Making quarter turns to the left.
12. Jump, making half turns to the right while in the air. Making half turns to the left.

HOPPING

Procedure: Do activities on one foot and then the other.
1. Hop in place.
2. Hop forward. Backward. Sideways.
3. Hop uphill and downhill.
4. Hop in and out of a hoop.
5. Hop to rhythm, two hops on the right foot and two on the left.

SKIPPING

Procedure
1. Step-hop on the right foot then step-hop on the left.
2. Skip in a straight line, forward and backward.
3. Skip around a circle.

LEAPING

Procedure
1. Leap forward.
2. Run and leap.
3. Leap sideways.
4. Leap over objects.

CLIMBING

Procedure
1. Climb steps.
2. Climb a ladder.
3. Climb on a jungle gym.
4. Climb on a cargo net.
5. Climb a vertical pole.
6. Climb a vertical rope.

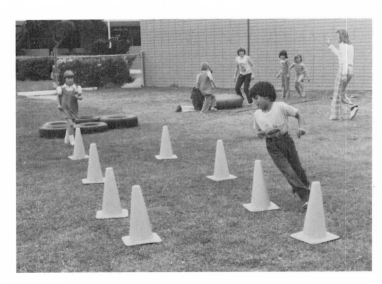

Fig. 14-7. Outdoor obstacle course.

7. Climb in and out of a box.
8. Climb on and off a tricycle.

OBSTACLE COURSE

Procedure: Obstacle courses are often painted on a surface, but for the greatest challenge and fun it is better to incorporate objects that the children can go on, over, or through (Fig. 14-7). Following are a few suggestions:

1. Footsteps to walk on forward and backward
2. Handprints to creep on forward and backward
3. Balance beam to walk on
4. Cones to crawl, creep, or run around
5. Barrels to creep through
6. Cardboard boxes to step in and out of
7. Up and down slant board to walk on
8. A ladder to walk or run between the rungs of
9. A bench to step up on and jump off

LOCOMOTOR MOVEMENT CHALLENGES

Behavioral objective: Respond successfully to locomotor challenges
Developmental goal: Controlled locomotor skills
Space and equipment: Outdoor or gymnasium area
Number of participants: Entire class
Test reference: V and VI
Procedure

Walking

1. Can you walk tall around the room?
2. Can you walk fast without touching your classmates?
3. Can you walk without touching your heels on the ground?
4. Show me the smallest steps you can take.
5. Can you walk quickly and quietly without touching anyone?
6. When you hear the signal, change directions.
7. When you hear the signal, change levels while walking.
8. Show me if you can keep hands high while walking low.
9. Can you walk like you are happy? Sad?
10. Show me how you would walk in a strong wind.

Running

1. Show me how fast you can run to the wall and back.

2. Can you swing your arms high when you run?
3. Can you run fast and freeze on a signal?
4. Show me how high you can lift your knees when you are running.
5. Show me how quietly you can run.
6. Can you change from low to high when you run?
7. Show me how loud you can run.

Jumping

1. Can you jump up and down in place?
2. Can you jump higher and higher?
3. Show me how you can jump forward. Backward. Sideward.
4. Can you jump over the beanbag on the floor?

Hopping

1. Show me who can jump on one foot.
2. Can you jump on the other foot?
3. Can you hop around a circle and change feet when you tire?
4. How low can you be when you hop?
5. Show me some big hops.
6. Can you hop softly?
7. Can you hop loudly?
8. Show me who can hop backwards.
9. Can you hop sideways?
10. Can you hop forward on one foot and back on the other?
11. Can you hop with your hands on your hips?
12. Show me who can hop with their arms on their heads.
13. Until the freeze signal, can you walk three steps and hop five?
14. Can you run ten steps, hop four times, and jump five times?

Skipping

1. Can you skip around the area without bumping into anyone?
2. Can you change direction?
3. Can you skip and hold your arms high?
4. Can you skip in a circle? Bigger? Bigger?
5. Can you skip fast? Slow? High? Low?

Leaping

1. Can you run and end with a leap?
2. Can you leap higher and higher?
3. Show me who can make the highest leap.
4. Who can show me how you leap for something high? Grab it.
5. Can you leap from side to side without moving forward?

Galloping
1. Can you walk forward keeping one foot in front of the other?
2. Show me who can go faster keeping the same foot in front.
3. Show me if you can go fast like a pony, hitting your hips as you gallop.
4. Can you gallop and change directions?
5. Can you gallop with a partner?

Sliding
1. Can you stand with your feet apart? Slide one foot over to the other.
2. Can you slide in one direction across the floor?
3. Show me how fast you can move sideways.
4. Can you slide four times to the right and then four times to the left?

Relay games

Relay activities introduce the child to competitive play in an enjoyable setting. Using learned motor skills, each child is challenged to introduce speed and accuracy to support a team effort. Relays lend themselves to squad organization and many can be conducted in a short play period. When presenting relays, the teacher should be certain that the activity is in line with the abilities of the children and that every effort has been made to equalize the teams. Safety should be emphasized; make sure the turn line is open and not up against a wall. Also, children in each squad should hold out their right arms to give direction to the returning players, thereby avoiding unnecessary contact during the activity.

RELAYS

Behavioral objective: To successfully perform locomotor skills in a relay activity
Developmental goal: Locomotor skills, speed, and agility
Space and equipment: Multipurpose play area
Number of participants: Six to eight students per team
Test reference: IV and V
Procedure
1. *Run down and back*
   The first person in line runs down to touch the turning line with the foot. After touching the line, the child returns to the starting line, touches the next player's left side, and goes to the end of the line. The relay continues until all participants have had a turn.
2. *Jump down and back*
   Repeat relay 1 substituting jumping for running.
3. *Hop down and back*
   Repeat relay 1, substituting hopping for running (Fig. 14-8).

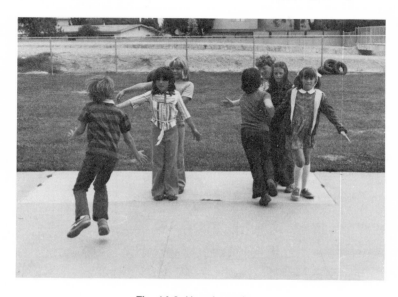

Fig. 14-8. Hopping relay.

4. *Gallop down and back*
   Repeat relay 1, substituting galloping for running.
5. *Skip down and back*
   Repeat relay 1, substituting skipping for running.
6. *Airplanes*
   A cone is placed on the turning line in front of each team. The first "airplane" in each line spreads its "wings" and, on the command "go," "flies" down to the turning line, circles the cone, and comes back. The relay continues until all participants have had a turn.
7. *Jump the brook*
   Parallel lines about 2 feet apart are placed parallel to and 10 feet in front of the starting line. (Jump ropes may be used to define the brook.) The first player runs and jumps across the brook, continues to the turning line, and returns to the starting line, jumping the brook on the way back, so the next player in line can proceed.
8. *Sore toe*
   The first player on each team stands on one foot and grasps with both hands the toes of the other foot. The player hops to the turning line, releases the foot, and runs to tag the next player. The second player should be standing on one foot ready to begin hopping when tagged.
9. *Skip around*
   The first person skips to the cone placed at the turning line, makes a complete circle around it, and returns to the starting line.

Tag games

When conducting tag games the teacher should always establish boundaries. One should adapt the rules to ensure that slower runners or less skilled players are not always "it." The creative teacher will observe unfair competition and adjust the game accordingly for full enjoyment. Most tag games are best played in a limited, marked area such as a basketball court.

SIMPLE TAG

Behavioral objective: To overtake and tag another child and to avoid being tagged

Developmental goal: Agility and endurance
Space and equipment: Multipurpose play area
Number of players: Entire class
Test reference: V
Procedure: One child is chosen to be "it." All children are scattered within a designated play area. "It" tries to tag another player. When a player is tagged and becomes "it," the game continues. A player who is tagged may not tag back the person who tagged him or her.

CIRCLE TAG

Behavioral objective: To move safely in a clockwise circle and to tag the one in front
Developmental goal: Endurance and directionality
Space and equipment: Multipurpose play area
Number of players: 10 to 12
Test reference: V
Procedure: The children stand in a circle formation with about 6 feet between each player (Fig. 14-9). On a signal, all the players run in a clockwise direction around the circle and attempt to tag the players directly in front of them. When a player is tagged, he or she takes two steps toward the center of the circle and sits down until only one player is left untagged. The last player left is the winner.

STOOP TAG

Behavioral objective: To tag and to avoid being tagged
Developmental goal: Endurance and flexibility
Space and equipment: Multipurpose play area
Number of players: 10 to 15
Test reference: III and V
Procedure: The children stand in an informal group within boundary lines. Children are safe from "it" when stooping. No child may stoop more than twice while one child is "it."

SKIP TAG

Behavioral objective: To overtake and tag another child while skipping
Developmental goal: Coordination and endurance
Space and equipment: Multipurpose play area
Number of players: 10 to 12
Test reference: V
Procedure: The children form a single circle and all face inward. A tagger is chosen and

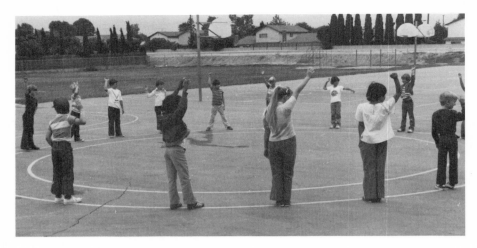

Fig. 14-9. Preparing for a circle tag game.

stands outside the circle. The tagger, while skipping around the outside of the circle, tags a circle player. The circle player skips around and tries to catch the tagger. If the tagger reaches the vacant space left by the circle player without being caught, the circle player becomes the tagger, and the game continues. The tagger remains the tagger if caught by the circle player. If the tagger is unable to take a circle player's space after two tries, the teacher should change directions or select another tagger.

Games of low organization

Games of low organization have few rules and are easily learned by young children. The opportunity to be daring and exhibit agility and speed in locomotor skills is brought forth in these activities. Children will select favorite games to play; however, the teacher should make sure a variety of activities are presented to ensure a balance of motor skill development.

COPY CAT

Behavioral objective: To mimic actions of group leader
Developmental goal: Locomotor and mimicry through visual cues
Space and equipment: Multipurpose area
Number of players: 10 to 12
Test reference: III, IV, and VI

Procedure: One player is chosen to be "it." All the other players line up in single file behind "it." As "it" leads them over a designated area of play, he or she performs certain actions, which the group mimics.

STOP AND START

Behavioral objective: To listen for a direction given by a leader and to move in the direction ordered
Developmental goal: Directionality and auditory awareness
Space and equipment: Classroom or multipurpose play area
Number of players: 4 to 12
Test reference: V
Procedure: The children stand about the room or field and watch the leader. When the leader points in any direction, the children must move in that direction. When the leader blows the whistle, the children must stop and turn in order to watch for the next direction. Children who fail to stop immediately or who fail to follow directions form a second group of players on the opposite side of the leader. The object of the game is to be the last player to remain in the original group.

DUCK, DUCK, GOOSE

Behavioral objective: To run around a circle without being tagged and to tag the runner
Developmental goal: Auditory perception and quickness
Space and equipment: Multipurpose play area

Number of players: 15 to 30
Test reference: IV and VI
Procedure: The children form a circle and face the center. The child who is chosen to be "it" runs around the outside of the circle, touching children on the shoulder and calling, "duck, duck, duck, goose!" All those who are called ducks squat and remain in their places. The one who is called goose chases "it," and if "it" gets to the vacant place in the circle before being caught by the goose, the goose becomes "it." If "it" is tagged before reaching the vacant place, he or she remains "it." "It" may say "duck" any number of times before saying "goose." All players stand again at the end of the chase.

CUT THE CAKE

Behavioral objective: To run around a circle in the opposite direction of a neighbor
Developmental goal: Directionality and quickness
Space and equipment: Multipurpose play area
Number of players: 6 to 12 in a group
Test reference: IV and V
Procedure: The children form circles and face the center and join hands. In each group the child who is chosen to be "it" is the knife and stands inside the circle. With both hands together the knife pretends to cut with a slicing motion just above the cake. When the knife taps the joined hands of two children hard in a cutting motion, these two children run in opposite directions around the circle. The two runners should stop when they meet and shake hands or perform some other stunt to avoid head-on collisions. The knife stands still and judges which one of the runners gets back to the place first. The winning runner is the next knife.

SQUIRREL IN THE TREES

Behavioral objective: To run safely to a different area before another person
Developmental goal: Auditory perception, agility, and speed
Space and equipment: Multipurpose play area
Number of players: Entire class
Test reference: V and VI
Procedure: The children stand in groups of three; two face each other and join both hands, forming the tree, and the third is the squirrel and stands inside the tree. The trees should be scattered around the playing area. There should be two or three squirrels without trees. When the leader calls, "Change trees," all the squirrels run to new trees. The teacher may blow a whistle to signal a change. The squirrels left without trees change places with children who are trees. All the children should have turns being squirrels.

OLD MOTHER WITCH

Behavioral objective: To listen for a signal and run safely to a designated area and to tag others
Developmental goal: Quickness, auditory perception, and endurance
Space and equipment: Multipurpose play area or grass with lines
Number of players: Entire class
Test reference: V
Procedure: The children stand in a single line side by side. One child is chosen to be Old Mother Witch and stands in front of the line, facing away from the other children. The witch starts walking away, saying the following verse:

"Old Mother Witch fell in a ditch,
Found a penny,
And thought she was rich."

The children in line follow as close behind as they dare. When finished with the verse, the witch turns around and says, "Whose children are you?" Someone from the line says any name, such as the Jones children or the Smith children. If three different names are given, the witch repeats the verse and continues on a few steps and then turns around again and asks the same question. As soon as someone calls out, "the old witch's children," the witch chases them back to the starting line. One person should be chosen to say, "the Old Witch's children." Any children who are caught join the witch and help to catch the others.

RED LIGHT

Behavioral objective: To move across to a finish line without being caught
Developmental goal: Auditory awareness and visual perception
Space and equipment: Multipurpose play area
Number of players: Any number
Test reference: V and VI
Procedure: One player is chosen to be the

leader and stands on the finish line. The leader counts very rapidly from one to ten while facing away from the players and then quickly says the words "red light" and turns around. The players move across the area during the counting and must freeze on the words "red light." Any player who is caught moving after the words "red light" have been said must return to the starting position. After the leader has sent back all who were caught, he or she turns around and begins counting. The players may move when the leader's back is turned. Once counting starts, the leader cannot turn around until the words "red light" have been called out. The first player to reach the finish line wins and becomes the leader for the next game.

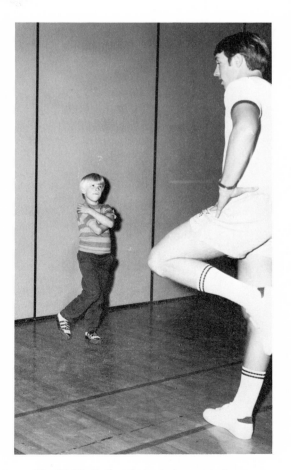

Fig. 14-10. Performing a balance challenge.

Balance activities

Balance involves the ability to keep the center of gravity over the base of support. Movements that change the center of gravity provide children with practice in regaining balance from a variety of positions. By involvement in different balance activities and introduction of balance stress through a variety of challenges, children experience practice in controlled balance actions. Basic balance is fundamental to successful participation in higher level activities (Fig. 14-10).

A. BALANCE CHALLENGES WITHOUT EQUIPMENT

Behavioral objective: To maintain balance in a variety of positions
Developmental goal: Balance
Equipment and space: Multipurpose play area
Number of participants: Entire class
Test reference: VI
Procedure

1. Can you stand on one foot with your hands on your hips?
2. Can you stand on one foot with your hands out to the side?
3. Show me how you can stand on the other foot with your hands out to the side.
4. Can you stand on one foot and touch your knee with the other?
5. Show me who can stand on one foot and hold the other foot with the hand.
6. Can you support yourself on your hands and feet looking at the sky?
7. While supporting yourself on your hands and feet face up can you raise your left leg high?
8. While supporting yourself on your hands and feet face up can you raise your right arm and keep your balance?
9. Can you stand with your arms out to the side and one leg back? One leg forward?
10. Who can stand on one leg with both arms out in front? In back?
11. Can you balance in a creeping position with one arm forward? With one leg back?
12. Can you balance in a creeping position with your left arm up and your right leg back? Right arm up and left leg back?

4. WALKING BEAM

Behavioral objective: To maintain balance while performing a variety of activities on a walking beam

Developmental goal: Balance

Space and equipment: Multipurpose area and a walking beam

Number of players: Groups of 4 to 6

Test reference: VI

Procedure: The walking beam, sometimes referred to as a balance beam, is a challenge to children and an excellent and inexpensive piece of equipment for improving balance. It must, however, be used with teacher direction since the tasks should be sequentially increased in difficulty if a child's interest and learning are to be maintained. Make certain that children walk slowly heel-to-toe with the feet in the center and the eyes focused on a target at the end of the beam. They should be able to feel the support without looking down. Children usually walk on the beam with their shoes on; however, kinesthetic awareness can be increased if they are in stocking feet.

Balance tasks are made progressively more difficult by placing obstacles on the beam, by having children balance or carry objects, or by turning the beam on its narrower side (Fig. 14-11).

1. Can you slowly walk forward on the beam with your arms out to the side? Hands on your hips?

2. Show me if you can walk backward with your arms out to the side. With hands on your hips.

3. With your hands on your hips can you walk to the center of the beam, turn, and walk sideways to the end?

4. With your arms sideways, can you walk to the middle of the beam, turn around, and walk backward?

5. Show me if you can walk across the beam leading each step with your right foot. Left foot.

6. Can you walk forward and step over a beanbag placed in the middle of the beam? Can you pick it up?

7. Can you walk to the center, kneel on one knee, get up, and go to the end?

8. Show me if you can walk across the beam with a beanbag balanced on your head.

9. Can you walk to the center, pick up the beanbag, put it on your head, and walk to the end? Can you pick it up, turn, and walk backward?

10. Can you walk forward and step through the Hula-Hoop?

11. Can you walk forward and step over my wand (6 inches high)? Backward?

12. Can you walk forward and go under

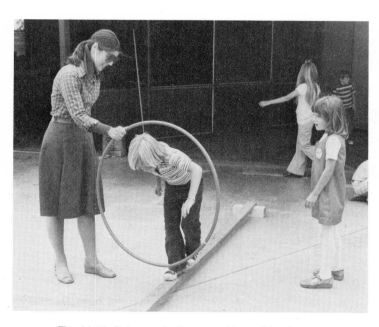

Fig. 14-11. Balance challenge on the walking beam.

my wand (36 inches high)? Backward?

13. Can you walk forward with your arms
out and balance a beanbag in the
palm of each hand? Backward?

14. Can you walk to the middle of the
beam and hop on one foot to the end?

15. Can you walk to the middle of the
beam, do a Mercury stand for 5
seconds, and then walk to the end?
(*To do a Mercury stand, stand on
either foot, bend the body forward
until it is at a right angle with the
supporting leg, bend the free leg
slightly upward from the knee, and
hold the head up and arms to the side
horizontally.*)

16. Show me a cat walk (on all fours).

17. Can you carry a weight in each hand
as you walk across the beam?

18. Show me if you can carry two weights
in one hand. Reverse hands. Can you
do it backward?

19. See if you can carry a ball as you walk
across the beam, bounce it once in
the middle, and then go to the end.

20. Can you bounce a ball with both
hands as you walk across the beam?

BALANCE BOARD

Behavioral objective: To maintain balance in a
variety of activities using a balance board

Developmental goal: Balance

Space and equipment: Multipurpose area and
24 inch by 24 inch balance board

Number of players: Groups of 4 to 6 for each
board

Test reference: II, III, and VI

Procedure: If the child encounters difficulty
when using a balance board, put up a target
at eye level several feet in front. It will help
if the child keeps looking at the target while
balancing on the board. Before beginning
challenges, have the child get "the feel" of
the board by rocking gently side to side and
back and forth (Fig. 14-12).

1. Can you look at the target while you
are balancing?

2. Can you look at someone else while
you are balancing?

3. Can you touch your knees? Shoulders? Hips? Head?

4. Show me if you can touch your feet
and then stand up without losing balance.

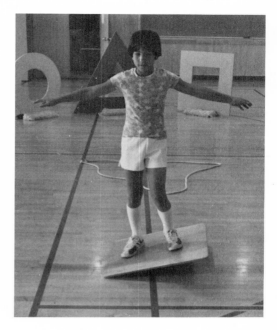

Fig. 14-12. Controlling the body on the balance
board.

5. Can you balance on one foot? On the
other foot?

6. Can you pick up a ball while balancing?

7. Can you bounce and catch it?

8. See if you can turn on the board and
face the other direction.

9. Can you balance with your feet wide
apart? Close together?

10. Show me something else you can do
on the balance board.

TIN CAN STILTS

Behavioral objectives: To maintain balance in a
variety of activities using tin can stilts

Developmental goal: Balance, body awareness
in space, and eye-hand and eye-foot coordination

Space and equipment: Multipurpose area and a
pair of cans for each child

Number of players: Entire class

Test reference: IV and VI

Procedure: To learn to balance while elevated,
a child begins by standing on tin can stilts
(Fig. 14-13). Once children are able to stand
straight without watching their feet and to
walk with smooth strides, they easily go on
to regular wooden or metal stilts. It is best to

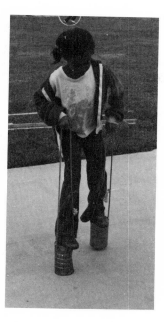

Fig. 14-13. Walking on tin can stilts challenges balance.

have a variety of can heights. Tuna, fruit (29 ounce), and juice (32 ounce) cans are all excellent because they have a large surface for foot placement. To use them, punch holes in opposite sides of the cans with a beer can opener. Thread clothesline through both holes and tie the ends at approximately the height of the child's waist. Following is a progression for learning to walk on tin cans:

1. Balance on the cans, holding the strings taut.
2. Walk, looking ahead and standing tall.
3. Use smooth strides.

Once these skills are mastered the child can try the following challenges:

1. Can you take ten steps forward with your stilts? Backward?
2. Can you use a taller pair and still take ten steps forward and backward?
3. Show me if you can walk around the square.
4. Can you walk sideways crossing one foot in front of the other?
5. Can you walk on the line placing one can in front of the other?
6. Can you walk on the line keeping your right foot in front all the time? Your left foot?

7. See if you can go through the obstacle course.
8. Can you balance on one can holding the other in the air?
9. See if you can kick the ball with a stilt.

CIRCULAR BALANCE BOARD

Behavioral objectives: To maintain balance in a variety of activities using a circular balance board

Developmental goal: Balance, directionality, and laterality crossing the midline

Space and equipment: Multipurpose area and circular balance board

Number of players: Groups of 4 to 6

Test reference: VI

Procedure: Unlike the regular balance board, this piece of equipment is not used to balance parallel to the ground but to balance on an angle while rotating the board in a complete circle (Fig. 14-14). The task is easiest if the feet are spread wide apart. The object is for all parts of the circle to rotate around and touch the ground in sequence. To do this, the hips must rotate and the feet not move. For those who cannot get the round-and-round feeling, it helps for the teacher to press down and around on the edges as the child attempts to rotate.

1. Can you go around three times to the right? Ten times?
2. Can you change and go around three times to the left? Ten times?
3. Can you bounce a ball as you go around?
4. Can you go to the right until I say change and then to the left?
5. Show me how close you can get your feet and go around ten times both ways.

TOOBER

Behavioral objectives: To maintain balance in a variety of activities using a Toober

Developmental goal: Leg strength and dynamic balance

Space and equipment: Multipurpose area, Toober (large innertube), and safety mat

Number of players: Groups of 4 to 6

Test reference: IV and VI

Procedure: When using a Toober, the child is propelled into the air, and so specific precautions must be taken. Always have a mat under the tube and someone holding the sides of the tube.

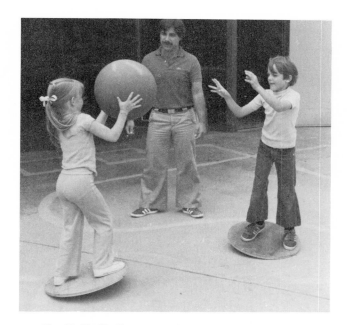

Fig. 14-14. Challenges on the circular balance board.

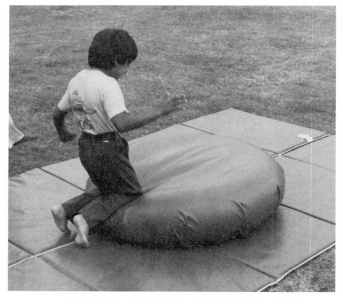

Fig. 14-15. Rebound activity on the Toober.

1. Can you walk around the edge of the Toober in a complete circle?
2. Show me how you can bounce on the edge and jump off onto the mat (Fig. 14-15).
3. Can you bounce on the edge and jump into the middle?
4. See if you can bounce to the other side and jump onto the mat.

Hula-Hoop activities

The Hula-Hoop can be used in a variety of ways. Children normally use it to experience continuous motion, but they can also roll it along the ground and use it in solving problems while working alone or with a partner. When using it in continuous motion, the child must have a certain amount of rhythm, balance, and practice to be able to keep it circling smoothly and for any length of time. Music is fun and helpful for children while they move the hoop around their bodies (Fig. 14-16, *A*). Once they master the trick, they can try new activities. The hoop is an excellent prop for creative movement. The teacher can challenge the children to attempt different movements with it (Fig. 14-16, *B*).

CONTINUOUS MOVEMENT

Behavioral objective: To circle a hoop around the body in a continuous motion
Developmental goal: Rhythm and coordination
Space and equipment: Multipurpose area and Hula-Hoops
Number of players: Entire class
Test reference: V and VI
Procedure: The teacher can challenge the child to do continuous-movement tricks by asking the following questions:

1. Can you spin the hoop around your body?
2. Can you spin it around another part?
3. Can you make it move slower or faster?
4. Can you make it move higher on your body?

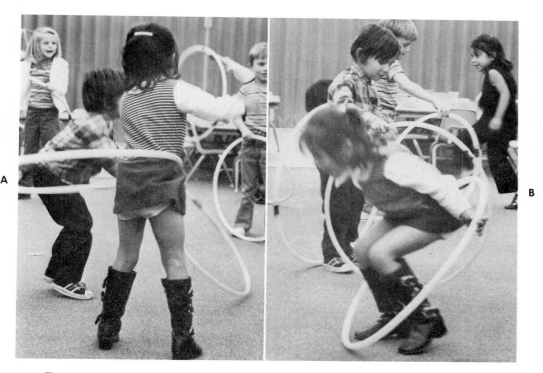

Fig. 14-16. A, Children twirling Hula-Hoops. **B,** Children experimenting with Hula-Hoops.

ROLLING ✓

Procedure: The teacher can challenge the child to do rolling tricks with the following questions:

1. Can you roll your hoop and jump through it?
2. Can you spin it like a top?
3. Can you roll it away and have it come back by itself?

PARTNERS ✓

Procedure: The teacher can challenge the child to do tricks with a partner with the following questions:

1. Can you roll it to your partner?
2. Can you help your partner crawl through, not letting the hoop touch the ground?
3. Can your partner jump through?

MANIPULATIVE SKILLS

Most of the lifetime sport activities include striking, throwing, and catching. When teaching basic manipulative activities, the teacher should emphasize proper form in each of these skills. The teacher should be aware of the theory of opposition in throwing activities and should stress rhythm and balance control in giving with the object in catching games. Refer to Chapter 8 for specific throwing and catching techniques.

✓ MANIPULATIVE BEANBAG SKILLS

Behavioral objective: To perform manipulative activities with beanbags

Developmental goal: Object manipulation and control

Space and equipment: Multipurpose area and a beanbag for each child

Number of participants: Entire class

Test reference: I and II

Procedure: When this level child practices catching and throwing skills, a beanbag is an excellent choice of projectile. It is relatively easy to throw and catch, and it does not hurt the child if it is missed. It also keeps play more continuous because a beanbag will not roll or bounce away, requiring time for the child to chase it (Fig. 14-17).

1. Can you walk around the room balancing the beanbag on your head? On your hand? On your other hand?
2. Can you keep the beanbag on your foot while you walk across the room?
3. Can you toss your beanbag in the air and catch it with two hands? One

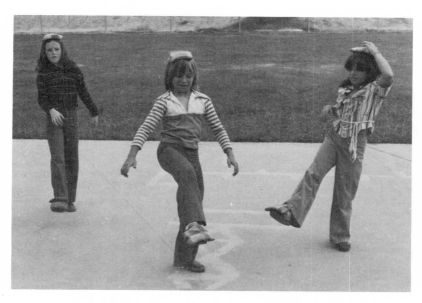

Fig. 14-17. "Can you balance a beanbag on your head and foot?"

hand? Alternating hands with each catch?

4. See if you can toss your beanbag from hand to hand.
5. Can you sit and throw your beanbag in the air then stand up and catch it?
6. Can you put your beanbag on your foot and kick it up and catch it? See if you can do this again but clap your hands before you catch it.
7. Can you pass a beanbag around the circle without dropping it? Can you pass two of them? Three?

Beanbag games

TARGET TOSS

Behavioral objective: To throw beanbags into designated targets

Developmental goal: Eye-hand coordination

Space and equipment: Multipurpose play area, beanbags, and Hula-Hoops

Number of participants: Entire class in groups of 3

Test reference: II

Procedure: Place three Hula-Hoops 3 feet apart with the throwing line 5 feet from the first hoop. A child stands at the throwing line and attempts to toss a beanbag into the first hoop, then the second, and then the third. The child receives three tries at each hoop. A beanbag landing in the hoop on the first try counts three points, on the second

try, two points, and on the third try, one point.

LADDER TOSS

Behavioral objective: To throw and catch with a partner

Developmental goal: Eye-hand coordination

Space and equipment: Multipurpose play area with ladder markings and beanbags

Number of participants: Entire class in groups of 2

Test reference: II and VI

Procedure: A child stands in the first square of the "ladder" and catches a beanbag thrown by a partner. After each successful catch, the child moves back one square. Score one point for the first square catch, two points for the second square catch, and so on. Catcher and thrower change places after a miss, and a new game is started.

PICKING DAISIES

Behavioral objective: To move an object quickly from one space to another

Developmental goal: Spatial relationships, speed, and flexibility

Space and equipment: Play area, indoors or out, and 15 beanbags

Number of participants: Groups of 4 to 6

Test reference: I, III, and V

Procedure: Place 15 beanbags on a line and ask a child to place them, one at a time, inside a circle 10 feet from the line. (Beanbags must be placed and not thrown.)

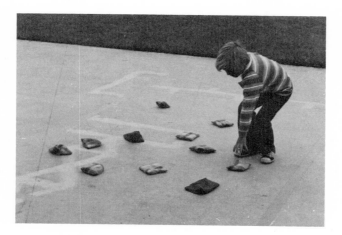

Fig. 14-18. Playing beanbag pickup.

BEANBAG PICKUP ✓

Behavioral objective: To collect and hold a number of beanbags in two hands

Developmental goal: Speed and agility

Space and equipment: Multipurpose play area and 15 beanbags

Number of participants: Entire class one at a time

Test reference: I and V

Procedure: Fifteen beanbags are scattered around a play area and one child is selected to pick up as many as possible in 15 seconds (Fig. 14-18). The rest of the children count off the seconds. The child collecting the most beanbags within the time limit is the winner.

CIRCLE PASS

Behavioral objective: To develop quickness and control in passing a beanbag

Developmental goal: Fine motor, eye-hand control

Space and equipment: Multipurpose play area and beanbags

Number of participants: 6 to 8 to a circle

Test reference: I and V

Procedure: Arrange children in two or more equal circles sitting down. Have children pass a beanbag around the circle. When it gets back to the starting point, the first child stands. The winning team is given one point.

SMOKESTACK RELAY

Behavioral objective: To pass a beanbag quickly and stack in a pile

Developmental goal: Object control and object balance

Space and equipment: Multipurpose play area and one beanbag for each child

Number of participants: 6 in each row

Test reference: I and II

Procedure: For this relay have the players seated in equal lines with six beanbags piled in front of the first player. On signal, the beanbags are passed back one at a time. The last player in the line lays the first beanbag on the floor and each succeeding beanbag on top of the one preceding it with only the first one touching the floor. The stack must stand without any assistance from the stacker. If the stack falls, it must be restacked. The first team to build the smokestack correctly wins the relay.

FOX AND SQUIRREL

Behavioral objective: To pass an object quickly

Developmental goal: Eye-hand coordination and quickness

Space and equipment: Multipurpose play area and beanbags

Number of participants: 10 to 12

Test reference: I and V

Procedure: Children stand or sit in a circle formation, and a beanbag called the squirrel is passed around the circle. A second beanbag, known as the fox, is started around in the same direction. When the fox catches the squirrel, the game is over. This same game may be played with two balls of different sizes.

BEANBAG TAG

Behavioral objective: To avoid being tagged while carrying the beanbag

Developmental goal: Agility, throwing skills, and speed

Space and equipment: Playground and beanbags

Number of participants: Entire class

Test reference: II and V

Procedure: One child is "it" and carries a beanbag as other children chase him or her. If "it" is tagged, the tagger takes the beanbag and becomes "it." "It" may toss the beanbag to another child who then becomes "it" and is chased by the others.

POISON BEANBAG

Behavioral objective: To pass the beanbag quickly to another person

Developmental goal: Quickness in object manipulation

Space and equipment: Playground or gymnasium and three beanbags

Number of participants: 10 to 12

Test reference: I and V

Procedure: Children stand or sit in a circle. Beanbags are handed rapidly clockwise or counterclockwise from player to player. When the signal is given, any player holding a beanbag is "poisoned" and drops out of the circle. As players leave the circle, decrease the number of beanbags used so the last two players are exchanging only one beanbag.

BEANBAG RING THROW

Behavioral objective: To throw accurately at a target

Developmental goal: Eye-hand coordination

Space and equipment: Multipurpose play area and three beanbags per team

Number of players: 8 to 40

Test reference: II

Procedure: The children divide into teams of four to six. The members of each team line up in squad formation behind that team's restraining line. At a signal, the captain of each team, while standing behind the restraining line, throws three beanbags in succession toward a circle. The distance between the restraining line and the circle can be varied according to the ability of the children. Any beanbag that touches the circumference of the circle cannot be counted in computing the score. After the score is recorded, the captain picks up the beanbags, carries them to the next player on the team, and then goes to the end of the squad.

DEVELOPMENTAL BALL SKILL PROGRESSION

1. Roll a large ball between two objects.
2. Roll a large ball to a partner.
3. Roll a large ball against a wall and catch it.
4. Bounce and catch a large ball with two hands.
5. Bounce a large ball with either hand.
6. Bounce a large ball while walking in a straight line.
7. Bounce a large ball while running in a straight line.
8. Bounce a large ball while moving in a figure-eight pattern.
9. Catch a large ball rolled from a partner.
10. Catch a large ball bounced from a partner.
11. Catch a large ball thrown from a distance of 5 feet.
12. Catch a softball thrown from a distance of 10 feet.
13. Catch a 9-inch ball thrown from a distance of 20 feet.
14. Throw a large ball to a partner with a two-hand, underhand toss.
15. Throw a large ball to a partner with a chest pass.
16. Throw a beanbag to a floor target with an underhand throw.
17. Throw a softball to a wall target with an underhand throw.
18. Throw a softball to a wall target with an overhand throw.
19. Throw a softball for distance and accuracy.
20. Throw a softball to a moving target.
21. Shoot a basketball from the chest.
22. Shoot a basketball underhand.
23. Dribble a basketball and shoot overhand.
24. Kick a stationary ball.
25. Kick a moving ball.
26. Run and kick a stationary ball.
27. Run and kick a moving ball.
28. Kick a ball for distance.
29. Dribble a ball in a straight line with both feet.
30. Dribble a ball in a zigzag line with both feet.
31. Stop a moving ball with one foot.
32. Hit a ball off a batting tee.
33. Hit a ball thrown underhand.
34. Hit a ball thrown overhand.
35. Serve a volleyball underhand.
36. Hit a volleyball underhand.
37. Hit a volleyball with a chest set.
38. Serve a volleyball overhand.
39. Throw a football to a partner.
40. Throw a football to a moving target.

Play continues until all have had a chance to throw the beanbags. Speed is not as important as accuracy in throwing. One point is earned for each beanbag that lands completely within the circle. The team wins that has the highest score after all the players have had a chance to throw the beanbags. Each squad should keep its own total score, making sure that only the beanbags that landed completely in the circle are counted. Wastebaskets can be used, if enough are available, to make it easier to know which throws earn points.

Ball skills

Once a child feels comfortable throwing and catching a beanbag, a ball, preferably a 7-inch utility ball, may be introduced. The developmental ball skill progression chart (see boxed material on p. 317) displays the progression of skill sophistication necessary for the child to compete successfully in advanced level games and sports. Level 2 children, through discovery challenges, should develop a base from which higher skills can be attained and honed through practice. When teaching ball skills, the teacher must provide a proper size ball in line with the developmental level of the child. A ball too large or too small or a challenge too great for the present ability level of the children will deter the ball skill learning process. Beginning skills usually involve a large ball and short distances for throwing and catching skills in which large muscles can be used. Advanced level activities use a smaller ball and greater distances, reflecting the requirements for traditional games such as baseball and football.

Throwing and catching skills

BALL HANDLING

Behavioral objective: To be able to control a ball in a variety of situations
Developmental goal: Eye-hand coordination in throwing and catching skills
Equipment and space: Multipurpose play area and a ball for each child

Number of participants: Entire class in small groups of 7 to 9
Test reference: II
Procedure
 1. Show me what you can do with your ball.
 2. Can you roll the ball to the wall (6 feet away)?
 3. Can you roll the ball, run ahead, and stop it?
 4. Can you toss the ball in the air and catch it?
 5. Can you bounce the ball along the line (Fig. 14-19)?
 6. See if you can toss the ball high, let it bounce, and catch it.
 7. Can you toss the ball high, let it bounce, clap your hands and catch it? How many times can you clap your hands and catch the ball?
 8. Can you toss your ball in the air and catch it while running?
 9. Can you toss your ball in the air, close your eyes, and catch it?

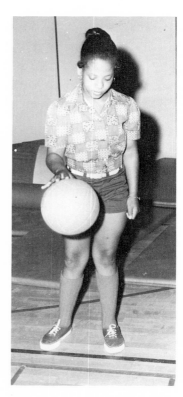

Fig. 14-19. Developing ball-handling skills.

10. Can you toss your ball from hand to hand?
11. Can you roll a ball to a partner?
12. Who can bounce the ball to a partner with one hand?
13. Can you throw the ball to a partner, using an overhand throw?
14. Show me a bounce pass to a partner.
15. Can you toss the ball high to a partner, using an underhand throw?
16. Can you bounce and catch your ball (Fig. 14-19).

LEADER AND CLASS

Behavioral objective: To throw and catch accurately
Developmental goal: Eye-hand coordination
Space and equipment: Multipurpose play area and playground ball
Number of players: 4 to 40
Test reference: II
Procedure: The children divide into groups of four to six. The members of each group stand side by side in a line. One end of the line is designated the head and the other, the foot. The member at the head of the line becomes the leader and faces the group, standing 8 to 10 feet in front of them (Fig. 14-20). The leader tosses a ball to each player in the group in turn, and each throws the ball back to the leader. A player who misses the ball must go to the foot of the line. The leader who misses a ball must go

to the foot of the line, and the next player at the head becomes the leader. If the ball goes around the group twice and the leader has not missed, the leader goes to the foot of the line, and the player at the head becomes the leader. In this game, volleyball, softball, football, or soccer skills can be used, according to the grade level and ability.

CIRCLE BALL

Behavioral objective: To throw and catch a ball
Developmental goal: Eye-hand coordination
Space and equipment: Multipurpose play area and playground ball
Number of players: 6 to 10 per circle
Test reference: II
Procedure: The children form circles. One child in each circle is chosen to be the leader and stands in the center of the circle. The leader tosses the ball to each circle player, who must toss it back. If the leader drops a well-tossed ball, the child who tossed it becomes the new leader. A different child should have a turn as leader after a complete revolution has been made and the leader has not missed a ball, and each child should have a turn as leader.

Kicking skills. Basically, American children play ball games with their hands, and few can compare with the sophisticated talent of their foreign counterparts when it comes to kicking skills.

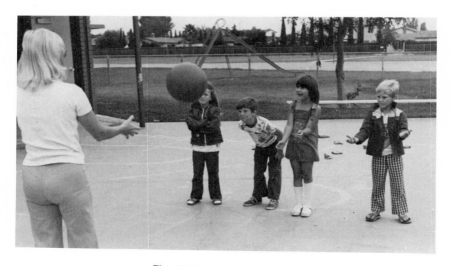

Fig. 14-20. Leader and class.

Challenges involving ball control, agility, and coordination must be presented to the child early in life to enhance progressive development in kicking and dribbling skills. Through guided practice in organized kicking activities, children can gain confidence and become as comfortable with eye-foot coordination skills as they are with eye-hand activities.

BALL KICKING AND FOOT DRIBBLING CHALLENGES (Fig. 14-21)

Procedure
1. Can you kick a stationary ball?
2. Who can kick a stationary ball and hit the target?
3. Can you run forward and kick a stationary ball?
4. Can you kick your ball to a partner?
5. Can you kick a moving ball?
6. Who can kick a rolling ball to a target?
7. Can you kick a stationary ball forward with the inside of your foot?
8. Who can kick a moving ball forward with the inside of the foot?
9. Can you kick a moving ball to your partner?
10. Show me how far you can kick the ball.
11. Can you dribble your ball to a line and back using the sides of your feet?
12. Who can dribble the ball around and between the cones using the sides of the feet?
13. Can you dribble the ball and pass it to a partner?
14. Can you stop the ball using the sole of your foot?

Lummi sticks

Children in level 2 enjoy beginning stick activities and have fun discovering what they can do with a stick. The following challenges offer beginning skills in object control. The inexpensive equipment is excellent for the development of eye-hand coordination, laterality, directionality, balance, and rhythmical play. If the activity is not familiar to the teacher, the use of records makes it easy to teach.

SINGLE STICKS

Behavioral objective: To be able to manipulate a stick with rhythm and control
Developmental goal: Eye-hand coordination, directionality, and balance
Equipment and space: Multipurpose area and one stick for each pupil
Number of participants: Entire class
Test reference: I and II
Procedure
1. Can you wave your stick in a circular motion?
2. Can you hold your stick straight up and walk your fingers up and down it? Change hands, and do it again.

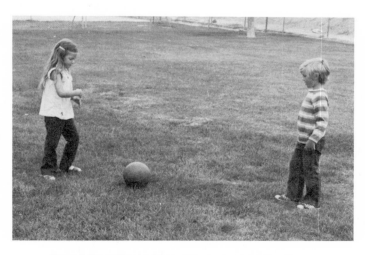

Fig. 14-21. Using kicking skills in a game situation.

3. Can you spin your stick flat on the floor? Spin it the other way.
4. Who can toss their stick from hand to hand?
5. Who can flip their stick in the air and catch it after one turn?
6. Can you hold your stick in front of you with two hands, drop it, and catch it before it hits the ground? Do it with one hand.
7. Who can drop the stick and catch it on the bounce?
8. Who can balance the stick on a part of the body?
9. Can you balance the stick on two fingers?
10. How many parts of your body can balance your stick on?
11. Can you pass your stick around your body? How fast can you go?

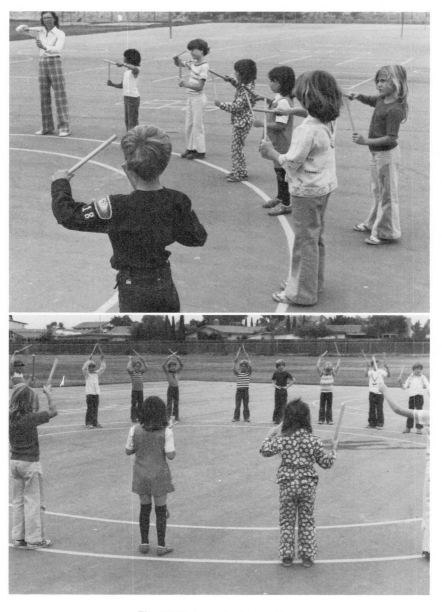

Fig. 14-22. Lummi stick routines.

12. Can you pass your stick around your body and then go the other way?

DOUBLE STICKS (Fig. 14-22)

Behavioral objective: To be able to hit one stick with the other with accuracy

Developmental goal: Eye-hand coordination, directionality, balance, laterality, and agility

Equipment and space: Multipurpose area and two sticks for each pupil

Number of participants: Entire class.

Test reference: I

Procedure

1. Use all of the single stick activities with double sticks.
2. Can you play "hammer the nail" with your sticks? Hammer with the other hand.
3. Can you hammer the nail with your eyes closed?
4. Show me who can hold the ends of both sticks together and hit them.

FITNESS ACTIVITIES

The fitness component should be incorporated into each physical education lesson. Each day children should participate in at least 3 to 5 minutes of warm-up exercises. The warm-up should begin with stretching and easy movements, move to increased intensity exercises, and then end in relaxation activities. The exercise program is suited to both the classroom and out-of-doors. Regardless of the lesson presented, fitness activities should be included to achieve the complete lesson. Refer to Chapter 10 for additional information.

EXERCISE PROGRAM FOR YOUNG CHILDREN

Behavioral objective: To develop total fitness in young children

Developmental goal: Flexibility, strength, and endurance

Space and equipment: Multipurpose area

Number of participants: Entire class

Test reference: III

Procedure

Arms and shoulders

ARM SWING: Stand with the feet apart, swing arms forward overhead, keeping the elbows straight, and then backwards. Arms can be swung in different directions.

ARM CIRCLES: Stand with the feet apart and the arms extended to the side at shoulder height. Rotate the arms in small circles, gradually increasing in size. Change direction.

KNEE PUSH-UPS: Start with the elbows close to the body then extend arms with back straight.

STRETCHER: Stand and raise the elbows to shoulder height with fists clenched and palms down. Thrust the elbows backward vigorously and keep the head erect.

Abdomen

SHOULDER CURL: Lie on the back with arms folded across the chest, and curl the head and shoulders forward.

SIT-UP: Lie on the back with the knees bent and sit up, touching elbows to knees.

Back

ARCH: Assume a sitting position with hands on the floor under the shoulders and fingers pointing to the back. Arch the back with the weight on the hands and feet. Lower the body and repeat.

SUPPORT BALANCE: Assume a back-support position with the face up and support the body as follows: on two hands and one foot, on two feet and one hand, on one foot and one hand on the same side of the body, and on one foot and one hand on opposite sides of the body.

Legs and pelvic girdle

BEND AND STRETCH: Stand with the arms raised over head and feet apart at shoulder width. Bend forward, reaching downward between the legs as far back as possible and keeping legs straight. Return to upright position and repeat.

JUMPING JACK: Stand with the feet together and hands to the sides. Jump up, landing feet in a wide straddle position, and touch hands above the head as the feet land apart. Jump up again and land with feet together and hands at the sides. Continue in rhythm.

TOE TOUCH: Sit on the floor with the feet together and hands on the thighs. Bend forward slowly and touch toes with fingers without bending the knees.

KNEE LIFT: Stand erect with the feet together and arms at sides. Raise the right knee as high as possible, grasping the leg with both hands and pulling the knee to the body. Return to the starting position and repeat with the left knee.

General body muscles

RUBBER NECK: Lower the head and rotate right, back, left, and down. Repeat changing direction.

TRUNK TWISTER: Stand with the feet apart and hands on hips. Twist trunk first to the right and then to the left. Repeat in rhythm.

SIDE BEND: Stand with the hands on the hips. Bend trunk sideways, first to the right and then to the left. Repeat in rhythm.

RUNNING: Children should run at least 300 yards daily. Running can be made more enjoyable by developing a fitness course along which exercise stations are positioned throughout. Participation in cross-country races and obstacle courses and maintaining individual records are good motivational aids. Children also like to take their heart rates before and after a race.

CARDIORESPIRATORY CHALLENGES

Behavioral objective: To experience continuous activities designed to develop stamina

Developmental goal: To develop cardiorespiratory endurance

Space and equipment: Multipurpose play area

Number of players: Entire class

Test reference: IV and V

Procedure: Arrange the class in a circle or informal group setting. Teacher and the class count the repetitions aloud together.

Endurance hops

1. Children hop on both feet continuously up to 200 times.

2. Children straddle hop continuously up to 200 times.
3. Children scissor hop up to 200 times.
4. Children hop on right foot up to 50 times.
5. Children hop on left foot up to 50 times.
6. Children squat-jump, touching hands to floor and springing upward again and again as long as possible. (Knees should be bent only half way during the squat.)

Children achieving the "magic" 50 or 200 in each activity can be given certificates of recognition.

Running in place

Have children run in place by lifting their knees as high as possible. Each arm should move rhythmically forward and back. Start the children running for a half minute and increase the time gradually until a 2 or 3 minute run is achieved.

Walk, trot, and sprint

Have children form a large circle. On the first whistle, the children begin to walk around the circle. The second whistle signals a change to a trot, and the third whistle signals a sprint. The fourth whistle signals the children to slow to a walk again. The teacher repeats the sequence until an acceptable workout has been completed.

CONTINUOUS RHYTHMICAL EXERCISE

Behavioral objective: To experience exercise through continuous rhythmical movement

Developmental goal: Cardiovascular development, strength, and flexibility

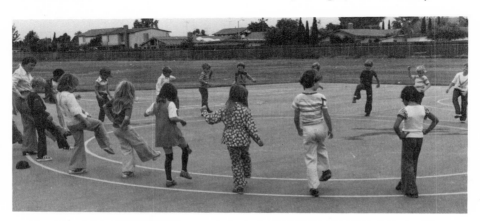

Fig. 14-23. Hopping during continuous rhythmical exercise.

Space and equipment: Multipurpose play area and painted circle

Number of participants: Entire class

Test reference: III, IV, VI, and VII

Procedure: The children begin by walking around in a circle. The teacher gives directions, such as walk fast, run, swing your arms, hop, or skip or any other locomotor skill. The teacher stops the movement periodically and gives directions for a specific exercise or stunt, such as a sit-up or jumping jack (Fig. 14-23). After completion of the exercises, children continue to walk or run in the circle formation. The activity can continue for 5 minutes without stopping. To end the exercise, the teacher can slow the circle to a stop and have the children take deep breaths, raising their arms high and exhaling with a forward bend.

FOLLOW THE LEADER

Behavioral objective: To lead children in a variety of motor challenges

Developmental goal: Climbing skills and agility

Space and equipment: Playground with permanent equipment

Number of players: Entire class

Test reference: IV, VI, and VII

Procedure: Have one child lead the group running around the play area. Use the permanent equipment and add obstacles so the children climb, hop, and go under, over, and around obstacles. Leaders can create their own fitness challenges for the children to follow.

Long jump rope

Probably no game is so universally accepted as jump rope. It takes a minimum of equipment for a maximum of fitness and fun (Fig. 14-24). It should begin to be taught at the five-year-old level and can progress to a degree of difficulty that adults find challenging.

LONG ROPE JUMPING

Behavioral objective: To be able to jump consecutively to ten

Developmental goals: Cardiorespiratory fitness, balance, and rhythm

Space and equipment: Multipurpose area and 10-foot ropes

Number of participants: 4 to 6 students per rope

Test reference: IV and VI

Procedure: Following is a progression for learning long rope jumping that has proved to be successful with beginning students.

1. Without a rope, the children bend their knees and jump straight up and down in place on the teacher's command to jump and wait.
2. The children jump in a 1-foot–square

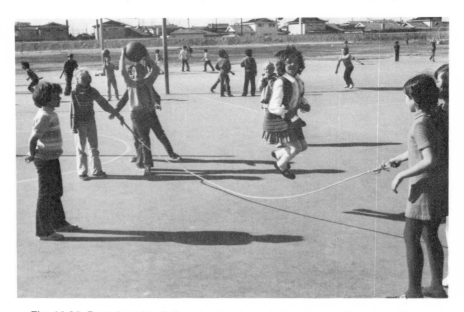

Fig. 14-24. Rope jumping is fun and develops rhythm and cardiovascular fitness.

"magic box" drawn on the playground area with chalk. They must be able to jump in this magic box five times in rhythm before progressing to jumping with the rope. The teacher should insist that the children wait after each command to jump, using the verbal command "jump, wait, jump, wait" and so on (Fig. 14-25). Learning to jump without the rope eliminates the lateral movement often learned from jumping side to side over a low rope, which is detrimental to efficient rope jumping.

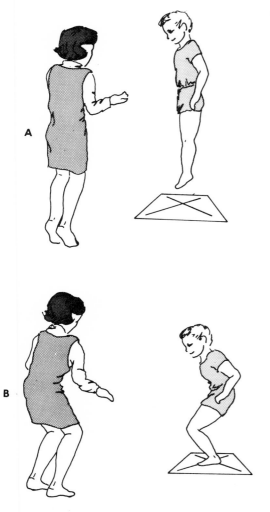

Fig. 14-25. Jumping in magic box to commands: **A,** jump and, **B,** wait.

3. During this initial stage of learning how to jump straight up and straight down, the child should learn (a) to keep the feet together, (b) not to jump too high, (c) to land easily on the balls of the feet, (d) to stay in one place, (e) to maintain correct rhythm to the jump-wait beat, and (f) to flex the knees.
4. The child should learn how to be a good turner. A full arm motion must be used so the rope will not be pulled back, causing "high water" for the jumper. A good turner must follow and stay even with the teacher.
5. The child should face the teacher and jump in the magic box drawn with chalk on the playground. The teacher, and not the feet, should be watched and a jump should occur only when the teacher indicates it by the jump-wait command (Fig. 14-26, A). Several practice calls of "jump" before the rope is actually turned will allow the teacher to see how fast the child reacts to the command. The teacher must adjust the speed of the call and the rope turn to the child's quickness or slowness of reaction time.
6. It is best to have no more than five beginners at one time using this technique. After a beginning practice period in which all have learned to jump, a heterogeneous group of children should jump together; this seems to speed the learning process, since the beginners pick up techniques from the more skilled students. The teacher should positively reinforce the learning of correct techneques of jumping rope by saying, for example, "How lightly you land on your feet," "Your knees are bent just right," or "What a fine turner you are; you stay right with me."
7. After each child has had a turn at jumping, time should be spent turning the rope. However, in the beginning, a competent turner makes the teacher's job easier, and the rotation can be delayed until all have accomplished the skill.
8. The child learns jumping skills in the following progression: (a) stand next to the rope and begin jumping; (b)

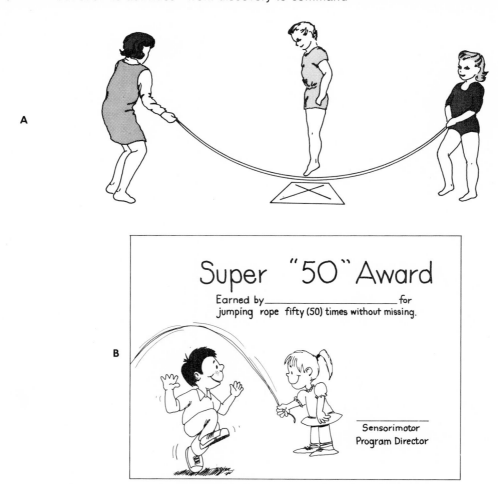

Fig. 14-26. A, Jumping successfully using the magic box technique. **B,** Awards such as the Super "50" help motivate children to improve their jumping skills.

run in while the rope is turning and jump; (c) run in and out, jumping in between; (d) run in and out without jumping; (e) turn around while jumping; (f) touch the ground between jumps; (g) jump with a partner; (h) change places with a partner while jumping; (i) pantomime rhymes while jumping; (j) run in the back door and continue to jump; and (k) jump double dutch (two ropes turning alternately in opposite directions).

It has been found that after a child learns to jump well when someone else is turning, it is easier for him or her to learn solo jumping, in which the additional skill of the hand coordination must be integrated with the jump. There are many different rhymes that children repeat as they jump rope. They encourage children to increase their jumping ability, maintain a regular tempo, and test individual progress in an enjoyable manner. Awards such as the Super "50" also help motivate children to improve their jumping skills (Fig. 14-26, *B*). Following are some of the favorites of elementary school children:

LADY AT THE GATE

Lady, lady at the gate, eating cherries from a plate
How many cherries did she eat? One, two, three, etc.

JOHNNY

Johnny over the ocean, Johnny over the sea,
Johnny broke a bottle and blamed it on me.
I told ma and ma told pa, Johnny got a lickin'
   so ha, ha, ha!
How many lickin's did Johnny get? One,
   two, three, etc.

KISSES

Down in the valley where the green grass
   grows,
There sat *(child's name)* as sweet as a
   rose.
She sang and she sang and she sang so
   sweet,
Along came *(child's name)* and kissed her
   on the cheek.
How many kisses did she get? One, Two,
   three, etc.

ABCs

Apples, peaches, peanut butter,
What's the initial of my true lover?
A, B, C, etc.

GYPSY

Gypsy, gypsy, please tell me
What my husband is going to be;
A rich man, a poor man, a beggar man, a
   thief,
A doctor, a lawyer, an Indian chief.

Verses that require that the child act
out a stunt while jumping are more difficult, since while doing them, a child
must either break rhythm or change the
balancing position of his body. Some of
these verses are as follows:

ARCHIE BUNKER

Archie Bunker went to France,
To teach the children how to dance.
First the heel, then the toe,
Turn around, and out you go.

TEDDY BEAR

Teddy bear, teddy bear, turn around,
Teddy bear, teddy bear, touch the ground.
Teddy bear, teddy bear, show your shoe,
Teddy bear, teddy bear, that will do.
Teddy bear, teddy bear, go upstairs,
Teddy bear, teddy bear, say your prayers.
Teddy bear, teddy bear, turn out the light,
Teddy bear, teddy bear, say good night.

SPANISH DANCER

Not last night, but the night before,
Twenty-four robbers came knocking at my
   door.
I ran out *(child runs out)* and they ran in
   (child comes in again)
And hit me over the head with a rolling pin.
I asked them what they wanted, and this is
   what they said:
Spanish dancer do the splits, Spanish
   dancer give a high kick,
Spanish dancer turn around, Spanish dancer
   get out of town.

HOUSE TO RENT

House to rent, inquire within.
As I move out, let Mary* move in.

IN SPIN

In, spin
Let Susie come in.
Out, spout
Let Susie go out.

LITTLE ORPHAN ANNIE

Little Orphan Annie
Hops on one foot, one foot.
Little Orphan Annie
Hops on two feet, two feet.
Little Orphan Annie
Hops on three feet, three feet.
   (Two feet and one hand)
Little Orphan Annie
Hops on four feet, four feet.
   (Two feet and two hands)
Little Orphan Annie hops out.

OLD MAN LAZY

Old Man Lazy drives me crazy.
   (Baby rope)
Up the ladder,
   (Overs)
Down the ladder,
   (Reverse rope; overs)
Old Man Lazy.
   (Baby rope)

RED HOT PEPPERS

Mabel, Mabel,
Set the table
And don't forget
The red hot peppers.†

---

*Name of next jumper.
†Rope is turned "peppers" (very fast).

CHANGING BEDROOMS

Changing bedrooms
Number one
Changing bedrooms
Number two
Changing bedrooms
Number three
etc.

(In this rhyme the rope is turned by two people, and two people are jumping at the same time. As each number is called, the jumpers exchange places in the rope without missing a jump.)

RHYTHMS AND DANCE

Since primitive times, rhythms and dance have played a major role in expressing the ideas and feelings of man in each civilization. Fertility rights, festive occasions, and preparation for war have all been expressed in some form of rhythmical activity. Today the many cultures throughout the world are recognized by the particular kind of dance activity associated with their culture or geographical area. Dancing usually expresses a joyous mood and is a pleasurable activity enjoyed by all.

To perform the creative movements or specific dance steps involved in a good rhythm program, the child needs to develop balance, coordination, poise, and self-confidence. Most children have a good sense of rhythm and enjoy moving their bodies to to the beat of a drum or other types of musical accompaniment. However, the degree to which a child learns rhythmical coordination depends a great deal on the emphasis placed on the dance program in the elementary school. Some suggestions for developing rhythm in children are as follows:

1. They can duplicate the rhythm by clapping their hands, snapping their fingers, stamping their feet, or using other rhythm instruments (Fig. 14-27).

2. By using a drum or clapping their hands to slow or fast rhythms, the children can learn to step on every beat.

3. They can develop ball skills and rhythm by bouncing a ball to the beat. Additional skills of running around the ball, turning and catching the ball, and throwing the ball into the air can be combined with the rhythmical pattern described.

4. They can jump rope to a rhythmical beat.

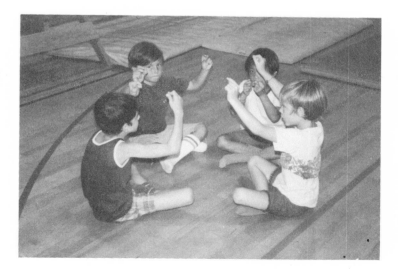

Fig. 14-27. Children developing rhythm through finger snapping.

Although it is desirable for the dance teacher to have the ability to play some type of musical instrument, it is not necessary for an effective lesson in rhythmical activities. There are many records available for each category of dance that offer excellent accompaniment during the lesson. In addition to this, percussion instruments can be made by the children that allow for greater involvement in the total rhythm program, such as rhythm sticks made from dowels, sandpaper blocks, and drums made from cans with drumheads from inner tubes. In most cases, materials for these instruments can be secured free of charge, and all children can participate in both construction and rhythmical activities.

Fundamental rhythms

Dance includes basic locomotor skills provided in various combinations and degrees of force. Most children come to school already knowing a variety of fundamental locomotor skills; however, in many cases the learning of these skills has been limited to uneven and nonrhythmical movements, and there is a definite need to develop smoothmess and rhythm in the execution of these skills. The following eight basic locomotor patterns serve as the basis for many of the more sophisticated dance steps.

Walk. The walking step is an even rhythmical movement involving transferring of the weight from one foot to the other. A rhythmical count or beat should be employed to develop a smooth walking step.

Run. The running step is an even rhythmical movement similar to the walk except that the speed is increased and the weight is carried on the balls of the feet. In the running step, both feet are momentarily off the ground at the same time (Fig. 14-28).

Hop. The hopping step is an even rhythmical movement that involves springing from the floor from one foot and landing on the same foot. The spring and landing are executed with the balls of the feet as in the running step.

Jump. The jumping step, an even

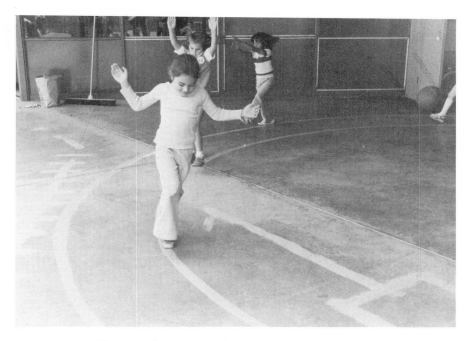

Fig. 14-28. Children learning to walk and run smoothly.

rhythmical movement, is a spring from the floor with both feet, in which the toes are used for pushing off and landing.

Leap. The leaping step is an even rhythmical movement that is an extension of the run. It differs from the run in that the knee bend at the beginning and end of the movement is exaggerated. One foot is used for pushing off and the other for landing. During the leap, both feet are off the floor at the same time.

Skip. The skipping step, an uneven rhythmical movement, is a fast step-hop with the foot. After each step-hop, the foot is extended forward in preparation for the next step-hop by the opposite foot.

Gallop. The galloping step, an uneven rhythmical movement, is the transferring of weight from the lead foot to the closing foot. The same foot remains the lead foot throughout the sequence of steps.

Slide. The sliding step is an uneven rhythmical lateral movement, in which the same foot continues to lead as in the gallop. The weight is transferred from the lead foot to the back foot in a sliding manner.

Following is a list of records that can be used to learn the fundamental rhythm skills:

Walk } Run }	Folkraft album 20 and RCA Victor album E-71, vol. 1
Hop	Childhood Rhythms, series I, nos. 101 and 102; Folkraft album 20 (fundamental steps and rhythms); and RCA Victor album E-71, vol. 1 (rhythmic activities)
Jump	Folkraft album 20 and RCA Victor album E-71, vol. 1
Leap	Childhood Rhythms, series V, nos. 501, 502, and 505
Skip	Childhood Rhythms, series II, nos. 202 and 205; Folkraft album 20; and RCA Victor album E-71, vol. 1
Gallop	Childhood Rhythms, series III, nos. 302, 303, and 305; Folkraft album 20; and RCA Victor album E-71, vol. 1
Slide	Folkraft album 20 and RCA Victor album E-71, vol. 1

Creative rhythms

Elementary school children enjoy creating their own movement patterns to music. Discovering how the body moves and determining what kind of movements can best describe an idea or feeling are enjoyable activities and develop rhythmical skills. Participation in creative activities is one of the major objectives of elementary physical education. Children should be encouraged to discover how they move and to understand their own physical capabilities and limitations. Through their imaginations they can describe in movement a variety of things in the world about them (Fig. 14-29).

In creative dance the teacher can present an idea and then allow the children to create movement patterns that express their feelings toward the idea. They may create a variety of rhythmical movement patterns in describing the wind, a flower, an animal, a mode of transportation, a feeling of joy or sadness, or a quality of strength or weakness. If all children are going to work on the same problem, the teacher often discusses it with the class as a whole, prior to beginning any activity. Positive reinforcement should be given at all times as the children attempt to solve the problem through creative movement. Recognition can be given to the most creative children in the class by allowing them to demonstrate their solutions to the problem. This often serves as a motivating factor to the more reserved children in the group.

Another approach to creating movement feelings in children is to have them listen to music and then construct dance movements that express their feelings regarding the particular type of music. The music should be played first while the children just listen and begin to develop ideas as to how they will move to the rhythmical tones involved.

Another activity that can help to develop rhythm and the recognition of rhythm is the beating of a drum. Children can discover the rhythm of their names by

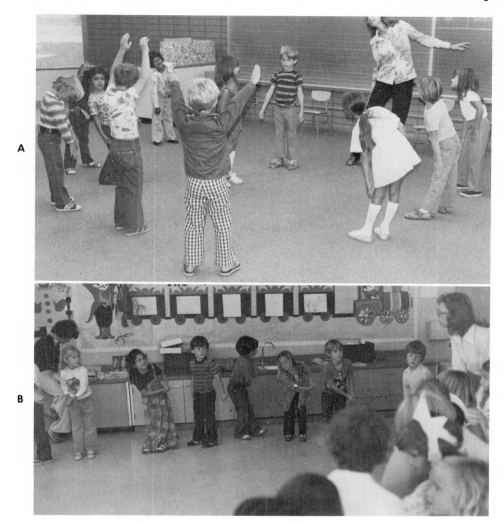

Fig. 14-29. Children creating rhythmical movements.

expressing each syllable with a corresponding drum beat. Children can also tell stories with the drum by increasing or decreasing the intensity or the tempo. They can learn to express ideas through variations of the rhythmical pattern and intensity of the drum beat. Children in the class also may listen and try to guess what story a child is telling. The drum can also be used for beating out rhythms that desribe the various modes of locomotion used in dance activities.

A game that is often played in rhythmical development is lock and key (Fig. 14-30). Lock and key is a game of recog-

nition of rhythmical patterns by either an individual or a group, using instruments made of materials such as metal, wood, and glass. The lock says, "Find the key, find the key," and circles around the group searching for a key. "I'm a wooden lock. To open the lock you must do the same as me." The lock offers a rhythmical pattern. The key listens carefully and with encouragement attempts to duplicate the rhythm with the same implement. The lock then asks, "Did he (or she) open the lock?" The group responds by chanting, "He (or she) opened the lock, he (or she) opened the lock," or "No,

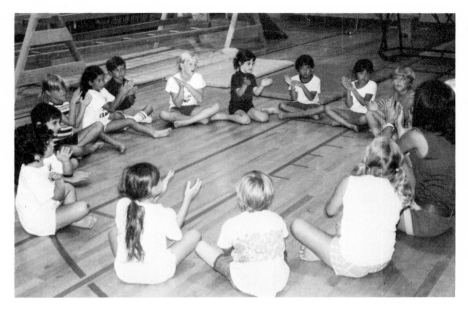

Fig. 14-30. Playing the rhythm development game of lock and key.

try again, try again." In this kind of game not only does the individual have to be able to identify the rhythm and duplicate it in order to open the lock, but also the group must determine whether the rhythm repeated by the key was an accurate reproduction of the original rhythm. Intricate or simple patterns may be used, depending on the level of the group. Although some children temporarily fail, they will eventually succeed and receive peer admiration.

The creative rhythm lesson is based on movement exploration activities. Discovering which movement activity best fits the beat gives much enjoyment to children and helps lessen the inhibitions often associated with creative movement. The teacher should allow children who are more timid to mimic others during the early stages of creative movement lessons. However, later on in creative movement activities, the teacher may select these individuals as the first to give their solution so that they receive proper peer recognition.

Following is a list of records that can be used to learn creative rhythm.

| Animals | Childhood Rhythms, series V, no. 501, and series I, nos. 102 and 103; RCA Victor rhythm series 45-5007, vol. 2; and MGM S-4264 |
| Nature and creative rhythms | Columbia C-30769; Atlantic 68002; and MGM S-4264 |

Successful student participation in a creative rhythm lesson requires a teacher who enjoys dance and is willing to become a part of the activities. The teacher must be quick to recognize excellence in student performance and to develop an atmosphere of freedom in which the children can express themselves in a creative mode.

The following activities are recommended for the level 2 developmental stage; however, one must realize there can be some overlap because of differences in maturational stages.

IMITATIVE AND INTERPRETATIVE RHYTHMS

Behavioral objective: To create individual rhythmical movement patterns
Developmental goal: Increase rhythmical abili-

ties through locomotor and nonlocomotor activities

Space and equipment: Multipurpose area, drum, and record player

Number of participants: Entire class

Test reference: III and VI

Procedure

Imitative rhythms

The children express themselves by trying to imitate something. They interpret this identity with appropriate movements accompanied by a suitable rhythm, such as clapping, beating a drum or sticks, or recordings. There are several ways to begin. The teacher can let the children hear the rhythm and then do what it makes them think if, or the children can decide what they wish to imitate and the music is then selected to follow their choice. Suggestions by the teacher must play an important part at this stage of development because children often have not had enough experience to make decisions on their own. The following are sample ideas:

Going places—shopping, market, picnic, and zoo

Animals—cat, dog, elephant, bear, monkey, kangaroo, and snake

People—mother, doctor, fireman, and clown

Transportation—car, boat, train, bicycle, and airplane

Nature—flowers, wind, and plants growing

Holidays—Halloween, Easter, and Christmas

Familiar actions—cleaning house, flying kites, and going to school

Interpretative rhythms

Interpretative rhythm is recreating an idea with movement. Through it children can show feelings and emotions. Familiar stories such as *Red Riding Hood* or *Goldilocks* provide good opportunities for expression. Another way to perform interpretative rhythms is to use feeling words, such as happy, sad, love, hate, brave, and hurt.

Singing action games. An integral part of childhood rhythms is participation in singing action games. A classic example is Farmer in the Dell, which children today still love and play spontaneously. Though these games are not creative in nature, their repetition in both verse and movements makes them easy to learn and fun to do and also gives children the security of knowing the basic framework so they can enjoy the rhythm and movements that are fundamental to these singing games.

TEN LITTLE INDIANS

Procedure: This may be played two ways: (1) the children step-hop around the "fire" while singing or (2) the children are given numbers from one to ten and each stands then sits when his or her number is sung.

One little, two little, three little Indians,
Four little, five little, six little Indians,
Seven little, eight little, nine little Indians,
Ten little Indian children.
Ten little, nine little, eight little Indians,
Seven little, six little, five little Indians,
Four little, three little, two little Indians,
One little Indian child.

ON MY PONY

Procedure: This is sung to the tune of Ten Little Indians. The action consists of galloping in time to the music.

Giddy-yap, Giddy-yap on my pony,
Giddy-yap, Giddy-yap on my pony,
Giddy-yap, Giddy-yap on my pony,
See me ride my pony.

TEAPOT

I'm a little teapot short and stout.
  (Sway from side to side.)
Here is my handle, here is my spout.
  (Put one hand on hip for handle, arch other hand for spout.)
When I get all steamed up, hear me shout.
  (Sway from side to side.)
Tip me over, and pour me out!
  (Tip over slowly like pouring.)

ROW, ROW, ROW YOUR BOAT

Row, row, row your boat,
  (Sit and pretend to row.)
Gently down the stream.
  (Wiggle hands together.)
Merrily, merrily, merrily, merrily,
  (Clap hands.)
Life is but a dream.
  (Put hand under cheek like sleeping.)

WRITING NUMBERS IN THE AIR

Procedure: This is sung to the tune of Here We Go Round the Mulberry Bush.

A line straight down and that is all
  (Repeat two times)
To make the numeral 1.
Around and down and to the right
  (Repeat two times)
To make the numeral 2.
Half around and half again
  (Repeat two times)
To make the numeral 3.
Down, across, and down again
  (Repeat two times)
To make the numeral 4.
Down, around, and make a flag
  (Repeat two times)
To make the numeral 5.
Half around and all around
  (Repeat two times)
To make the numeral 6.
A line across and then slant down
  (Repeat two times)
To make the numeral 7.
Curve around and then back up
  (Repeat two times)
To make the numeral 8.
All around and then straight down
  (Repeat two times)
To make the numeral 9.
A line straight down and circle round
  (Repeat two times)
To make the numeral 10.

LOOBY LOO

Formation: The children form a single circle, facing in.

Music: Folkraft 1184 and RCA Victor 45-5067 and 41-6153

Procedure: During the singing of each verse, the children stand still and dramatize it. Then, after each verse, they sing the chorus, during which they join hands and slide, skip, run, or walk to the left or right (Fig. 14-31).

1. "I put my right hand in, I put my right hand out;
   I give my right hand a shake, shake, shake
   And turn myself about, Oh,"

Chorus
   "Here we go looby loo, here we go looby light.
   Here we go looby loo, all on a Saturday night."

2. "I put my left hand in," etc.
3. "I put my two hands in," etc.
4. "I put my right foot in," etc.
5. "I put my left foot in," etc.
6. "I put my head 'way in," etc.
7. "I put my whole self in," etc.

DID YOU EVER SEE A LASSIE?

Formation: The children form a single circle, with their hands joined. The child who is "it" stands in the center of the circle.

Music: Folkraft 1183; RCA Victor 45-5066; and Pioneer 3012

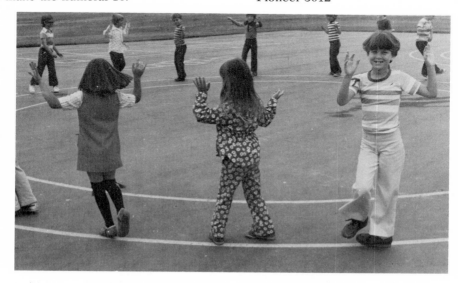

Fig. 14-31. Looby loo—"and turn myself about."

Procedure: All the children sing as they walk to the right in a circle:

> "Did you ever see a lassie [or laddie], a lassie, a lassie,
> Did you ever see a lassie do this way and that?"

"It" thinks of some movement. All the children drop hands, face the center of the circle, watch the leader's movement, and imitate it, singing:

> "Do this way and that way, do this way and that way,
> Did you ever see a lassie do this way and that?"

The leader chooses a replacement, and the game is repeated.

LONDON BRIDGE

Formation: Two players with uplifted hands joined form an arch representing the bridge. A line of children pass under the bridge, each holding onto the waist of the person in front of him or her.

Music: RCA Victor E-87 and 45-5065 and Decca 9-Du 9000 (45-73572)

Procedure: The children pass under the bridge and sing, and on the word "lady," the guardians of the bridge lower their arms and catch the player directly underneath.

> "London Bridge is falling down, falling down, falling down,
> London Bridge is falling down, my fair lady."

They continue singing as the bridge sways back and forth.

> "Take the key and lock her up, lock her up, lock her up,
> Take the key and lock her up, my fair lady."

All the children sing as the guardians of the bridge take the prisoner off to the side.

> "Off to prison she must go, she must go, she must go,
> Off to prison she must go, my fair lady."

They ask the prisoner whether he or she wants a bag of gold or a bag of diamonds, or they ask some equivalent question. The guardians have already privately agreed on which of the two objects they each represent, and according to the prisoner's choice, they place the prisoner behind one of the two guardians. When all are caught, the side with the most players wins. A tug of war also

may be used to determine which side is the winner, once all players are caught.

FARMER IN THE DELL

Formation: The children form a single circle, hands joined with a "farmer" in the center.

Music: Folkraft 1182; RCA Victor 21618, Basic singing games; and RCA Victor Album E-87.

Procedure: The children circle to the right singing:

> The farmer in the dell,
> The farmer in the dell,
> Heigh-o the dairy-o,
> The farmer in the dell.

The farmer in the center chooses a "wife" as the children sing:

> The farmer takes a wife,
> The farmer takes a wife,
> Heigh-o the dairy-o,
> The farmer takes a wife.

The wife then chooses a child, and the song continues, with each child in turn selecting the character they are singing about.

> The wife takes a child, etc.
> The child takes a nurse, etc.
> The nurse takes a cat, etc.
> The cat takes a rat, etc.
> The rat takes the cheese, etc.
> The cheese stands alone, etc.

The cheese then chooses the farmer for the next round.

THE MUFFIN MAN

Formation: The children stand in one large circle, with their hands joined. One child is chosen to stand in the center.

Music: Folkraft F-1188 and RCA Victor 45-5065.

Procedure: The children skip to the left and sing:

> "Oh, have you seen the muffin man,
> the muffin man, the muffin man,
> Oh, have you seen the muffin man, who
> lives in Drury Lane?"

One child stands in the center and looks for a partner from the big circle, as they sing:

> "Oh, yes we've seen the muffin man, the muffin
> man, the muffin man,
> Oh, yes we've seen the muffin man, who lives
> in Drury Lane."

The center child skips toward the chosen one and offers both hands. Then the two occupy the center and skip in a circle to the right, as the children sing:

"Two have seen the muffin man," etc.

These two then choose partners from the outside circle and all four join hands and circle to the right, as they all sing:

"Four have seen the muffin man," etc.

This procedure is followed until all are chosen. Then they sing:

"All have seen the muffin man," etc.

RECORDS—LEVEL 2

There are numerous records available to assist the teacher in presenting a well-rounded and creative physical education program. The following are samples of those that have proved to be of great value and to be most enjoyable for the children.

1. Clap, Snap and Tap—Brazelton EA 48.
2. Fun Activities for Fine Motor Skills—Stewart.
3. Fun Activities for Perceptual Motor Skills—Stewart, Kim 9071.
4. Heel, Toe, Away We Go—Stewart, Kim 7950.
5. Homemade Band—Palmer AR 545.
6. Learning Basic Skills Through Music, vols. 1 and 2—Palmer AR 521 and AR 522.
7. Moving—Palmer AR 546.
8. Multipurpose Singing Games—Palmer.
9. Simplified Lummi Stick Activities—Johnson K 2015.
10. Walk Like the Animals—Stewart.

15

Level 3: Expanding

The activities in level 3 require intermediate skills and prepare the child for the more advanced games presented in the upper grades. Lead-up games that require specific skills serve as the foundation for sophisticated team games and sports. The activities in this section challenge the student's cognitive powers, since more advanced strategies are involved, and teamwork and cooperation are necessary for successful performances. The child's motor abilities are tested, since the games involve a higher level of agility, balance, endurance, and eye-hand coordination.

Some children in the lower levels may be ready for the challenge of the activities in this section. The teacher should determine the activity level to use on the basis of the needs and abilities of the children in the class based on the information received from the administration of the Basic Motor Ability Test, Chapter 2. Organizational information for tag games, relays, games of low organization, and ball skills is presented in level 2.

PERCEPTUAL-MOTOR ACTIVITIES

Perceptual activities in level 3 involve combinations of movement skills. Locomotor activities stress sequential memory tasks and require cognitive decisions. Perceptual-motor activities are designed to challenge the senses through figure-ground discrimination, auditory identification, and kinesthetic awareness. Necessary sequential memory tasks challenge the child to increase the ability to continue with the task or to increase concentration. The challenges at this level build on the skills developed in level 2 and serve as lead-ups to level 4 sports and games through the introduction of partner activities.

Walking activities

1. Walk lightly with your shoulders and your toes pointing forward without touching anyone.
2. Walk in one direction and, when you hear the second signal, change direction. Stop when you hear the third signal.
3. Begin walking as small as you can, and slowly change to walking as tall as you can.
4. Walk forward and backward with your hands hanging below your knees.
5. Walk forward, backward, and sideways without touching anyone.
6. Walk forward raising your knees high and slapping them with your hands.
7. Clap your hands slowly and walk to the rhythm. Increase the tempo from slow to fast.
8. Walk in different directions, clapping your hands first in front and then in back of your body.

Running activities

1. Run forward without bumping into anyone, and stop when you hear the signal.
2. Run forward, and change directions each time you hear the signal.
3. Run forward lifting your knees as high as you can.
4. Run quietly on tiptoe.
5. Begin running slowly and increase your speed until you hear the signal to stop.
6. Run in small circles and then in large circles.
7. Run in a zigzag pattern, and stop on the signal.
8. Run quickly, and freeze on the signal, holding your position.
9. Run quickly, stop on the signal, and lower yourself to a sitting position as slowly as you can.

Jumping activities

1. Jump as high as you can and land with your knees bent.
2. Jump forward as far as you can, swinging your arms high.
3. Jump as high as you can, and land very lightly on your feet.
4. Jump two jumps forward, two backward, three to the right, and three to the left.
5. Jump and make a quarter turn to the right and then make a half turn, three-quarter turn, and finally a full turn. Do the same, turning to the left.
6. Jump forward and back and then leap to the right and back to the left.

Skipping activities

1. Skip, changing directions without bumping into anyone.
2. While skipping, make a square, circle, triangle, and rectangle.
3. Skip as high as you can and then as low as you can.
4. Skip in a zigzag pattern, stop on the signal, and skip in a circle when you hear the next signal.
5. Skip holding hands with a partner.
6. Skip as fast as you can and then as slow as you can.

Locomotor partner activities

1. Walk away from your partner, and return without bumping into anyone.
2. Skip away from your partner, and gallop back without bumping into anyone.
3. Walk away from your partner using large high steps, and return using low small steps.
4. Run away from your partner. One of you hop back and the other jump back.
5. Run away from your partner, and return skipping backwards.
6. Play leap frog with your partner, taking three jumps each and then sitting down (Fig. 15-1).

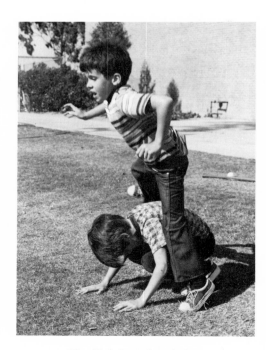

Fig. 15-1. Leap frog is fun.

Ball activities with a partner

1. Toss the ball to your partner using a two-hand, underhand throw.
2. Toss the ball to your partner using a one-hand, underhand throw.
3. Toss the ball to your partner using a two-hand, overhead throw.
4. Toss the ball to your partner using a one-hand, overhand throw.
5. Bounce the ball to your partner using two hands.
6. Bounce the ball to your partner using one hand.
7. Throw the ball underhand as high as you can to your partner.
8. Bounce the ball back and forth to your partner, counting the times you catch it without a miss.

Ball dribbling activities

1. Walk forward, and dribble the ball with one hand.
2. Dribble the ball in place three times with the right hand and then three times with the left.
3. Walk forward, and dribble the ball five times with the right hand and then five times with the left.
4. Run forward, and dribble the ball with either hand.
5. Walk forward, and dribble the ball without looking at it.

6. Dribble the ball forward, and stop on a signal; then dribble it backward on the next signal.
7. Dribble the ball in square, circle, and triangle shapes (Fig. 15-2).

Hoop activities (Fig. 15-3)

1. Lay the hoop on the floor, and stand in the center, balancing on one foot.
2. Stand in the center of the hoop, and balance on three body parts, four body parts, and five body parts.

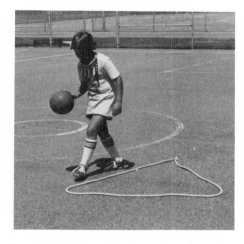

Fig. 15-2. Ball dribbling in a triangular pattern.

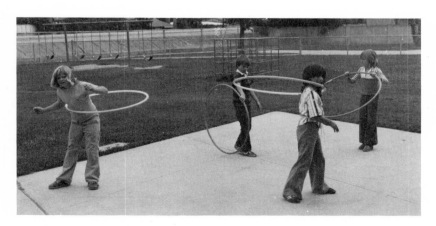

Fig. 15-3. Show me what you can do with your hoop.

3. Stand in the hoop, and balance with two body parts inside the hoop and two body parts outside the hoop.
4. Stand in the center of the hoop and hop five times and stop.
5. Jump forward into the hoop and then backward out of the hoop.
6. Turn your hoop around three different parts of your body.
7. Run, and roll the hoop with your hand.
8. Spin the hoop on the floor like a top.
9. Hold your hoop with two hands, and use it like a jump rope.
10. Flip the hoop away from you, and make it spin back.

Rope activities

1. Place your rope in a straight line, and walk on the rope from end to end.

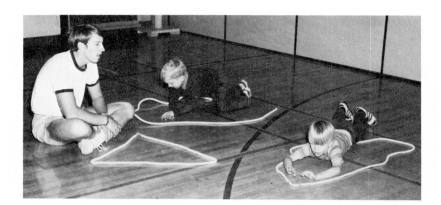

Fig. 15-4. Making geometric shapes.

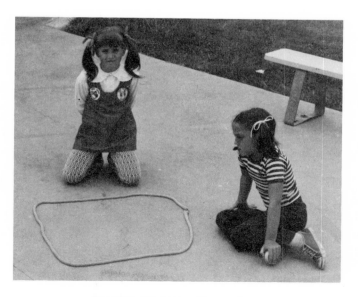

Fig. 15-5. Working with a partner.

2. Make your rope into a circle, and walk around it with one foot inside and the other outside.

3. Make a circle, square, triangle, and rectangle with your rope (Figs. 15-4 and 15-5).

4. Make as many numbers as you can with your rope.

5. Make as many letters as you can with your rope.

6. Place your rope in a straight line, jump back and forth over it, and then hop back and forth over it.

7. Make your rope into a circle, hop around the inside, and then skip around the outside.

8. Place your rope in a straight line, and walk forward crossing over with your feet. Walk backward crossing over the rope.

Visual discrimination

Same shape. Children are asked to touch everything in sight in the room that is the same shape as the shape shown by the teacher. It can be a square, circle, rectangle, or triangle. To limit the game, the teacher can ask for a specific number of objects.

Name it. The teacher draws in the air a large outline of a letter, number, or some object in the room. Children are asked to look around and guess what was drawn. Using letters and numbers is an easy way to begin. The child can then progress to objects.

What goes where? Three to five objects are arranged in a row behind a curtain. (A student can hold up a towel or piece of material for a curtain.) The curtain is removed for a few seconds, making the objects visible, and then replaced again. One student is called on to name the objects in order. The teacher should rearrange the objects before continuing with the game.

What is missing? The teacher arranges six to nine objects in a row as the children watch and, placing a curtain in front so no one can see, remove one or two objects. The curtain is removed and a child is then asked what has been taken away.

Who was touched? The teacher goes around the room touching four or five people. A child is asked to tell who was touched, giving the names in correct order. If the child can't remember, hints may be given, such as a color the child is wearing. This game may be varied by touching objects rather than children.

Auditory discrimination

Finishing rhymes. The teacher repeats a rhyme. The second time it is repeated the children come in with the last words as the teacher stops. For example, Humpty Dumpty sat on a (children say "wall"). Humpty Dumpty had a great (children say "fall"). Succeeding times the teacher leaves out more of the ending words until he or she say only the first word, with children saying the rest of the rhyme.

Finding treasure. The teacher asks who would like to find the treasure and mentions four things, for example, a pencil, a book, a piece of paper, and a ball (the number can be increased for more difficulty). The chosen child then gets the things in order. It sometimes helps for the students to repeat the objects aloud as they are first mentioned by the teacher.

Listening and moving. The teacher gives movement directions to a child or class, and they respond in the correct order, for example, hop on one foot, walk two steps forward, turn around, and clap twice.

Tapping the rhythm. The teacher or a child taps a rhythmical beat with pencils or sticks. One child, and then the whole group, copies the beat. Clapping also is very effective.

Who is it? The teacher describes a child in class. All the children try to guess who has been described.

Do what I say. In the beginning the children imitate the actions and directions of the teacher, such as "hands on head, on shoulders, on knees." Then the teacher says one thing but does another, and the children must follow what they hear, not what they see.

Kinesthetic discrimination

Find the object. The teacher goes around the room holding up objects and placing them in a bag. One child is asked to name one of the objects in the bag, and another child is chosen to feel for and locate the correct object.

Guess what. The teacher draws a shape, number, or letter on a student's back and has the student name what was drawn. The difficulty can be increased by using spelling words.

Feel and say. The teacher hands a child an object behind his or her back and has the child identify it by feel only.

TAG GAMES

TOP HAT TAG

Behavioral objective: To balance a beanbag while tagging and being tagged
Developmental goal: Posture and balance
Space and equipment: Multipurpose play area
Number of players: Entire class
Test reference: V
Procedure: The children are scattered within a designated area. One child is chosen to be "it" and another to be the runner. The runner and "it" place beanbags on their heads, and they do not use their hands to hold the beanbag. "It" chases the runner and tries to tag him or her. The runner may transfer the beanbag to the head of any other player, who then becomes the runner. If the runner is tagged, he or she then becomes "it." If the beanbag falls off the head of the runner, the runner becomes "it" and the former "it" becomes the runner.

NOSE AND TOES TAG

Behavioral objective: To tag and to avoid being tagged

Developmental goal: Flexibility, agility, and endurance
Space and equipment: Multipurpose play area
Number of players: Entire class
Test reference: V
Procedure: A child chosen to be "it" attempts to tag any one of the other children who then becomes "it." A child who is tagged holds up one hand for a moment to show the others who is "it." A player may escape being tagged by grasping the nose with one hand and the toes of one foot with the other hand. Each child should be allowed a maximum of three escapes by grasping the nose and toes.

COMMANDO TAG

Behavioral objective: To devise ways of breaking out of the circle and to avoid being tagged
Developmental goal: Agility, cooperation, and endurance
Space and equipment: Multipurpose play area
Number of players: 8 to 10 in each circle
Test reference: V and VII
Procedure: The children form circles. One child is selected to be "it" and stands in the middle of the circle. The circle players join hands. On a signal, "it" tries to break through the circle by crawling under or over joined hands or by breaking the handholds of the players. If "it" breaks through, the two circle players who "it" breaks through chase "it," and the one who tags "it" becomes the new "it."

HOOK-ON TAG

Behavioral objective: To tag and to avoid being tagged and to work together as a unit
Developmental goal: Coordination, cooperation, and endurance
Space and equipment: Multipurpose play area
Number of players: Groups of 2, 3, or 4
Test reference: V and VII
Procedure: The children line up one behind the other, each grasping the waist of the one in front. The player at the front of each line is called the engine, and the one in the rear is the caboose. One child is chosen to be "it." "It" tries to hook onto the caboose of any group. When "it" succeeds, the engine of that group becomes the new "it." There

may be more than one "it" at the same time if the group is large.

ANIMAL TAG

Behavioral objective: To respond to auditory signals and avoid being tagged

Developmental goal: Speed and agility

Space and equipment: Multipurpose play area

Number of players: Entire class

Test reference: IV and V

Procedure: A "den" is marked off in each of two corners of the playing field. Each den is large enough to accommodate all the players. Children are named after a variety of animals. Several children may represent one animal if the group is large. All the children stand in one den. One child, the "chaser," stands between the two dens. The chaser calls out the name of an animal, for example, "lions." All the lions attempt to run across the playing area to the other den without being tagged by the chaser. Any players caught become chasers.

WILD HORSE TAG

Behavioral objective: To avoid being tagged while in a confined area

Developmental goal: Running skills and agility

Space and equipment: Multipurpose play area

Number of players: Entire class

Test reference: IV and V

Procedure: A circular "corral" 15 feet in diameter is marked with chalk on the ground to one side of the "play area, or range." Three to six of the children are "cowhands," and all the others are "wild horses." One of the cowhands is designated the "foreman." When the foreman calls out "wild horses," the horses must run into the range. The horses must stay within the boundaries of the range until they are caught by one of the cowhands. When the horses are caught, they go to the corral. The last child caught becomes the new foreman and chooses the players to be cowhands. A child may be a cowhand only once until all have had a turn.

LINK TAG

Behavioral objective: To work as a team in tagging others

Developmental goal: Cooperation and teamwork

Space and equipment: Multipurpose play area

Number of players: 8 to 20

Test reference: IV

Procedure: The children are scattered about the area. Two children are selected to be the taggers. They link hands and attempt to tag other players with their free hands. As players are tagged, they take their place between the two original taggers; the chain grows longer with each additional player tagged. Only the end players may tag. The players being chased may break the chain if they are pressed too closely. If they break the chain, the chain players must unite again before they may continue tagging. Tired runners who are not being chased may retire to the sideline to rest, remaining there until they are ready to reenter the game. The last two players tagged become the taggers for a new game.

HOT POTATO

Behavioral objective: To tag a person who is holding an object and to avoid being caught while holding an object

Developmental goal: Visual perception and agility

Space and equipment: Multipurpose play area and beanbag

Number of players: Entire class

Test reference: I and V

Procedure: The children are scattered in a designated area. One child is selected to be the runner and is given the beanbag, or "hot potato." Another child is selected to be "it." To start the game, "it" begins to chase the runner with the hot potato. The runner may at any time give the hot potato to another player who then becomes the runner. If "it" tags the runner with the hot potato, the runner becomes "it." The new "it" must count to five before chasing anyone.

SPOT TAG

Behavioral objective: To move quickly to tag another person

Developmental goal: Agility and endurance

Space and equipment: Multipurpose play area

Number of players: Entire class

Test reference: V

Procedure: One child is chosen to be "it." All the children are scattered within a designated play area. "It" tries to tag another player. When a player is tagged, he or she becomes "it" and must place one hand on the spot that was tagged and hold it there while attempting to tag another player.

RELAY GAMES

OBSTACLE RELAY

Behavioral objective: To successfully run in and out of markers as quickly as possible

Developmental goal: Agility, endurance, self-control, and team loyalty

Space and equipment: Classroom or multipurpose play area, and chairs or rubber cones

Number of players: 6 to 8 on each team

Test reference: V

Procedure: The children line up in squad formation. Chairs or markers are placed 6 to 10 feet apart and directly in front of each team. The first player runs in and out around the chairs and back to the starting position and then taps the next team member. The relay is continued until the last player in each squad has had a turn. The first squad to finish is the winner.

STUNT RELAY

Behavioral objective: To run and touch a designated line, turn, and remember to do a stunt

Developmental goal: Self-control and memory

Space and equipment: Multipurpose play area

Number of players: 6 to 8 on each team

Test reference: V and VI

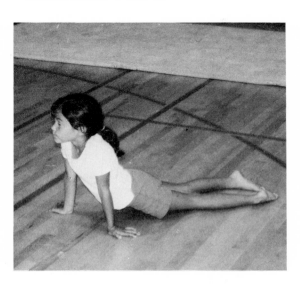

Fig. 15-6. Demonstrating the seal walk.

Procedure: The children stand in squad formation behind a starting line. A turning line is drawn about 30 to 40 feet away. On a signal, the first player runs to the turning line and on the way back performs a stunt designated by the teacher (Fig. 15-6). The teacher should select the stunt according to the abilities of the children involved.

SHUTTLE RELAY

Behavioral objective: To run across an area and tag a team member

Developmental goal: Endurance and self-control

Space and equipment: Multipurpose play area

Number of players: 6 to 8 on each team

Test reference: V

Procedure: The children divide into teams, and each team divides in half. The team halves line up on either side of two restraining lines, spaced approximately 20 feet apart, in file formation. The first player runs across the designated area to the other half of the team and tags the right hand of the first player in line. The tagged player runs back to the opposite side and tags the next player in line, and so on, until all have had a turn. The teacher may substitute locomotor or ball skills for straight running.

OBJECT-PASSING RELAY

Behavioral objective: To pass a beanbag along a line of players without dropping it

Developmental goal: Eye-hand coordination and laterality

Space and equipment: Multipurpose play area

Number of players: 6 to 8 on each team

Test reference: I and II

Procedure: The children form teams, with no more than eight players to a team, and they stand side by side in squad formation. Each captain is given a beanbag. At a signal, the children pass the beanbag along the line as rapidly as possible to the end of the line. The last player touches the beanbag to the floor and starts it back toward the beginning of the line. The bag may be passed in different ways, such as with the right hand, the left hand, or both hands. If a bag is dropped or is not passed according to the selected method, it must be returned to and restarted by the captain. The team wins who first returns the beanbag to the captain in the prescribed manner.

WALK, RUN, OR HOP RELAY

Behavioral objective: To perform a designated motor skill quickly

Developmental goal: Endurance and coordination

Space and equipment: Multipurpose play area

Number of players: 6 to 8 on each team

Test reference: IV, V, and VI

Procedure: The children line up in teams. The teacher draws a turning line 20 to 40 feet away from the starting line, the distance depending on the age and ability of the children. The first player of each team performs any specified locomotor movement (run, walk, hop, leap, skip, slide, or gallop) to the turning line and back. When the first player returns, the next team member takes his or her turn. The relay is continued until each team member has had a turn.

LOCOMOTION RELAY

Behavioral objective: To move fast against an opponent in a competitive situation

Developmental goal: Endurance and coordination

Space and equipment: Multipurpose play area

Number of players: 10 to 40

Test reference: IV and V

Procedure: The children form squads of four to six players. The first player on each team runs forward and to the left around a marker, runs back, tags the right hand of the next player, and goes to the end of the team. The next player must wait behind the starting line and must not run until his or her right hand is tagged. When every player on a team has had a turn, the whole team sits down. The first team to sit in a straight line wins. A variety of locomotor skills and stunts can be incorporated into this game in their entirety or in combinations, such as the skip, hop, gallop, crawl, crab walk, wheelbarrow, and swagger walk. The distance for the relay should be in relation to the difficulty of the skill involved and the age level of the children.

OVER AND UNDER RELAY

Behavioral objective: To pass an object to another person quickly and accurately

Developmental goal: Coordination and teamwork

Space and equipment: Multipurpose play area and playground ball or beanbags

Number of players: 10 to 40

Test reference: I and III

Procedure: The children form squads of six to eight players. The first player on each squad passes the ball overhead with both hands to the next player, who passes it between the legs to the next player, who passes it overhead, and so on to the last player, who receives the ball and runs down the right-hand side of the team to the front (Fig. 15-7). Then all the players move back one space from the starting line, and the relay continues, the first player always passing the ball overhead to the next player. The

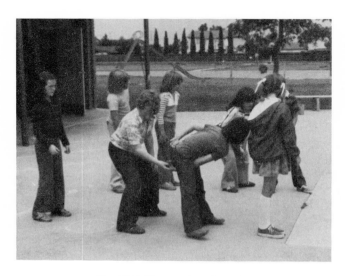

Fig. 15-7. Over and under relay.

team that returns first to the starting position wins. When a team completes the relay, all the team members should sit down to make it easier to judge which team finishes first. For variation, the children can all pass the ball overhead or all roll or pass the ball between their legs.

DIZZY IZZY RELAY

Behavioral objective: To run fast and to control the body with an added stress factor
Developmental goal: Balance and endurance
Space and equipment: Multipurpose play area and bats
Number of players: 6 to 40
Test reference: V and VI
Procedure: The children divide into teams, with no more than six to a team. The teams line up in squad formation behind a restraining line. Each captain is given a baseball bat. At a signal, each captain runs forward to a line 25 feet away and, when beyond the line, places the bat in an upright position on the ground, places the forehead on the end, and in that position runs around the bat three times. He then runs back to the team and hands the bat to the second runner. Play continues until one team wins by being the first to have all its members complete their turns. Adequate space must be allowed between teams, since some children get dizzy and have difficulty running a straight line.

CARRY AND FETCH RELAY

Behavioral objective: To run fast and to carry an object to a designated area
Developmental goal: Endurance
Space and equipment: Multipurpose play area and beanbags
Number of players: 6 to 40
Test reference: I and IV
Procedure: The children form teams of six to eight players and line up in squad formation in back of the starting line and opposite a circle. Each team leader is given a beanbag. At a signal, the team leader runs forward, places the beanbag in a circle, and runs back to the rear of the squad, tagging the first player in the row as he or she passes. The second player dashes forward, grabs the beanbag, runs back, and hands it to the third player. The third player returns the bag to the circle. Play continues until all the team

members have run. A beanbag may not touch the circumference of a circle. The team wins whose captain first receives the beanbag from the last runner or is tagged by the last runner, provided that no beanbag contacted the circumference of the circle during the race.

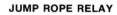

JUMP ROPE RELAY

Behavioral objective: To jump rope and to travel forward as fast as possible
Developmental goal: Endurance and coordination
Space and equipment: Multipurpose play area and jump ropes
Number of players: 5 to 6 on each team
Test reference: V and VII
Procedure: The children form teams and line up in squad formation behind a starting line, with the first player on each team holding a jump rope. The teacher draws a turning line about 20 feet away. On a signal, the first player jumps rope to the turning line and back (Fig. 15-8). The relay continues until the last player in each squad has had a turn. (Individual jump rope is covered later in this chapter.)

RESCUE RELAY

Behavioral objective: To run quickly to a line and return with a partner
Developmental goal: Endurance and cooperation
Space and equipment: Multipurpose play area
Number of players: 6 to 8 on each team
Test reference: IV and V
Procedure: The children form teams and line up in squad formation behind a starting line. Each team captain stands opposite the team behind a second line drawn parallel to and 20 feet in front of the first line. On a signal, the captain runs to the first member of the team grasps hands, and runs back with the teammate to the turning line. The player whom the captain brought over returns and brings the next player back. The relay continues until the last person has been "rescued" and brought over to the captain's line.

CIRCLE BEANBAG RELAY

Behavioral objective: To run and carry an object to be given to another player
Developmental goal: Speed, agility, and object management

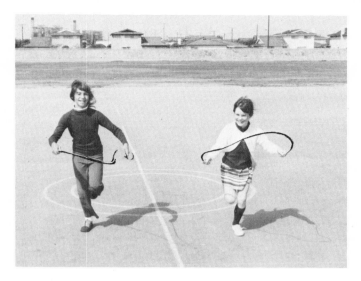

Fig. 15-8. Jump rope relay requires rhythm and coordination.

Space and equipment: Multipurpose play area and beanbags

Number of players: 6 to 10 in each circle

Test reference: I and IV

Procedure: Teams are arranged in a circle formation rather than single file lines. Each team forms its own circle. The first player holds a beanbag and runs around the outside of the circle. As the runner completes the circle, the beanbag is handed to the second player, and the first player sits down in place. The winning team is the first one to have all players seated in their circle formation.

RUN AND KNOCK DOWN RELAY

Behavioral objective: To manipulate objects with the hand and foot

Developmental goal: Hand and foot control and speed

Space and equipment: Multipurpose play area

Number of players: 6 to 8 in each squad

Test reference: I and IV

Procedure: Bowling pins are placed on the turn line opposite each team. The first player runs to the pin, knocks it down with the foot, immediately resets the pin, and returns to tag the next player.

BEANBAG BALANCE RELAY

Behavioral objective: To move quickly without dropping a beanbag balanced on the head

Developmental goal: Balance and coordination

Space and equipment: Multipurpose play area and beanbags

Number of players: Entire class in groups of 6

Test reference: VI

Procedure: Place a beanbag on the head of the first player. On a signal the first player runs to the turn line and back, placing the beanbag on the head of the second player. Players may not touch the beanbag with the hands while moving. If the beanbag falls, the player must stop and replace the beanbag before continuing to move.

ROLL-A-BALL RELAY

Behavioral objective: To move a ball accurately with the hand

Developmental goal: Eye-hand coordination and object control

Space and equipment: Multipurpose play area and 7-inch playground ball for each group

Number of players: Entire class in groups of 6

Test reference: III

Procedure: Cones are placed on the turning line. Each team is given a ball. Each player on the team must roll the ball around the turn marker and back to the starting line using the hands only (Fig. 15-9) before tagging the next player.

TIGHT ROPE RELAY

Behavioral objective: To walk successfully on a narrow base

Developmental goal: Balance and control

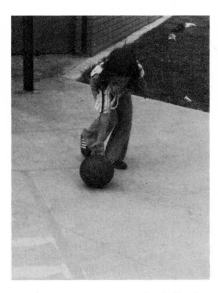

Fig. 15-9. Preparing for roll-a-ball relay.

Space and equipment: Multipurpose play area and long jump ropes
Number of players: Entire class in groups of 6
Test reference: VI
Procedure: Long jump ropes are placed lengthwise in front of each team. Each player must use the heel-toe walk to travel the length of the rope and back before tagging the next player.

BEANBAG IN CAN RELAY

Behavioral objective: To accurately place or retrieve an object from a receptacle
Developmental goal: Object control and quickness
Space and equipment: Multipurpose play area, beanbags, and cans
Number of players: Groups of 6
Test reference: I and IV
Procedure: An empty can is placed on the turn line. The first player runs, places a beanbag in the can, and returns to tag the next player. The second player runs to the turn line, retrieves the beanbag from the can, and returns it to the third player.

LOW ORGANIZATION GAMES

JUMP THE BROOK

Behavioral objective: To successfully jump increasing distances

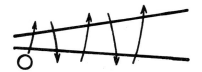

Fig. 15-10. Jump the brook.

Developmental goal: Leg strength and coordination
Space and equipment: Multipurpose play area
Number of players: Entire class
Test reference: IV
Procedure: Two lines are drawn about 2 feet apart at one end and 6 feet apart at the other end. The children stand in single file formation about 10 to 15 feet away from the lines, which represent the sides of a brook. Each child in turn runs forward and jumps across the brook and continues to jump in line, increasing the width each turn. The child jumping at the widest part without stepping in the brook is the winner. Failure is kept to a minimum, since the children pick their own width for the jump. The children should be encouraged to try to increase their jumps each time the game is played (Fig. 15-10).

TWO DEEP

Behavioral objective: To tag a person and to avoid being tagged
Developmental goal: Endurance and agility
Space and equipment: Multipurpose play area
Number of players: 10 to 30
Test reference: V
Procedure: The children form a single circle and face the center, standing an arm's length apart. One child is chosen to be the runner, and another, the chaser. The chaser tries to tag the runner, who tries to escape being tagged by running around the outside of the circle *for a short distance* and then stopping in front of a circle player, where he or she is safe from the chaser. The runner plus the player in front of whom he or she has taken refuge make the circle two persons deep at that point; the player at the rear therefore becomes the runner (Fig. 15-11). If caught, the runner becomes the chaser and the chaser becomes the runner. If a chaser is unable to tag a runner, the teacher may change directions, making the chaser

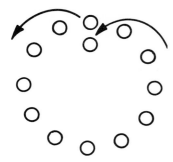

Fig. 15-11. Two deep.

the runner and thus allowing him or her to become safe by being two deep.

TOUCHDOWN

Behavioral objective: To transport an object across an opposing team's goal line without being tagged

Developmental goal: Strategy and cooperation

Space and equipment: Multipurpose play area

Number of players: 10 to 30

Test reference: V

Procedure: The children form teams. The teams stand in single lines on opposite goal lines and face each other. The members of one team go into a huddle and decide who will carry an object, such as a small rock, stick, or chalk, to the opposite goal line. The children hold their hands as if they were carrying the object. On a signal, the members of the team with the object run toward the opposing team's goal line and the opponents run forward to tag them. When a child is tagged, both hands are opened to show whether or not the object is being carried. If the child carrying the object gets to the opponents' goal line without being tagged, and calls out the word "touchdown" he or she scores one point for the team and then the team gets another turn. If the child is caught, the object is given to the other team and play is repeated, with the members of the other team going into a huddle to decide how to get the object across the field.

STEALING STICKS

Behavioral objective: To retrieve an object and to avoid being tagged

Developmental goal: Agility, speed, and strategy

Space and equipment: Multipurpose play area and sticks or beanbags

Number of players: 6 to 20

Test reference: I and V

Procedure: The children divide into two equal teams. The team members stand in their own territory scattered between the center line and their own goal and face the opposing team's goal. Each team selects a captain, who may appoint some of the players as runners and some as guards to protect their own goal. The guards may not stand closer than 12 feet to their own goal, but they may approach it if they are attempting to tag an opposing runner.

The object of the game is for members of a team to run to their opponents' goal and secure their opponents' sticks. Runners are allowed to take only one stick a trip. Players may be caught as soon as they have both feet in the enemy's territory. To escape being tagged, they may return to their own side of the center line as often as they desire. If caught, players are taken to their captors' prison and must stand there until rescued by someone from their own team. While prisoners, they may reach out toward the approaching runners but must keep both feet behind the prison lines. Runners may not take any sticks from their opponents' goal while any member of their team is in prison; the prisoners must be rescued first. If the runners reach the prisoners without being tagged, prisoners and their rescuers return to their own side in safety. Runners may rescue only one prisoner each trip. Runners successful in reaching their opponents' goal, take a stick and return to their own side in safety. The game is won by the team whose members first carry away all of their opponents' sticks.

STREETS AND ALLEYS

Behavioral objective: To tag and to avoid being tagged

Developmental goal: Auditory perception and agility

Space and equipment: Multipurpose play area

Number of players: 20 to 30

Test reference: V and VI

Procedure: The children stand in four to six parallel lines, an arm's length apart in all directions. A runner and a chaser are chosen. The children all face the same direction and join hands with those on each side, forming streets between the rows. To form alleys, they drop hands, turn sideways, and grasp hands in the opposite direction. The chaser tries to tag the runner; they go up and down the streets but cannot break through or go under arms. The leader aids the runner by calling for streets or alleys at the proper time so that passage is blocked for the chaser. When the runner is caught, the chaser and the runner choose two other children to take their places.

STEAL THE BACON

Behavioral objective: To retrieve an object and to return home safely

Developmental goal: Agility and strategy

Space and equipment: Multipurpose play area and beanbag, eraser, or similar object

Number of players: 10 to 30

Test reference: I and V

Procedure: The children form two teams and line up facing each other. The team members are numbered consecutively from 1 to 15. A beanbag or eraser, "the bacon," is placed in the center between the two lines. The teacher calls a number, and the players with that number from opposing teams try to retrieve the bacon without being tagged by the opposing player. If player 2 from team A picks up the bacon first, player 2 from team B tries to tag the team A player before he or she crossed the team A home line. A point is scored each time the bacon is retrieved safely. So that there is more activity and participation, a number of games with smaller teams can be played simultaneously.

TREASURE ISLAND

Behavioral objective: To retrieve an object and to avoid being tagged

Developmental goal: Agility and strategy

Space and equipment: Multipurpose play area and beanbag, towel, ball, or other object

Number of players: 8 to 20

Test reference: I and V

Procedure: The children form a circle around a smaller circle. One child is chosen to be the pirate and stands in the smaller circle near the treasure (beanbag) while the rest of the children stand outside Treasure Island (the smaller circle). Players run onto the island at will to try to take the treasure and get off the island without being tagged by the pirate either before or after taking the treasure. If tagged, the player is eliminated from the game. The player who succeeds in getting the treasure off the island without being tagged becomes the pirate. The game starts again with those who were tagged rejoining the game.

ANIMAL CHASE

Behavioral objective: To run at a specific signal and to tag or avoid being tagged

Developmental goal: Auditory awareness, endurance, and strategy

Space and equipment: Multipurpose play area

Number of players: Any number

Test reference: V

Procedure: The children stand on a line facing the teacher. Together they choose five animal names. Each child is then given one of the animal names. A hunter is chosen, who stands in the middle of the playing area. When the hunter calls the name of an animal, all children who have that name try to run to a line opposite them without being caught. If they are caught, they are put in the cage, which is an area marked off outside the end boundary line. The hunter continues to call the names until they have all been called. The hunter then counts the number that have been caught and chooses someone to be the hunter who has never been one. The same animal names may be used, or new ones may be chosen.

PUSSY WANTS A CORNER

Behavioral objective: To get into an empty circle

Developmental goal: Alertness, quickness, and cooperation

Space and equipment: Multipurpose play area with a number of circles—one less than the number of children

Number of players: 10 to 15

Test reference: V and VI

Procedure: Each child stands with at least one foot touching a circle. The child who is the pussy stands anywhere outside the circles. The pussy moves around the play area saying, "Pussy wants a corner." The other children try to change places without being noticed. If the pussy can get into an empty circle, the child who just left that circle becomes the pussy. Occasionally the leader calls, "Everyone change." At this call, everyone runs to a new circle, including the pussy, and the child left without a circle becomes the pussy.

CENTER RING

Behavioral objective: To imitate designated animals

Developmental goal: Imagination and creative movement

Space and equipment: Multipurpose play area

Number of players: Entire class

Test reference: VI

Procedure: The children stand in a circle, with one child in the center, who is the ringmaster. The ringmaster moves about the center of the circle pretending to crack the whip and calls out the names of various animals. The circle players then imitate the animals. If the ringmaster calls out, "All join the parade," the children may imitate any animal they wish. The ringmaster selects the child who best imitates the animal to be the next ringmaster.

FOX AND RABBIT

Behavioral objective: To successfully pass an object quickly to another person

Developmental goal: Object control

Space and equipment: Multipurpose play area and two small balls

Number of players: 8 to 10

Test reference: I and VI

Procedure: One ball is the "rabbit" and the other the "fox." The teacher stands in the center of the circle and hands the rabbit to a child who immediately passes it around the circle. The teacher then quickly hands the same child the fox, which is passed after the rabbit around the circle. The children try to pass the rabbit to the starting point before the fox overtakes it.

HILL DILL

Behavioral objective: To successfully avoid being tagged while running

Developmental goal: Agility

Space and equipment: Multipurpose play area

Number of players: Entire class

Test reference: V

Procedure: "It" calls out, "Hill dill, come over the hill!" and the players run to the opposite goal while "it" tags as many as possible. All of those tagged assist "it." The last player tagged becomes the new "it."

RINGMASTER

Behavioral objective: To dodge effectively around obstacles and avoid being tagged

Developmental goal: Agility and stretching

Space and equipment: Multipurpose play area

Number of players: Entire class

Test reference: V

Procedure: The girls are the "tigers" and the boys are the "lions." The caller is the "ringmaster" standing in the middle of the circus grounds. The ringmaster may call tigers and lions seperately or both at the same time. The object for the tigers and lions is to get to the other goal line without being tagged by the ringmaster. Those tagged must sit on the ground at the spot where they were tagged and help the ringmaster from a sitting position. The game continues until there is only one tiger or lion left.

COME HOME CHICKENS

Behavioral objective: To avoid being tagged while running to opposite side of tag area

Developmental goal: Agility and speed

Space and equipment: Multipurpose play area

Number of players: Entire class

Test reference: IV and V

Procedure: The children line up behind the line at one end of the court. One child is chosen to be the "farmer" and stands on the opposite end line. Another child, the "weasel," stands in the middle of the area. The game begins by the farmer calling "Come home chickens." The children, the "chickens," answer, "We can't, the weasel will get us." The farmer replies, "Come home anyway, you naughty chickens." The chickens run to the other end and the weasel tags as many as possible. Those tagged help the weasel. The farmer goes to the other end, and the game is repeated.

DOG CATCHER

Behavioral objective: To avoid being tagged

Developmental goal: Auditory recognition

Space and equipment: Multipurpose play area

Number of players: Entire class

Test reference: V

Procedure: Divide the children into four groups. Select one child to be the "dog catcher." Each group must decide on a kind of dog, for example, bulldog, German shepherd, collie, cocker spaniel, or poodle. The dog catcher will call the name of one of the groups and they try to run across the area without getting tagged. Any dog caught must go to the "dog pound." After the dog catcher has called all of the groups, the number of dogs caught is counted, and another catcher is selected. The one catching the most dogs is the winner.

BACK TO BACK

Behavioral objective: To change partners quickly
Developmental goal: Agility and balance
Space and equipment: Multipurpose play area
Number of players: 20 to 25
Test reference: V
Procedure: The children stand with their backs together spaced throughout the room. Another player is "it." When "it" yells "catnip" everyone runs and must seek a new partner quickly. The person left without a partner becomes the next caller.

FIRE ENGINE

Behavioral objective: To listen for a specific number and to run quickly to a designated line
Developmental goal: Auditory awareness, endurance, and quickness
Space and equipment: Multipurpose play area
Number of players: Any number
Test reference: IV
Procedure: All the children stand on a line at the end of the playing area. They count off by fives. The fire chief stands at the side of the court halfway between the end lines. The chief calls, "Fire! fire! station number (1 to 5)." The children whose number is called run to the opposite end line and back to the middle line. The first one back becomes the new fire chief, and the game continues.

MIDNIGHT

Behavioral objective: To listen for a specific word and to run to home before being tagged
Developmental goal: Auditory awareness and fast reaction
Space and equipment: Multipurpose play area
Number of players: Entire class
Test reference: IV and V
Procedure: The children stand in a single line side by side on a line called home. One child is chosen to be the "old man" and

stands, facing them, about 30 feet away. The children leave their home and, as they approach the old man, keep asking him, "What time is it?" The old man answers, "8 o'clock," "10 o'clock," and so on. The old man may tag the children only at midnight; therefore, if the reply is any time except midnight, they are safe. When the old man says "midnight," the children must run for their home. The old man chases them, trying to catch as many as possible. Any who are caught must go with the old man and help him or her catch the others. The last child caught becomes the old man for the next game.

⅄ FOX AND SQUIRRELS

Behavioral objective: To tag and to avoid being tagged
Developmental goal: Endurance, agility, and sportsmanship
Space and equipment: Multipurpose play area
Number of players: Entire class
Test reference: IV and V
Procedure: The children stand in groups of three; two face each other and join both hands, forming the tree, and the third child, the squirrel, stands inside the tree. Trees should be scattered around the playing area. One squirrel without a tree and one fox are chosen to start the game. The fox attempts to catch the squirrel. To avoid being caught the squirrel may run inside a tree, forcing out the squirrel in that tree. If the fox catches the squirrel, they exchange roles. After several chases, the trees and squirrels should change places. The game should be repeated until each child has had a chance to be a squirrel.

BEAR IN THE PIT

Behavioral objective: To break through a circle
Developmental goal: Strength, strategy, endurance, and agility
Space and equipment: Multipurpose play area
Number of players: 15 to 35
Test reference: VII
Procedure: The children stand in a circle and face the center with their hands joined. One child is chosen to be the bear in the center of the pit (circle). The bear attempts to get out by diving under or over the other children's arms or between their legs or by breaking through their arms. Once the bear

is free, all the players chase it. The one who tags it becomes the next bear.

FAIRIES AND BROWNIES

Behavioral objective: To chase and tag others on a signal

Developmental goal: Quickness, endurance, and auditory perception

Space and equipment: Multipurpose play area

Number of players: 13 to 30

Test reference: V

Procedure: The children are divided into two equal groups of fairies and brownies. Each group stands behind a line. The lines should be about 60 feet apart. The fairies turn their backs toward the brownies. A leader or lookout watches the game and gives the necessary signals. The brownies creep forward quietly. The fairies are not permitted to look over their shoulders while the brownies are approaching. When the brownies are near enough for the fairies to tag players, the lookout calls, "Look out for the brownies!" The fairies then turn and chase the brownies, tagging as many brownies as possible before the brownies cross their safety line. All the brownies who are tagged become fairies and join that group. The game is repeated with the brownies turning their backs. The winning side is the one having the greater number of

players at the end of the available time period.

CROWS AND CRANES

Behavioral objective: To chase and tag others on a given signal

Developmental goal: Auditory perception and endurance

Space and equipment: Multipurpose play area

Number of players: 12 to 30

Test reference: IV and V

Procedure: The children stand side by side in two single lines facing each other about 60 feet apart. The children in one line are crows, and those in the other are cranes. A child chosen to be the leader stands in the middle. The teams walk toward each other, and the leader calls out the word "cr-r-r-rows" or "cr-r-r-ranes," holding the word until the teams are close together (Fig. 15-12). If the word is "cranes," the cranes run back to their line and the crows try to tag them. All who are tagged join the other side. The calls should be drawn out as long as possible, to add to the suspense and uncertainty of the game.

NEW ORLEANS

Behavioral objective: To act out an occupation and to guess it and then to chase and tag

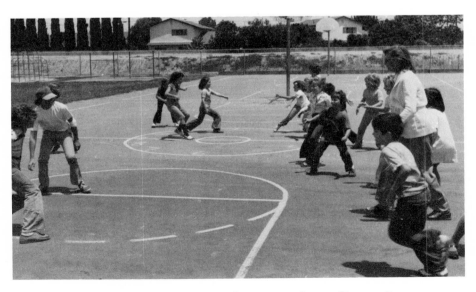

Fig. 15-12. The game crows and cranes requires auditory acuity.

Developmental goal: Imagination, cooperation, and endurance

Space and equipment: Multipurpose play area

Number of players: 12 to 30

Test reference: IV

Procedure: The children stand side by side in two single lines facing each other about 60 feet apart. Team 1 decides on some trade it will represent and approaches team 2, and the teams have the following dialogue:

Team 1	Team 2
Here we come.	Where from?
New Orleans.	What's your trade?
Lemonade.	Show us something if you're not afraid.

The members of team 1 act out motions illustrating their trades, and those of team 2 guess what it is. When someone from team 2 guesses what it is, the members of team 1 run for their goal and those of team 2 try to tag them. All those who are tagged go with team 2.

RED ROVER

Behavioral objective: To tag others

Developmental goal: Auditory perception, endurance, and agility

Space and equipment: Multipurpose play area

Number of players: Entire class

Test reference: IV

Procedure: The teacher draws three parallel lines, each 20 feet apart. The children stand on one end line and face the center line. One player is chosen to be "it" and stands on the center line. "It" says, "Red Rover, Red Rover, let Jim, Jane, Bill, and Sue (any four or five players) come over." The players who were called run to the opposite end line, and "it" attempts to tag as many as possible before they reach the line. The child who is "it" should be allowed to have three or four turns, and then another child should be chosen to be "it." The player who catches the most children wins the game.

UNCLE SAM

Behavioral objective: To listen for a signal and to identify specific colors and to run to another side

Developmental goal: Color identification, speed, and agility

Space and equipment: Multipurpose play area

Number of players: Entire class

Test reference: V

Procedure: The teacher draws two parallel lines 30 to 40 feet apart. The children stand along one line. The other line is called the river. One child is chosen to be Uncle Sam and stands in the center of the play area. The children standing behind the line call out, "Uncle Sam, may we cross your river?" Uncle Sam says, "Yes, if you have blue (or any color)." All children wearing that color must run to the opposite side. Uncle Sam tries to tag as many as possible before they cross the opposite end line. Those who are caught must help Uncle Sam. The last person to be caught wins the game.

SIMPLE BALL GAMES

GALLOPING LIZZIE

Behavioral objective: To pass a ball before being tagged and to tag a person who has a ball

Developmental goal: Eye-hand coordination, quickness, and endurance

Space and equipment: Multipurpose play area and a ball

Number of players: 6 to 12

Test reference: I and V

Procedure: The children stand in a circle fairly close together and face the center. One child stands outside the circle. The ball is given to a circle player. The ball is passed from player to player or is thrown across to an opposite player. The outside player tries to tag a circle player while the circle player holds the ball. When the outside player is successful in tagging a player, they change places. If a circle player drops the ball, he or she becomes the tagger and the former tagger takes over as a circle player. More than one ball may be used to make tagging easier.

CENTER-BASE BALL

Behavioral objective: To throw and catch a ball and to tag another person

Developmental goal: Agility and strategy

Space and equipment: Multipurpose play area and playground ball

Number of players: 6 to 16

Test reference: II

Procedure: The children stand in a single circle and face the center. They should stand at least 4 feet away from each other. One child stands in the center holding a ball. The center player throws the ball to a circle player and leaves the circle immediately. The one to whom the ball was thrown must catch it, take it to the center, place it on the ground, and then chase the first player. The center player tries to return to the ball and touch it without being tagged. If tagged, the center player joins the circle players and the circle player becomes the thrower. If the center player succeeds in reaching the ball without being tagged, the ball is thrown again, as before.

WONDER BALL

Behavioral objective: To pass a ball quickly to another person

Developmental goal: Eye-hand coordination and quickness

Space and equipment: Multipurpose play area and playground ball

Number of players: 6 to 10 per circle

Test reference: I

Procedure: The children form circles. They pass the ball around the circle from person to person while they say the following verse:

"The wonder ball goes round and round,
To pass it quickly you are bound,
If you're the one to hold it last
You—are—OUT!"

The child holding the ball on the word "out" is eliminated from the game. The children should pass the ball quickly but avoid wild throwing.

CALL BALL

Behavioral objective: To throw a ball and to catch a ball on one bounce

Developmental goal: Auditory perception and ball skills

Space and equipment: Multipurpose play area

Number of players: 6 to 10 per circle

Test reference: II and V

Procedure: The children form a circle. One child is chosen to be "it" and stands in the center. "It" tosses the ball into the air and calls a player's name. The child whose name is called must run in and catch the ball before it bounces more than once (Fig. 15-13). If successful, that child becomes "it." If not, the original "it" tosses the ball again. To make the game harder, the children can be required to catch the ball *before* it bounces. The children also may be given numbers or colors to which they must respond.

BALL PASSING

Behavioral objective: To pass and receive an object accurately

Developmental goal: Eye-hand coordination, teamwork, and quickness

Space and equipment: Multipurpose play area and balls or beanbags

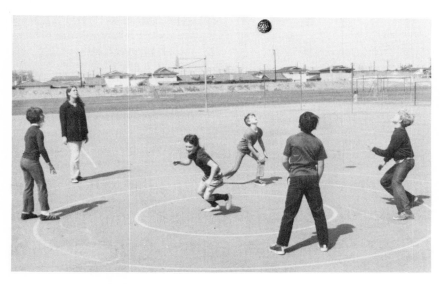

Fig. 15-13. Developing skills in a call ball game.

Number of players: 6 to 40
Test reference: I
Procedure: The children divide into two or more teams, depending on the number of children playing. Each team is given a name or number. The players of each team form a single circle and face the center. The teacher starts an object around each circle and then additional objects or balls until five or six are being passed. The game is played for a given number of minutes, with as many repetitions as desired. Those children who miss an object or ball must retrieve it and put it into play as soon as possible. The player must call loudly the name or number of the team when an object is missed. Each time the object is dropped or missed, a point is scored for the team, but the player remains in the game. The team with the lowest score at the end of the playing time wins. The game is more exciting when the objects passed vary in size and type.

WALL BALL

Behavioral objective: To keep the ball in play longer than one's opponent
Developmental goal: Eye-hand coordination and quickness
Space and equipment: Any smooth surfaced wall and eight playground balls
Number of players: 2
Test reference: II and V

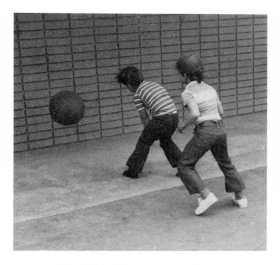

Fig. 15-14. Wall ball competition.

Procedure: The first player bounces the ball against a wall. The second player is allowed one bounce before he or she must hit it (Fig. 15-14). Shots are alternated until one player misses. The game requires no lines.

TEAM DODGE BALL

Behavioral objective: To hit a moving target with a ball
Developmental goal: Agility and coordination
Space and equipment: Multipurpose play area and playground ball
Number of players: 10 to 30
Test reference: II and V
Procedure: The children form two teams. One team forms a circle, and the other team stands inside it. The children on the circle team attempt to hit players in the middle of the circle with the ball. Soft playground balls should be used rather than soft soccer balls. Only hits below the waist count. Play continues for a specified length of time (2 to 4 minutes), and then teams change places. The team with the most players left in the circle wins. A variation can be played in which each player who is hit joins the circle as a thrower and the last remaining child is the winner.

EXCHANGE DODGE BALL

Behavioral objective: To change places with another person without being hit by a ball
Developmental goal: Auditory perception and agility
Space and equipment: Multipurpose play area and playground ball
Number of players: 12 to 20 in a group
Test reference: II, IV, and V
Procedure: The children divide into groups. Each group forms a circle with one child who is chosen to be "it" in the center. The children number off by fours or fives so that there are three or four children who have the same number. The center player also has a number that is used when he or she is not "it." The center player has a ball that is laid at his or her feet. The center player calls a number, and all the children with that number exchange places. The center player picks up the ball and tries to hit one of the children exchanging places. The center player remains "it" until one of the children is hit below the waist.

KEEP AWAY

Behavioral objective: To throw a ball to a teammate and to keep the ball away from an opponent

Developmental goal: Endurance and eye-hand coordination

Space and equipment: Multipurpose play area and playground ball

Number of players: 8 to 16

Test reference: II and V

Procedure: The children divide into two teams of equal size, and members of both teams scatter around the playing area. The teacher hands the ball to one player. On a signal, the players pass the ball, trying to give it to teammates and to keep it away from opponents. There is a limit of 5 seconds on how long players may hold the ball before passing it to another teammate, so that one player cannot keep the ball out of play. There is no scoring. The object is to see which team has the ball when time is called.

Fouls: Tripping, pushing, holding, kicking, or any other outstanding roughness is a foul and results in the ball's being given to the opposite team. A player is eliminated from the game if his or her play continues to be rough.

TWO SQUARE

Behavioral objective: To successfully hit a ball into an opponent's square

Developmental goal: Eye-hand coordination, agility, and strategy

Space and equipment: Two square markings and a playground ball

Number of players: 2

Test reference: II

Procedure: Two 5 foot by 5 foot squares are marked on the playground. One is marked A and the other B. The player in square A starts the ball by bouncing it into the other player's square. After the ball bounces, the opposing player returns it by hitting the ball with one or two hands with the palms up. The two players keep hitting the ball back and forth until one of them hits the ball out of the square. If the A player misses the ball the players change squares. The object is to remain in the A square.

FOUR SQUARE

Behavioral objective: To bounce a ball accurately into another square

Developmental goal: Eye-hand coordination

Space and equipment: Four square markings and playground ball

Number of players: 4 to 8 per square

Test reference: II and V

Procedure: The four squares are labeled A, B, C, and D. One child stands inside each square, and the other children line up outside square D. The serve always starts from square A. The child serves the ball by

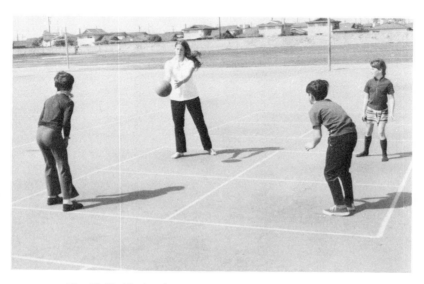

Fig. 15-15. Playing four square with a cross-age teacher.

dropping it and serving it underhanded on the bounce. The server can hit the ball to any one of the other three squares. The player receiving the ball must keep it in play by striking it after it has bounced once in the square (Fig. 15-15). He or she directs it to another square with an underhand hit. Play continues until one player fails to return the ball or commits a foul. If a player in squares A, B, or C misses or commits a foul, he or she drops back a square and the player in the next square moves up. If the player in square D misses or commits a foul, he or she goes to the end of the waiting line and the player at the head of the waiting line moves into square D. The player in square A at the end of the period is declared the winner.

Fouls: The fouls are as follows:
1. The player hits the ball with the side of the arm or overhand.
2. The ball lands on a line between the squares.
3. The player steps in another square to play the ball.
4. The player catches or carries a return volley.
5. The player allows the ball to touch any part of the body except the hands.

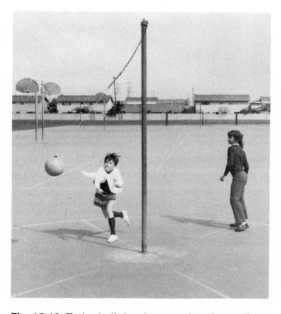

Fig. 15-16. Tetherball develops eye-hand coordination.

TETHERBALL

Behavioral objective: To hit a moving target with the hand and to wind a ball around a pole

Developmental goal: Eye-hand coordination

Space and equipment: Tetherball court and tetherball

Number of players: 2

Test reference: II

Procedure: One child stands on each side of the pole. The server puts the ball in play by standing in the service area, tossing the ball in the air, and hitting it in the direction he or she chooses. The opponent hits the ball back in the opposite direction. Each player tries to hit the ball so that the rope winds completely around the pole in the direction he or she has been hitting the ball and above the mark on the pole about 4 feet from the top (Fig. 15-16). Whenever a player commits a foul, the opponent receives a free hit. The free hit is taken like the serve, with the exception that the rope may not be unwound more than one-half turn before the hit is taken. The winner of the game serves to the next opponent.

Fouls: The fouls are as follows:
1. The player hits the ball with any part of the body other than the hands or forearms.
2. The player catches or holds the ball during play.
3. The player touches the pole.
4. The player hits the rope with the forearm or hand.
5. The player throws the ball.
6. The player winds the ball around the pole below the mark.
7. The player steps into the neutral area around the pole.
8. The player reaches into the opponent's court.

BATTLE BALL

Behavioral objective: To kick a ball across an opposing team's goal line and to stop the ball from crossing one's own goal line

Developmental goal: Coordination and teamwork

Space and equipment: Multipurpose play area and soccer ball

Number of players: 10 to 12 on each team

Test reference: IV

Procedure: The teacher draws two parallel

lines 20 feet apart. The children divide into two teams. One team stands on each line, and the players hold hands. Team 1 tries to kick the soccer ball across team 2's goal line, then team 2 tries to stop the ball and kick it back across team 1's goal line, and so on. When a team kicks the ball over the opposing team's line, it receives one point. If a player touches the ball with the hands, the team loses a point. If a player kicks the ball too high (over the heads of the other team), one point is deducted from his or her team's score. The team that first reaches a score decided on by the teacher wins the game.

BOUNDARY BALL

Behavioral objective: To throw a ball across an opposing team's goal line and to keep the ball from crossing one's own goal line

Developmental goal: Catching and throwing skills

Space and equipment: Multipurpose play area and playground balls

Number of players: 8 to 16

Test reference: II

Procedure: The children divide into two teams. The players on each team occupy the area between their own goal line and the center line. The size of the court should be adjusted to the ability of the children. At a signal, the members of each team attempt to throw the ball so that it will bounce or roll across their oppponents' goal line. The players try to prevent balls from crossing their own goal line. They may move about freely on their own side of the playing area but may not enter their opponents' territory. After the first throw, balls are thrown back and forth at will. Additional balls may be used to increase the activity. A player with the ball may not pass it to a teammate but must throw it. A player may run with the ball to the center line before throwing it. After a goal is made, the ball is returned to the captain of the team that threw it and is put into play again.

Each ball that rolls or bounces over a goal line scores one point. Balls that cross a goal line on the fly or that pass outside the width of the goal line do not score. If a player steps on or across the center line, one point is given to the opponents. The team wins that has the higher number of points at the end of a specified time period.

LINE DODGE BALL

Behavioral objective: To hit a moving target with a ball

Developmental goal: Agility and throwing skill

Space and equipment: Multipurpose play area and playground balls

Number of players: 3 to 30

Test reference: II and V

Procedure: The teacher draws two parallel lines about 20 feet apart. Halfway between the lines, a box about 4-feet square is drawn. One child is chosen to stand in the box. Half the children stand on one line, and half on the other line. The object of the game is to hit the player in the box at or below the waist with a ball. The center player may not step completely out of the box but may step out with one foot. When hit, the center player changes places with the one who threw the ball. In order that each child may have an opportunity to throw, the ball should be started at one end of the line, and as it is returned from the other side, the next person in line should have a turn. Additional balls may be used to make the game more active.

SPORTS LEAD-UP GAMES

CAPTAIN BALL

Behavioral objective: To develop passing and defensive skills as lead-up skills to basketball

Developmental goal: Eye-hand coordination and teamwork

Space and equipment: Basketball court and basketball

Number of players: 24

Test reference: II and IV

Procedure: The children divide into two teams and use pinnies or colored arm bands to distinguish their teams. Half the players of each team are forwards and the other half are guards. The forwards station themselves in the circles, and the guards stand near the forwards of the opposite side (Fig. 15-17). The ball is put into play in the center by the teacher, who tosses it to a guard of one team and thereafter to alternate teams if no score is made or to the team scored against when a point is scored. The guards try to get the ball and pass it to one of their forwards. The forwards try to pass it to their captains. One

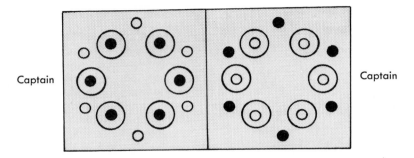

Fig. 15-17. Captain ball court. Players inside the circles are forwards, and players outside the circles are guards.

Fig. 15-18. Nine court basketball court. Opposing players are represented in each court area.

point is scored each time a successful pass is made from a forward to the captain. Forwards rotate one position clockwise, changing captain, and guards one position counterclockwise each time a point is scored or after every 3 minutes if no score is made, so that the children have the chance to play in all positions on the court. The game is played in halves with the guards and forwards changing places at the half.

NINE COURT BASKETBALL

Behavioral objective: To develop shooting, passing, and defensive skills as lead-up skills to basketball

Developmental goal: Teamwork, sportsmanship, and eye-hand coordination

Space and equipment: Basketball court and basketball

Number of players: 18 to 30

Test reference: II and IV

Procedure: The children divide into two teams and use pinnies or colored arm bands to distinguish the teams. They arrange themselves as indicated in Fig. 15-18. The teacher starts the game by tossing the ball to

one of the players in the center and thereafter to alternate teams in the center if no score is made or to the team scored against when a point is scored. The center player attempts to pass the ball to the forwards (players closest to basket), who then attempt to shoot for a basket. Each basket that is made counts two points. The players rotate one court after each score or approximately every 2 to 3 minutes if no score is made.

Violations: The violations are as follows:
1. The player steps out of his or her own court.
2. The player takes more than one step with the ball in the hand.
3. The player bounces the ball more than once.

The penalty for a violation is that the ball is given to the opposite team out of bounds.

Fouls: Pushing, charging, tripping, and other rough play involving personal contact are personal fouls. The penalty for a foul is one free throw awarded to the team against whom the foul was made. The free throw is taken by the forward in the center court. If a forward is fouled in the act of shooting for a basket and misses the basket, two free throws are awarded. If the basket is made in spite of the foul, only one free throw is awarded.

SPACE BALL

Behavioral objective: To throw a ball over the net out of the reach of an opponent and to catch a ball

Developmental goal: Eye-hand coordination and agility

Space and equipment: Volleyball court and volleyball

Number of players: 10 to 15 on each team

Test reference: II

Procedure: The teacher lowers a volleyball net down to about 6 feet or strings a rope between two standards. The net height may be adjusted according to the skill level of the children. The children divide into two teams, and one team stands on each side of the net in a scattered formation. One team throws the ball over the net and the other team tries to catch it before it hits the ground and to return it over the net. When a team drops the ball or when a ball hits the court surface in bounds, the other team receives a point.

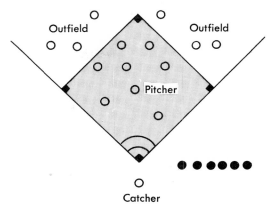

Fig. 15-19. Kickball diamond.

BASES ON BALLS

Behavioral objective: To kick for distance and to run to bases

Developmental goal: Eye-hand coordination and speed

Space and equipment: Softball diamond and playground ball

Number of players: 12 to 24

Test reference: IV

Procedure: The children divide into two teams, and they are numbered consecutively on each team. Team A players stand behind the line connecting third and home bases, and player 1 goes to field balls within the diamond. Team B players line up behind the line connecting first and home bases, and player 1 stands behind home plate. The player at home base places the ball on the surface of home plate and, taking one step, kicks the ball and immediately starts running around the bases. The runner tries to reach home base before the fielder returns to home plate with the ball. As soon as the fielder touches home plate with a foot or the ball while the ball is in the hand, the runner must stop. The bases that were touched are recorded. The run is finished and the runner retires to the end position on the kicking team. Player 2 on the kicking team then steps to home plate, and player 2 of the fielding team enters the diamond. When all members of the team have had a chance to kick the ball, the other team has its turn.

A ball that travels within the area outlined by home plate and first and third bases is a fair ball. If a fielder catches a fly ball, no score is made by the kicker, and new players from each team take their positions. A player is allowed a second kick if the first try fails to send the ball within the official boundaries. On a second failure, the player is retired to the end position on the team. The kicking team scores for each base reached before the fielder contacts home plate, as follows: one point for first base; two points for second base; three points for third base; and four points for home base. The team wins that has the highest number of points at the end of the playing period.

KICKBALL

Behavioral objective: To kick for distance and to run to bases

Developmental goal: Eye-foot coordination, speed, and sportsmanship

Space and equipment: Softball diamond and playground ball

Number of players: 8 to 20

Test reference: IV

Procedure: The children divide into two teams. One team stands behind the first base line, and each member takes a turn trying to kick the ball and run around the bases. The other team goes to the field, with a pitcher and catcher elected by the members (Fig. 15-19). After three members of the kicking team have been put out, the kicking team members go to the field and the fielding team members become the kickers. The game may be modified so that each team member has a chance to kick before the team goes to the field. The players rotate positions on the field so that all eventually have a chance to be pitchers and catchers.

The game is played according to softball rules, with the following exceptions:

1. The pitcher *rolls* the ball to the waiting kicker, who attempts to kick the ball into the field. To speed up play, each kicker may be allowed only one roll. If the player kicks the ball, he tries to run to first, second, third, and home bases before being tagged or thrown out by the other team. A player may not steal or play off bases while the pitcher has the ball in his hands in preparation for rolling it.

2. A base runner is out if tagged out or thrown out before reaching first, second, third, or home plate. A player is tagged out if the ball is in the hands of the baseman or fielder when the base runner is tagged. The runner is thrown out if the base is touched before the runner reaches it, either by the ball that is in the hands of a baseman or fielder or by some part of the body of a baseman or fielder who is holding the ball.

Each successful run to home plate scores one point. The team wins that has the higher score at the end of the time period.

OVERTAKE BALL

Behavioral objective: To run to bases quickly and to throw and catch accurately

Developmental goal: Speed, accuracy, and eye-hand coordination

Space and equipment: Double softball diamond and softball

Number of players: 6 to 30

Test reference: II

Procedure: The children divide into six equal groups of base runners, pitchers, catchers, first basemen, second basemen, and third basemen. If, for example, there were 24 children in the class, there would be four in each group. Eight bases are placed around a diamond to form a double diamond (one base inside the other) (Fig. 15-20). On a signal, base runner 1 runs, using the inside diamond, to first base and continues on around until he or she arrives back at home plate. On the same signal, pitcher 1 throws the ball to catcher 1, who then throws it to first baseman 1, and so on, around the outside diamond. The object is for the runner to

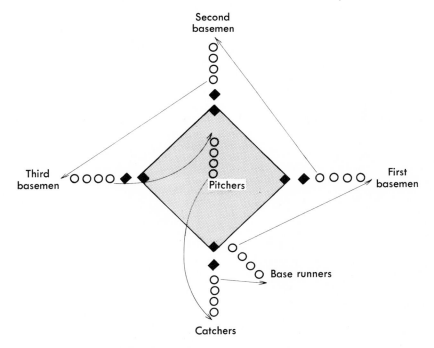

Fig. 15-20. Overtake ball diamond.

get home before the ball does. If the ball overtakes the runner at any base, the runner is out. After an out or a run is made by players 1, they all go to the end of their own lines and players 2 continue the game. It is important for basemen to use the outside diamond for throwing the ball in order to avoid hitting the runner with the ball. After all the players in each group have had their turn, each group rotates to a new position as shown in the diagram in Fig. 15-15 and as follows: Pitchers become catchers; catchers become base runners; base runners become first basemen; first basemen become second basemen; second basemen become third basemen; and third basemen become pitchers.

FRISBEE ACTIVITIES

Frisbee activities involve a different type of throw with an object that varies its speed and has unique flight characteristics. It is an excellent alternative to ball activities for developing eye-hand coordination and has great motivational potential. When beginning activities, it is best to use a backhand throw. However, advanced level players can throw both

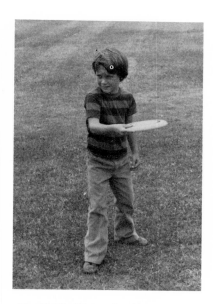

Fig. 15-21. Frisbee backhand throw.

forehand and backhand (Fig. 15-21) in game situations.

Frisbee skill progression

Throwing
1. Throw with an underhand grip from in front of the body.
2. Throw with an underhand grip from the hip.
3. Throw to a target from 15 feet away.
4. Throw for distance with an underhand grip.
5. Throw so that the Frisbee skips off the ground.

Catching
1. Catch with both hands in front of the body, chest high.
2. Catch with both hands overhead.
3. Catch with one hand in front of the body.
4. Catch with one hand to either side.
5. Catch with one hand behind the back.

Partner catching and throwing
1. Throw the Frisbee from waist level and catch it at waist level from 15 feet away.
2. Throw the Frisbee and catch it at eye level from 15 feet away.
3. Throw the Frisbee and catch it from farther away than 15 feet.
4. With a partner standing next to you, throw the Frisbee high in the air. The partner runs to catch it as it is coming down.
5. Throw the Frisbee back and forth to a partner while running alongside each other.

Frisbee games

Horseshoes. Two posts are set up 20 feet apart. Each player throws the Frisbee and the toss that lands closest to the post receives one point; a hit receives two points. The game ends when a player scores ten points.

Basketball. Place an open 2 foot by 2 foot box 10 feet away from the throw line.

Each player throws four Frisbees, trying to put the Frisbees in the box. Five points is received for each Frisbee in the box, and one point for hitting the box. A game is 25 points.

Baseball throw. Stack six foam or paper cups on top of a box, three on bottom, two in the middle, and one on top. Each player throws three Frisbees from a point 10 feet away. Each cup knocked over counts one point. A game is 50 points. If all cups are knocked over on the first throw, 10 points are scored.

Frisbee lag. The players toss Frisbees to a line 30 feet from the throw line. Each player throws one Frisbee. The player closest to the line receives five points. A game is 50 points.

Frisbee golf. A nine-hole course of varying lengths is set up. The players throw to a 5-foot circle with a flag in the center and throw from that circle to the next hole. The number of throws required to complete the course is totaled. The player using the least amount of throws to complete the course wins. Children can play in twosomes, threesomes, or foursomes and can start on different holes.

Precision throwing. Two 3-foot circles, 20 feet apart are made. One player stands in each circle and throws the Frisbee to the other player. Players should not step outside their circles to catch the Frisbee. Five points are scored for the thrower for each Frisbee caught inside the circle. If the catcher has to step outside the circle but still makes the catch, five points are scored for the catcher. If the catcher misses a good throw, five points are scored against the catcher.

Ultimate Frisbee. Ultimate Frisbee is a combination of soccer and basketball played with a Frisbee. The playing area is a soccer or football field with a circle 5 feet in diameter at each end of the field. The object of the game is to pass the Frisbee down the field and score a goal by tossing it into the 5-foot circle. There are six players on a team. The rules are:

1. Players may not run with the Frisbee. If they do, the Frisbee is given to the opponent.
2. If a player drops a passed Frisbee, the Frisbee is given to the opponent.
3. Players may hold the Frisbee for a maximum of 5 seconds before passing it. If they hold it longer, the Frisbee is given to the opponent.

STUNTS AND SELF-TESTING

Stunts and self-testing activities are those forms of physical education in which the child tests the individual ability to accomplish movement skills. The satisfaction that is gained through the successful accomplishment of these skills is a strong motivating factor for lengthy practice. Growth in skill, flexibility, strength, and agility is the basis for participation in some of the more complex activities in group situations. One of the better ways of giving recognition to the child for accomplishing these activities is to have a self-testing chart from which recognition can be given for each skill accomplished (Fig. 15-22). Although

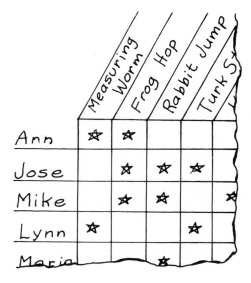

Fig. 15-22. Self-testing chart.

children always seem to compare themselves with other children in the class, they can also strive to accomplish as many of the stunts listed as possible within their own individual capabilities. When the teacher offers self-testing activities, it is best that a variety of stations be established in order to provide activity for many children in the class. Care should be taken to offer activities that range from the simple to the complex so that all children can achieve success and be challenged to progress to the more difficult stunts.

Stunts

Measuring worm. While on all fours, the child walks with the feet, up to the hands, keeping the hands on the floor; then the child walks with the hands, away from the feet (Fig. 15-23). As a variation, the procedure can be done backward.

Frog hop. From a squatting position, the child hops and lands on hands first and then feet (Fig. 15-24).

Rabbit jump. The child assumes a bent-knee squat position, with hands on the floor in front of and closer together than the feet. The child leaps forward by pushing with the feet and bringing the feet forward on the floor outside the hands (Fig. 15-25).

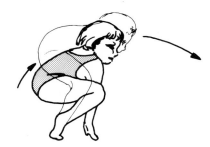

Fig. 15-25. Rabbit jump.

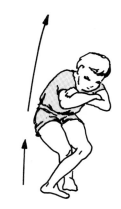

Fig. 15-26. Cross leg stand up.

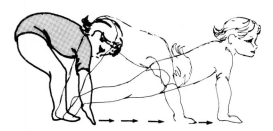

Fig. 15-23. Measuring worm.

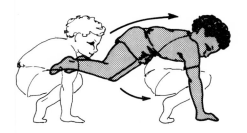

Fig. 15-24. Frog hop.

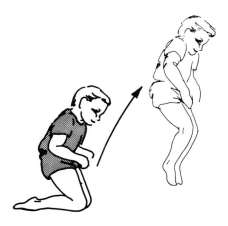

Fig. 15-27. Knee stand to standing position.

Cross leg stand up. The child sits with the legs crossed and then stands without pushing with the hands (Fig. 15-26).

Knee stand. From the kneeling position with the toes out flat behind, the child jumps in one motion to a complete stand (Fig. 15-27).

Bouncing the ball. The child jumps up and down from a squatting position while another child bounces him or her (Fig. 15-28).

Crab walk. Keeping the body straight and head up, the child walks forward on the hands and feet, with the back toward the floor (Fig. 15-29).

Wicket walk. The child takes hold of both feet with the hands and walks forward, keeping the knees straight (Fig. 15-30).

Balance on one foot. The child stands on one foot with the eyes closed for 30 seconds (Fig. 15-31).

Wheelbarrow. Keeping the body straight, the child walks forward on the

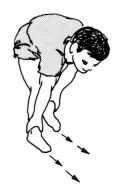

Fig. 15-30. Wicket walk.

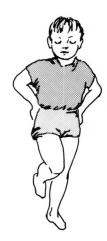

Fig. 15-31. Balance on one foot.

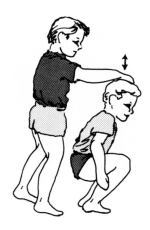

Fig. 15-28. Bouncing the ball.

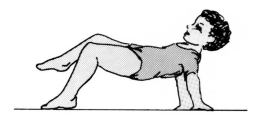

Fig. 15-29. Crab walk.

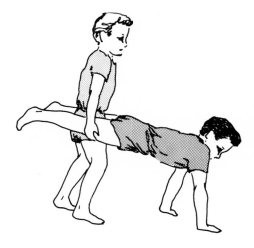

Fig. 15-32. Wheelbarrow.

hands while a partner holds the thighs instead of the ankles to eliminate too much lateral motion (Fig. 15-32).

Partner get-up. Two children sit back to back with their arms locked and push against each other to a standing position (Fig. 15-33).

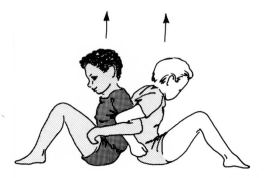

Fig. 15-33. Partner get-up.

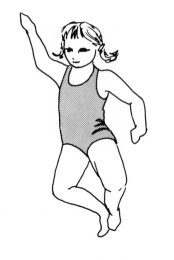

Fig. 15-34. Heel knock.

Heel knock. The child jumps in the air, clicking the heels to the side (Fig. 15-34).

Jump through arms. The child curls the hips forward, and tucks the knees and jumps through the arms (Fig. 15-35).

Human top. From a standing position, the child jumps into the air and turns around, facing the opposite direction on landing (Fig. 15-36).

Swagger walk. The child walks forward swinging the right foot around behind the left foot as far forward as possible and placing it close beside the left foot. As the right foot is placed flat on the floor, the child lifts the left heel and bends the left knee. Then in like manner the child swings the left foot around the right foot. The child makes progress by alternating the action of the right foot and left foot in rhythm in a swaying motion (Fig. 15-37).

Corkscrew. The child puts an object outside the left heel and winds the right arm behind the right leg, in front of the left leg, and around to get the object (Fig. 15-38). The heels may be raised if necessary.

Mercury stand. The child stands on either foot and bends the body forward until it is at right angles with the supporting leg, bending the free leg slightly upward from the knee and holding the head up and arms to the side horizontally. The child holds this position for 5 seconds without wavering (Fig. 15-39).

Twister. Two children face each other, holding their right hands. One child lifts the left foot over their clasped hands at the same time that the other child lifts the right foot over their hands; then they turn

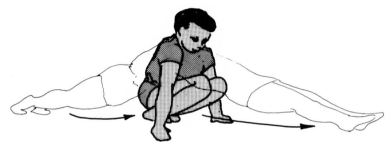

Fig. 15-35. Jump through arms.

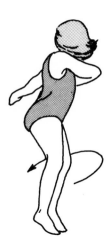

Fig. 15-36. Human top.

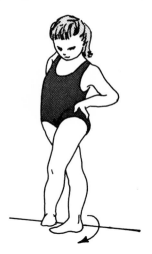

Fig. 15-37. Swagger walk.

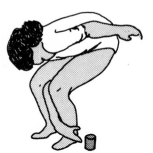

Fig. 15-38. Corkscrew.

back to back, keep on turning, lift their other leg over, and come back to the original position (Fig. 15-40).

Forward roll. The child squats, with the knees apart and the hands on the floor between the knees. Placing weight on the hands and the back of the shoulders, the child tucks the head so that the roll is on the shoulders (Fig. 15-41). The head does not need to touch the floor at all. The child keeps the tucked position and returns to the standing position.

Backward roll. The child assumes a squatting position and, placing the hands at the sides of the head and keeping the head tucked all the way over, rolls the body over backward (Fig. 15-42).

Knee dip. The child stands on one foot and grasps the other foot behind the back with the hand on the same side. The child bends the knee of the supporting leg and touches the knee of the nonsupporting leg to the ground and stands again (Fig. 15-43).

Through the stick. The child grasps a wand or rope with both hands behind the back, keeping the palms forward. The child brings the stick over the head to a position in front of the body, keeping the arms straight and still grasping the stick. The child lifts the right foot, swings it around the right arm and through the

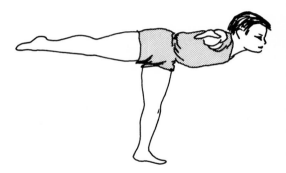

Fig. 15-39. Mercury stand.

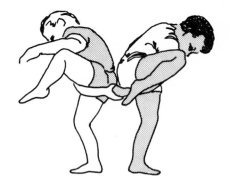

Fig. 15-40. Twister.

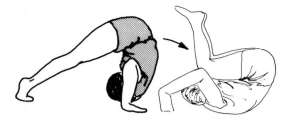

Fig. 15-41. Forward roll.

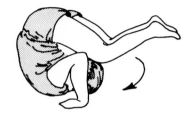

Fig. 15-42. Backward roll.

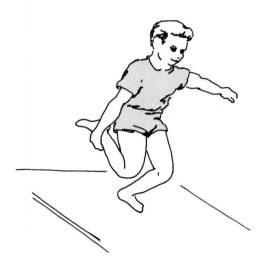

Fig. 15-43. Knee dip.

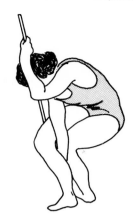

Fig. 15-44. Through the stick.

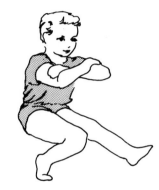

Fig. 15-45. Single leg squat.

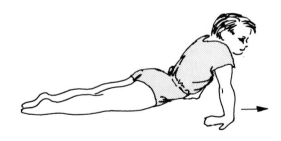

Fig. 15-46. Walrus walk.

hands from the front over the stick. He or she crawls through the stick head first by raising the stick with the left hand over the head (Fig. 15-44). The child then passes the stick down over the back, lifts the left foot off the floor, and steps backward through the stick. The child may slide the hands along the stick but may not let go of it.

Single leg squat. The child stands on one leg, with the other leg out straight. Then he or she squats on the supporting leg and stands again (Fig. 15-45).

Walrus walk. The child walks forward on the hands, dragging the feet and keeping the body straight (Fig. 15-46).

Jackknife. The child stands with the feet slightly apart, the arms back of the body, and the elbows bent; the child then jumps, bending the trunk forward and touching the toes before returning to the standing position (Fig. 15-47).

Human ball. The child sits with the knees bent close to the chest but separated, puts the arms down between the legs and around the outside of the shins, and clasps the hands in front of the ankles. The child may cross the feet if

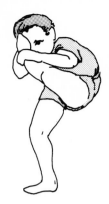

Fig. 15-50. Greet the toe.

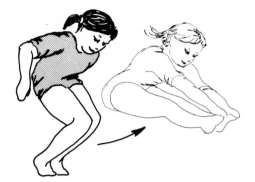

Fig. 15-47. Jackknife.

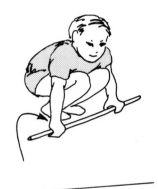

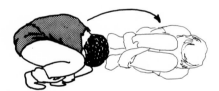

Fig. 15-48. Human ball.

Fig. 15-51. Jump the stick.

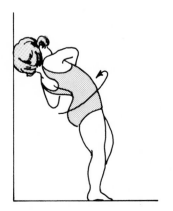

Fig. 15-49. Crane twist.

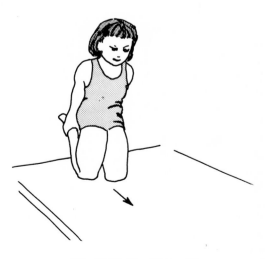

Fig. 15-52. Short leg walk.

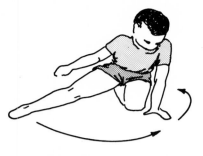

Fig. 15-53. Wind the clock.

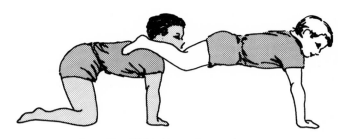

Fig. 15-54. Caterpillar walk.

desired. Then he or she rolls to the left side, over on the back, to the right side, and up to the sitting position again (Fig. 15-48).

Crane twist. A line is marked about 2 feet out from a wall. The child places the front of the head against the wall and, using the head as a pivot, turns the body around completely without moving the head from the wall and without stepping within the line (Fig. 15-49).

Greet the toe. Standing on one foot, the child grasps the other foot in both hands and touches the toe to the forehead (Fig. 15-50).

Jump the stick. The child holds a stick or rope in front of the body, with palms facing upward. He or she jumps and pulls the stick under the legs and then jumps back through to the starting position (Fig. 15-51).

Short leg walk. The child walks on the knees, holding the ankles in back. The child should keep the weight well forward, throw the chest up, and keep the back well arched (Fig. 15-52). Do this activity only on a mat.

Wind the clock. The child squats, bending the left knee and extending the right leg sideways. He or she puts the right hand on the floor between the knees and the left hand on the floor beside the left knee and then swings the right leg to the left, jumping over it with the right hand as it swings in front of the body and with the bent left knee as it swings to the left side, and brings it back to the starting place (Fig. 15-53).

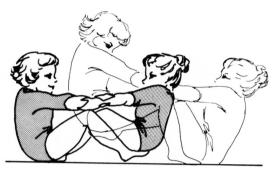

Fig. 15-55. Scooter.

Caterpillar walk. One child walks on the hands and places the feet on the back of a second child who is on all fours (Fig. 15-54). Then they walk forward, keeping in step with their hands and feet.

Scooter. Two children facing each other sit on each other's feet and join hands. They scoot forward as they bend their knees and one child lifts the partner about a foot off the floor (Fig. 15-55).

Simple pyramids using stunts learned

A variety of patterns and designs can result from combining stunts into simple pyramids. Children should be encouraged to create their own formations. In order to avoid injury, a child should not be allowed to bear the full weight of another child. The fun of pyramid building should be in the variety of designs created rather than the height achieved. An excellent demonstration program can be developed when pyramids are per-

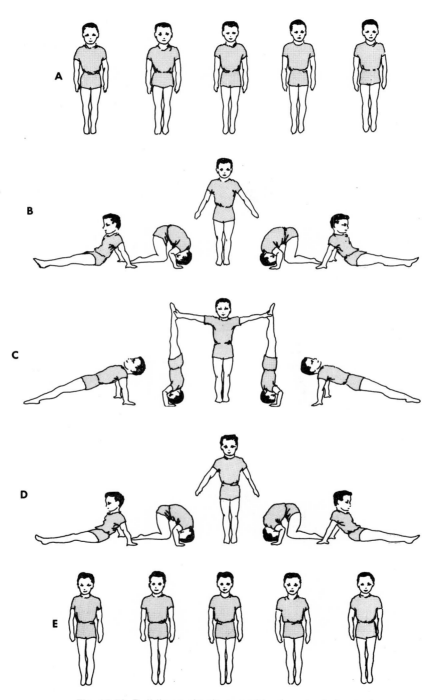

Fig. 15-56. Building a simple pyramid using stunts learned.

formed to a count. A designated person counts as follows as the children form the pyramid as illustrated in Fig. 15-56:

1. All children stand side by side *(A)*
2. They move into a ready position for the pyramid *(B)*
3. They execute their stunts to form the pattern *(C)*
4. They return to the ready position *(D)*
5. They return to the standing position *(E)* ready to perform another pattern, such as that illustrated in Fig. 15-57.

Trampoline activities

Trampoline activities provide the child with a feeling of exhilaration and fun; however, they must be conducted with extreme caution. At all times a child must be physically supported when executing a new or difficult task and must be spotted from all points around the trampoline.

Lead-up to trampoline activities should progress from jumping up and down on a mat, to jumping from a height, to bouncing on a springboard. When a child is on the trampoline, the teacher must be in direct physical control or provide a minimum of two spotters on each side of the trampoline. Lead-up procedures to the standing trampoline jump are as follows. The child:

1. Performs a side roll on the trampoline bed.
2. Crawls around the edge of the trampoline bed.
3. Walks on the bed of the trampoline forward, sideward, and then backward.

When a child has a fear of bouncing, even with manual support, the following sequence should be instituted before more advanced skills are attempted:

a. The teacher bounces the child on the back while both are on the trampoline bed. The teacher straddles the child and holds his or her outstretched hands.
b. The teacher straddles the child and bounces him or her on the right side and then on the left side.
c. The teacher bounces the child on the stomach, being careful not to jerk the child's head.
d. The teacher bounces the child on the knees, supporting the child from either the front or the rear position. In the front position, the child and the teacher encircle each other with their arms. In the rear position, the teacher supports the child under the arms.
e. The teacher bounces the child in a standing posture, gradually relinquishing support, and takes a spotting position off the trampoline bed.

The child:
4. Executes the basic rebound jump with the feet comfortably spread to provide a stable base of support, the knees slightly bent, and the arms bent with the hands about waist level; performs the jump by extending the knees, bringing the feet

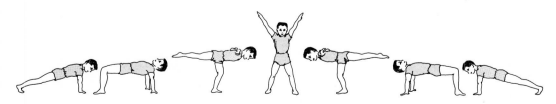

Fig. 15-57. Pyramid variation.

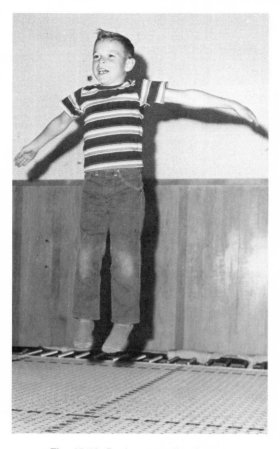

Fig. 15-58. Basic trampoline jump.

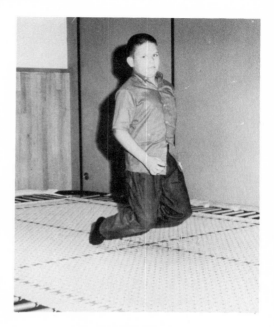

Fig. 15-59. Knee drop.

together, and reaching upward with the hands (Fig. 15-58); and then returns to the starting position and repeats the rebounding action. To stop a jump, the child bends the knees and hips on making contact with the trampoline bed.

5. Performs the two-foot jump.
6. Performs the two-foot jump and stops at will.
7. Jumps with one foot forward, alternating first the left foot and then the right foot.
8. Jumps and moves to the right one-fourth turn, then one-half turn, three-fourths turn, and finally a full turn.
9. Jumps and moves to the left one-fourth turn, then one-half turn, three-fourths turn, and finally a full turn.

Basic trampoline stunts. When a child can easily rebound and make a full turn in the air in either direction, he or she is ready for basic stunts, some of which are as follows:

Knee drop. The child, while airborne, bends both knees so that the legs are at right angles to the thighs (Fig. 15-59). In this position, the child lands on the knees on the trampoline bed, keeping the thighs and back straight, and then rebounds to the fully extended posture. Before going on to more difficult stunts, the children should be able to execute a knee drop at will. To increase the difficulty of the knee drop, he or she performs turns or twists while in the air in either direction. To facilitate the twist, the child first turns the head and then twists the shoulders in the desired direction. When able to perform a full twist the child is ready to progress to the next stunt. *Caution should be taken to maintain the trunk in line with the thighs to avoid low-back strain.*

Seat drop. The child flexes the hips and extends the legs while airborne. In an L

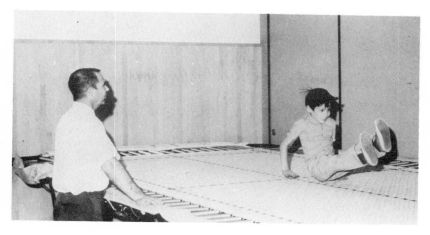

Fig. 15-60. Seat drop.

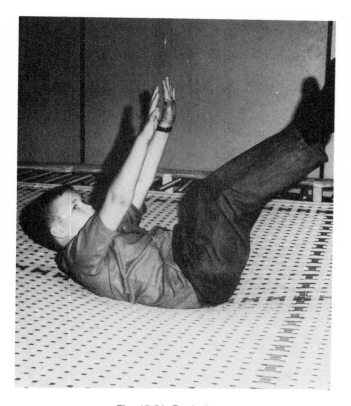

Fig. 15-61. Back drop.

position, the performer lands on the bed (Fig. 15-60) and rebounds back to the upright position. To receive the most advantage from the spring of the trampoline bed, the child must land with all parts of the legs and thighs contacting the bed at the same time and must keep the back straight. However, the child can use the hands for balance and rebounding by placing them palms down next to the hips. Adding a midair twist to the seat drop increases its difficulty to a great extent. The half and full twist are common additions; in both, the child raises one arm over the head and at the same time brings the arm across the chest as the rebound occurs. Simultaneously the child turns the head and rotates the hips in the direction of the twist. After completing the twist, the child immediately plants the feet on the trampoline bed.

Front drop. The child rebounds from the trampoline bed, lifting the hips even with the head. While falling back to the bed, the child straightens the body, raises the arms to shoulder level, and bends the elbows at right angles. He or she makes contact with the bed first with the abdomen. *Care should be taken not to hyperextend the back.* If contact is made properly, the child will rebound straight up from the bed, and can then flex the hips, bring the feet toward the bed, and extend the back into the full upright posture.

Back drop. After springing into the air, the child flexes the hips, lifts the legs so that the feet are higher than the head, and falls back, making contact with the bed on the upper back and keeping the head forward (Fig. 15-61). After making contact, the child snaps the legs forward to return the feet to the bed. Care should be taken to avoid landing on the neck; therefore, it might be best to progress into this stunt by starting from a squat position and then graduating to the full upright posture.

Development of a routine. Once children have learned the four basic trampoline stunts, they can develop routines. Children may put the four stunts together in any combination, adding half and full twists to increase the difficulty of the routine. Mastery of the basic stunts usually leads to more difficult moves such as the forward flip (Fig. 15-62), and back flip followed by layouts combined with midair twists.

Variations of stunts. Besides being used for stunts, the trampoline may be used for a variety of cognitive as well as motor functions. The child:

1. Jumps and lands on specified spots on the trampoline bed. This activity may be used to challenge the child to solve unique movement problems, such as landing on specific spots that the teacher names. The spots may be letters or numbers so that the child must solve cognitive problems while jumping.

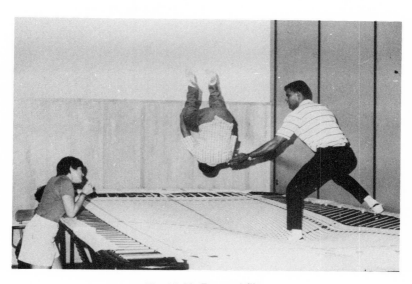

Fig. 15-62. Forward flip.

2. Jumps rope on the trampoline.
3. Catches various objects while on the trampoline.
4. Throws objects at a target while jumping on the trampoline.

Parachute play

Parachute play is a relatively new and exciting activity for all levels of children in the elementary physical education program. The cloth part, or canopy, is all that is used, and the strings must be removed or cut away. An entire class can participate successfully in continuous, vigorous activity at one time. The children, evenly spaced apart, grip the parachute firmly around the outside and, on a given signal, raise it and make it undulate or balloon high in the air. The objective of parachute play is to improve arm and shoulder strength, cardiorespiratory endurance, and movement skills through group cooperation and interaction.

For safety's sake, the following rules must be established before play begins:

1. If at all possible, the children play on a grass area.
2. They are spaced at even intervals around the parachute. It is helpful to have a parachute with alternate colored panels.
3. The teacher establishes a loud signal to start and stop a stunt—a whistle is usually preferred.
4. The teacher demonstrates the methods of holding the parachute—overhand grip, underhand grip, and alternate overhand and underhand (one hand on the top and one hand on the bottom). If a firmer grip is desired, the children can roll the edge of the parachute two or three times toward the center.
5. The teacher limits beginning activity to 10 to 15 minutes so that the children's hands do not get sore.

To begin the activity, the children stand an equal distance apart around the parachute and grip the edge.

Inflating the parachute. The children stretch the parachute tight at waist level and then all together bring the parachute edge to the ground (Fig. 15-63). On the teacher's command "up," the children should stretch high to complete the inflating. At the whistle, the parachute should be brought to the waist-level position.

Ballooning the parachute. The children inflate the parachute and then take three steps toward the middle. As the parachute starts to descend, the children back out.

Variations of parachute play
Change of places. While the parachute is ballooning, the teacher tells two chil-

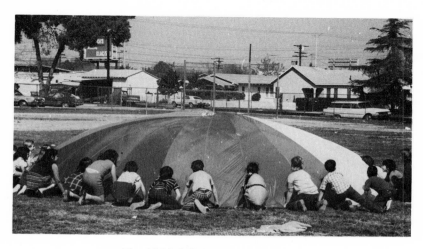

Fig. 15-63. Inflating the parachute.

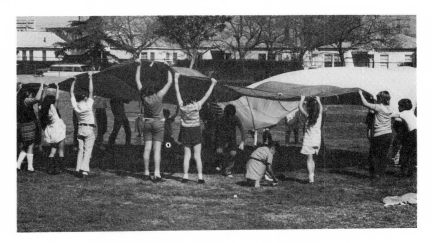

Fig. 15-64. Changing places in parachute play.

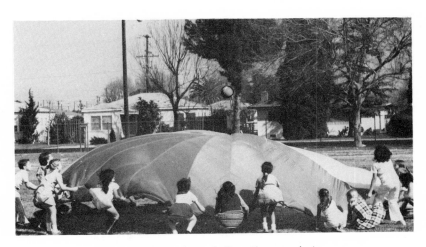

Fig. 15-65. Bouncing a ball on the parachute.

dren on opposite sides to change places, by running under the parachute (Fig. 15-64).

Tag. While the parachute is ballooning, the teacher tells a child to catch another child.

Steal the bacon. The teacher places a small object such as a beanbag under the parachute in the center. The class is divided into teams, each child having a number. The children inflate the parachute, and when it is at its highest point, the teacher calls a number and the players with that number from each team must attempt to grab the beanbag and get back to their position without being tagged by the other players with the same number. One point is awarded for a successful attempt. No point is awarded if the parachute descends on the players.

Ball bounce. The class is divided into two teams, which are placed on opposite sides of the parachute. A ball or balls are thrown into the center of the parachute (Fig. 15-65). Each team attempts to bounce the ball off the other team's side of the parachute. The children may not use their hands to keep the ball from leaving the canopy. A team is awarded a point each time they bounce a ball onto the ground on their opponents' side.

Bottoms up. The children inflate the

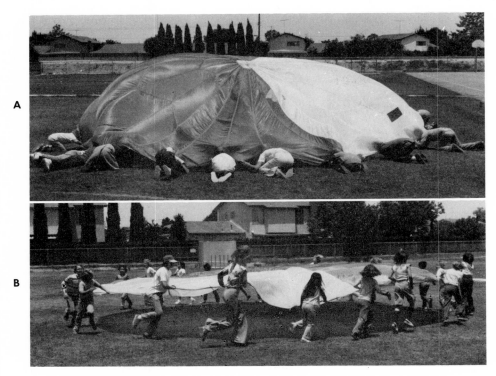

Fig. 15-66. A, Bottoms up. **B,** Developing locomotor skills using the parachute.

parachute and, on command, kneel down and bring the parachute tight around their necks and on the ground. The children see only heads inside of the parachute (Fig. 15-66, *A*).

Parachute challenges

1. Grip the parachute tight. On a signal walk to the right. When you hear the signal, change directions and walk to the left.
2. Next, run to the right, and change directions when you hear the signal (Fig. 15-66, *B*).
3. This time skip to the right and then back to the left when you hear the signal.
4. Can you hold the parachute with both hands and slide eight steps to the right and then eight steps to the left?
5. When you hear the signal make small waves by shaking your hands up and down.
6. Can you make large waves by moving your arms up and down?
7. Let's see if we can inflate the parachute. Release your hands and grasp it again before it reaches the ground.
8. Show me how you can move the parachute to the left while standing in one place and then back to the right.

Crazy legs

Crazy legs is played on a heavy canvas with rope handles around the outside. One child is chosen to stand in the center of the canvas while the others hold up the canvas (Fig. 15-67). In this activity some of the same techniques required in parachute play and the trampoline are used. For the child in the middle, the game provides a moving platform for fun, space perception, and balance skills. For the children on the outside holding up the canvas, it offers heavy activity for strengthening the legs and upper body as well as the opportunities for strategy and teamwork.

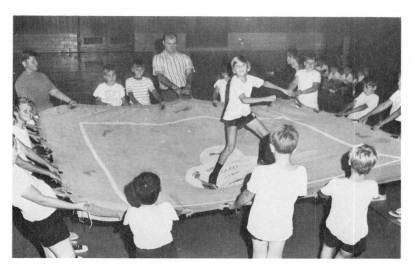

Fig. 15-67. Children playing crazy legs. (Courtesy James W. Grimm.)

The object of the game is for the person on the canvas to stay on his or her feet as long as possible. In order to make the task more difficult, the crazy legs platform is moved up and down in a waving motion and rotated slowly and fast. The activity should be performed over a padded area to provide a safe environment.

Physical fitness activities

Although children at this developmental level are often quite active and ready to play a variety of games, it often becomes necessary to motivate them to participate in specific physical fitness activities. Since children are eager to discover how they relate to the others in the class, it is necessary to untilize an evaluation tool to determine individual and group status. Through the administration of the Oregon Physical Fitness Test described in Chapter 10 or the AAPHER Fitness Test in Appendix B, the teacher can inform children of their current fitness status and plan activities in line with the needs identified by the test. Physical fitness testing provides the teacher with a base that can be used to determine needs and check improvement throughout the year. Children meeting established standards can receive recognition through the development of an awards system. Each school can develop its own standards and award programs or may adopt the physical fitness awards distributed by the President's Council on Physical Fitness and Sports. By posting records, giving awards, and publicizing outstanding performances schools can continually motivate children to improve their performance in fitness activities.

Developmental exercises. At this developmental level children are able to effectively participate in group exercises, such as push-ups, jumping jacks, windmills, sit-ups, and stretchers. (See Chapter 10.) Much pride can be achieved when a class is able to begin an exercise together, count the cadence in loud, sharp voice, stay together for the time required, and end sharply by clapping or standing at attention or in some other position. This type of general exercise program is best suited for group warm-ups. It ensures that all parts of the body are utilized in some form of fitness activity on a daily basis. Exercises of this type, prior to participation in a specific daily lesson, can be accomplished in squad formation and

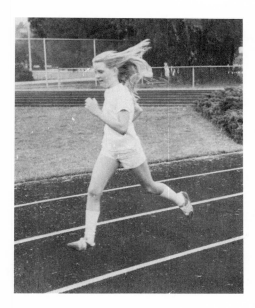

Fig. 15-68. Cross-country running style involves rolling from heel to toe.

completed in a short time period of 3 to 5 minutes.

Cross-country course. It is always more fun to run in an environment that is natural and in a setting that is conducive to exercise (Fig. 15-68). Running activities should be expanded from the normal playground area to include courses that are laid out on nearby parks or through the countryside. If your school is not located in this type of environment, then a couse can be marked around the general school site that will take children through trees and grass areas in addition to the regular playground. Posting yardages and keeping records of times or numbers of circuits completed can encourage children to run the course both during and outside of class time.

Circuit training. Circuit training, or participation in activities by stations, allows children to move from one fitness activity to another after completing the designated activity at each station. The exercise task to be completed at each station should provide for beginning, intermediate, and advanced levels. The total circuit should include fitness activi-

ties that encompass strength, endurance, agility, and flexibility. Through the completion of the proper number of repetitions at each station, each child will experience a well-rounded physical fitness workout. One advantage of the circuit training approach is that students may start at different stations, which provides for small group participation rather than large group exercise. The circuit can be developed indoors in a gymnasium setting or, in areas where weather is not a problem, outdoors. The number of stations can be adjusted to the space and equipment available and may be changed according to the needs of specific groups participating. An expansion of the circuit training approach is the development of the Parcourse, which came to this country from Europe and is becoming increasingly popular on school sites (see p. 418). Courses of this nature are available for children and families to use after school hours and as a part of the regular school program. The development of the Parcourse in an outdoor setting encourages children to participate whenever they have free time.

Jogging. Jogging for enjoyment and fitness is an excellent activity for children of the level 3 developmental group. Jogging consists of a slow, flat-footed running style performed in an almost completely upright posture. Running in this easy, relaxed manner enables individuals to participate in continuous movement over long periods of time. When initiating a jogging program, it is important that the children begin at a slow pace and not attempt to run too far before proper conditioning is achieved. They may begin by walking and then jogging until the need to walk again is felt. Each day the length of the jog should be increased until the children are able to run extended distances without undue fatigue. To motivate children in this activity, the teacher can keep records of heart rates and begin teaching elementary lessons in exercise physiology, showing the children how cardiovascular efficiency is achieved through proper development of the heart muscle and lungs. Marking distances on a course map and posting suggested times or course records along with average performances should be a part of the jogging program. Keeping records on total miles run by a class over a semester or year can result in enormous mileage figures and makes an excellent press release.

Obstacle course. The development of an obstacle course provides challenges for elementary school children that require high levels of physical fitness. The course may include commercially offered equipment or may be designed by the teachers in the school, often utilizing such items as telephone poles and concrete pipes, which can be obtained for little or no charge. Each obstacle course should include running, vaulting, agility, and balance activities; climbing skills; and explosive movements. Outdoor courses are usually of a permanent nature whereas indoor courses often are styled differently according to the equipment and space available as well as the inter-

ests and needs of the children. Regardless of the approach taken, the obstacle course is an excellent way to provide fitness activities for large groups (Fig. 15-69).

Continuous rhythmical exercises. The continuous rhythmical exercise program described in Chapter 14 can be expanded to meet the needs of intermediate children since the basic idea is the same. The program usually starts in the circle formation with the teacher giving directions, such as "Jog in a circular fashion." Swinging the arms may be used to stretch the shoulders in a general warm-up. For level 3 students the teacher need only increase the degree of difficulty of the exercises required and extend the length of time in which the children participate continuously up to 15 or 20 minutes. It should be noted that although this exercise program is primarily designed to utilize regular developmental exercises, many fun activities can be incorporated into the program in order to maintain interest and provide enjoyment. Such things as making funny faces while swinging the arms and chanting exercise rhymes while participating in vigorous

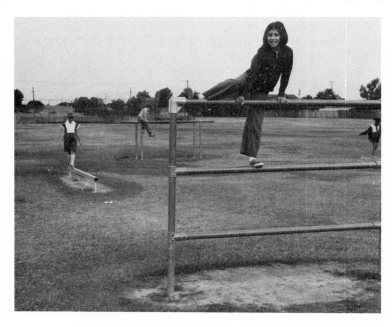

Fig. 15-69. Fitness obstacle course.

activity often provide the necessary motivation for a child's continued participation and enjoyment. The activities or exercises utilized in the continuous rhythmical exercise program are usually left up to the leader, and the pattern taken is seldom the same in any given day. Vigorous exercises should be alternated with recovery activities in order to maintain continuous movement for extended periods of time.

Individual jump rope

Jump rope skills were introduced in level 2, using the long rope and a variety of rhymes. Level 3 children are able to accept the challenge of the individual jump rope in which more extensive routines can be developed. There is no end to the individual creativity of children in developing jump rope routines.

The teacher can introduce a run with a skip, a jump backward, and other techniques to challenge the better students in the class. Caution should be taken not to progress so fast that the slow learners are discouraged. Jumping on one foot, jumping with alternate feet, and jumping with both feet together, combined with a variety of rope skills, can develop into an excellent individual jump rope routine (Fig. 15-70).

Direction change. While jumping forward, the child brings the arms together overhead and moves them to one side of the body. The rope is allowed to continue its arc while a one-half turn is made with the body. At the completion of the turn, the arms are separated above the head as the backward turn is in progress. It is important that the jumper maintain the same rhythm throughout the stunt. The same procedure is followed in order to return to the forward jumping position.

Double jump. Increased speed and timing are essential in executing the double jump. At the completion of a single jump, the child begins to anticipate the double jump as the rope comes around by increasing the speed of the rope and executing a higher jump. Many students will be able to master the double jump quite easily, and a few will progress to the triple jump, which is more difficult but can serve as an incentive to all.

Front cross. As the rope starts upward

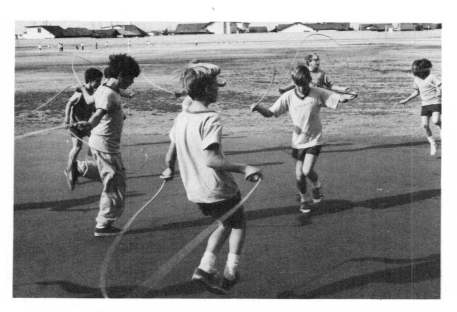

Fig. 15-70. Practicing individual jump rope routines.

behind the child, the arms are crossed, making a loop to jump through. After completing the cross jump, the child uncrosses the arms and makes the succeeding jump in the normal manner. A slightly higher jump is necessary for the successful accomplishment of this skill since the rope becomes shorter as the arms are crossed.

Jump rope routines. After the children have learned the individual rope skipping techniques, they may begin to develop their own routines. For example, a routine might include forward jumping, front cross, change to back jumping, return to front jumping, double jump forward, and front cross. Children can follow the leader and attempt to duplicate the jump rope routines as presented.

Hopscotch

Typical hopscotch. The traditional hopscotch design can be used either by following the numbers consecutively or by using a lagging object. This design is the most commonly used hopscotch activity.

Hopscotch circles. Hopscotch circles are designed to develop laterality. The student begins on one end of the circle and hops with both feet if circles are side by side, selecting the dominant foot for the circle in the center and the other foot for the side of the circle, according to the design. The teacher may look for difficulties the children have in moving through the circles in the most efficient manner.

Jumpscotch court. The jumpscotch court is designed for children to jump with both feet consecutively from one number to the next. The object is to reach number 10 without making an error. The teacher can observe the students for efficiency in moving, body agility in turning, and knowledge of consecutive numbers.

Question mark hopscotch. Question mark hopscotch is designed to be played in the same manner as regular hopscotch with the additional stress being that the children lean in one direction to make the turn in a continuous manner. The object is to progress all the way through the question mark and return to the dot without making an error. A lagging object can be used if desired.

Snail hopscotch. In snail hopscotch the child begins from the outside of the snail

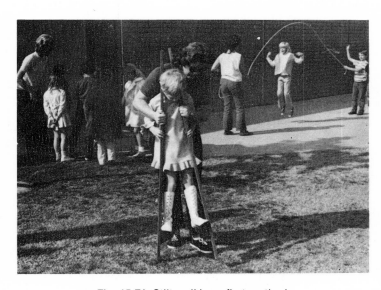

Fig. 15-71. Stilt walking—first method.

and jumps to the center, attempting to maintain balance while continuing along a pattern of smaller circular patterns. As the circle gets smaller, it is increasingly difficult to maintain balance and eliminate errors.

Wooden stilts

There are two ways of taking hold of the tall stilts. In the first method, a person holds the stilts 12 inches ahead of the child and a shoulder width apart. The child then grasps the stilts with the palms facing inward in front of the body (Fig. 15-71). In the second method, the child stands directly between the stilts and places them behind the shoulders. The stilts are grasped with the palms of the hands facing forward (Fig. 15-72). With either method, the child mounts by placing one foot at a time on the footrests. The second position has proved to be the easiest way for children to learn to balance when they go on their own because the shoulders act as an extra holding point.

When a child is learning to walk on stilts, an adult or older child should be stationed behind the beginner and hold the stilts while the child mounts and walks. The helper can tap with the foot on the back of the stilt that is to be moved next so that the child gets the left-right sequence. Once the child easily lifts and walks in rhythm, the helper can release the hold. From this point on, the child must practice mounting and working alone.

Some suggestions for this activity are as follows:

1. Stand as upright as possible, not looking at the feet.
2. Walk on grass or a nonslip surface with the tall stilts.
3. Lift the foot and hand at the same time, keeping pressure on the stilt with the foot.
4. Take small steps, being careful not to get the feet too far apart.
5. When mounting alone position the stilts and the hands first; next tip the stilts slightly backward and gently get the feet up; tip forward and walk with a slightly rocking motion from side to side.

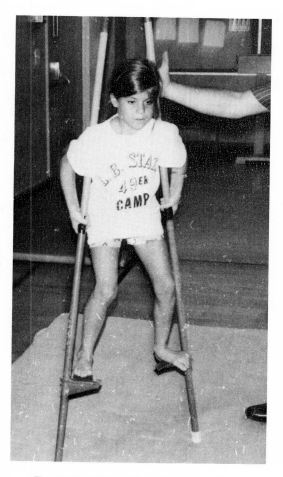

Fig. 15-72. Stilt walking—second method.

Stegel activities

In recent years the German Stegel and similar apparatus have become popular in the United States, mainly because of their simplistic design and unlimited possibilities for a variety of movement skills (Fig. 15-73). The Stegel is particularly adaptable to the needs of young children,

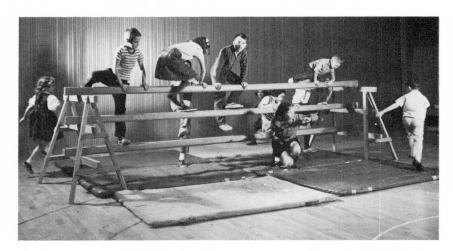

Fig. 15-73. Variations of Stegel climbing. (Courtesy Lind Climber Company, Evanston, Ill.)

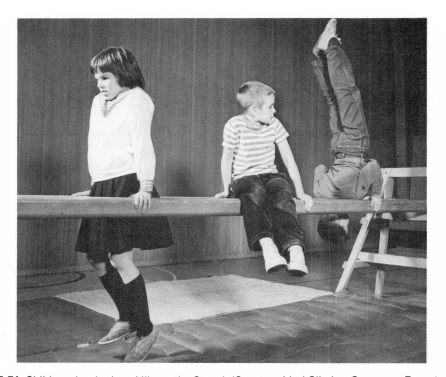

Fig. 15-74. Children developing skills on the Stegel. (Courtesy Lind Climber Company, Evanston. Ill.)

providing opportunities for movement exploration, imaginative play, and physical fitness activities.

The Stegel apparatus usually includes two sawhorselike supports, three wooden beams, an inclined wooden slide, and a ladder. All major parts are movable so that different equipment combinations can be used, depending on the needs of the participants.

The Stegel apparatus lends itself to low-level basic motor skills and also to high-level stunts and physical fitness activities (Fig. 15-74).

Stunts and physical fitness activities
Parallel bar arrangement
1. Dip
2. Hand travel
3. Straddle seat
4. Push-up
5. Shoulder stand

Beams and ladders
1. Front vault
2. Squat vault
3. Straddle vault
4. Rear vault
5. Chin-up
6. Forward roll
7. Backward roll

Variations of stunts
1. Obstacle course, for which there are innumerable possible obstacles for children to overcome, such as running up the slide, walking the balance beam, crawling in and out of the rungs of the ladder, and jumping off the end of the horse to a mat
2. Partner activities such as passing one another while traveling on the beam or ladder and playing catch while balancing
3. Performance of stunts with the Hula-Hoop, such as arm circles, neck circles, body circles, and jumping through

Creative rhythmical dance

As children progress toward physical maturity, they are ready to move from isolated fundamental rhythmical movements as described in Chapter 14 to a sequence of movements that express feeling or ideas. If children at this level have not been exposed to creativity in movement, a hesitancy to participate is quite common and the creative movement activities described in Chapter 9 should be used.

Teacher attitude determines a successful activity for the children. The need for an enthusiastic approach cannot be overemphasized. A selection of materials and confidence in one's ability to help children express themselves freely are also essential. Many teachers will not encourage movement of a creative nature because they fear the activity may get out of hand. This type of lesson should incorporate the same planning—goals, objectives, and evaluation—as any other physical education lesson. Because the children are using free-flowing movement in a restricted area, it is doubly important that standards for safety and control be established. These standards should include starting and stopping signals, space limitations, and tempo control and awareness and should be planned and reinforced by the children and teacher together.

Props. Props are helpful when first beginning these activities because use of a prop focuses attention on the object rather than the person. Props are excellent aids in getting children to begin exploring ways their bodies can move in a more uninhibited manner. Pieces of material, scarves, or streamers that flow when pulled through the air are of great value. Other items that are often used are balls, hoops, boxes, and sticks.

Instruments. Another aid is the use of different instruments. A child or groups of children can respond to a specific instrument such as bells. The second group can respond to sand blocks and a third group to a tambourine. By having the instruments played in sequence, the teacher can cause specific movements done to the individual sounds to be blended together to form a dance. Several instruments can then be played together with children responding to "their" instrument simultaneously. At this point, the instructor can establish that dance is a continuous flow of movement.

Other aids. Stories, poems, folk tales, and historical and current events can be used as a basis for dance, encouraging children to react with movement. Choice of the material can come from the regular curriculum and enhance the work done in the classroom. Meeting student interests in this manner serves as a catalyst to encourage creative dance.

FOLK DANCES AND SINGING GAMES

Folk dances and singing games can provide understanding and appreciation of the people of different cultures of the world and are readily integrated with lessons in history and geography.

The nature of folk dances and the provision for changing of partners keep the reluctance to dance with a member of the opposite sex to a minimum. The children should not choose their partners for dance activities. Any technique in which partners are arranged ahead of time should be used to ensure that no one is selected last. Although holding hands is not a problem with children in the primary grades, children in the intermediate levels often are self-conscious and feel uneasy during dance activities. For the most part, the teacher should make little issue of this matter; if partners are changed often and if the teacher shows enthusiasm for the activity and presents dance in a positive manner, few problems will result.

Folk dances provide vigorous activity and involve a variety of intricate foot patterns. Individuals who become well skilled in these activities not only ad-

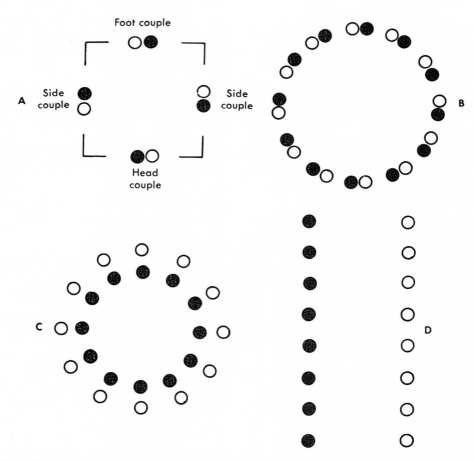

Fig. 15-75. Dance formations: **A,** square; **B,** circle; **C,** double circle; and **D,** double line. The dark circles represent the boys, and the light circles, the girls.

vance in their knowledge of the social graces but also increase their balance and coordination, all of which develop a favorable self-image. The following progression should be used for teaching folk dances:

1. The children listen to music.
2. The teacher demonstrates the dance step involved.
3. The children practice the dance step without the music.
4. They practice the step with the music.

The following dance formations are used in most dances (Fig. 15-75):

1. Square
2. Circle
3. Double circle
4. Double line

The following basic dance steps are used in the majority of dances in the elementary physical education program.

Step-point. The child performs the step-point by stepping on the left foot and pointing the right foot in front. He or she then repeats the motion, stepping to the right.

Step-hop. The child performs the step-hop by stepping on the left foot and hopping on the same foot. The movement is repeated, stepping on the right foot.

Step-swing. The child performs the step-swing by stepping on the left foot and swinging the right foot across in front of the left foot. The motion is repeated stepping on the right foot.

Bleking step. The child performs the bleking step by taking a hop on the left foot and extending the right leg forward with the heel touching the floor. The motion is repeated hopping on the right foot with the left leg extended. The left heel and right heel are changed in a rhythmical pattern.

Balance step. The child performs the balance step by stepping forward with the left foot and closing with the right foot, rising to the balls of the feet. The balance step can be done in any direction.

Schottische step. The child performs the schottische step by taking three running steps, beginning with the left foot, and then hopping on the left foot. The motion is repeated, beginning with the right foot.

Polka step. The child performs the polka step by stepping to the right and closing left to right and then stepping to the right again with a hold. The motion is repeated, stepping first with the left foot.

Buzz step. The buzz step is usually performed with a partner. Keeping the weight on the inside foot, the child pushes against the floor with the outside foot, as in riding a scooter, and revolves around the pivot foot.

Grapevine step. The grapevine step can be done in either direction to the side. The child crosses the right foot over in front of the left foot, takes a step on the left foot, brings the right foot behind the left foot, and then takes a step on the left foot.

Dances and singing games

HOKEY POKEY

Formation: The children form a single circle and face the center. If couples are used, the girl stands to the right of her partner.

Music: MacGregor 699 and Four Star 1505

Procedure: The children place their right foot forward into the circle and sing:

"You put your right foot in."

They place their right foot back away from the circle and sing:

"You put your right foot out."

They shake their right foot toward the center of the circle and sing:

"You put your right foot in and you shake it all about."

They place their palms together above their head and rumba their hips and sing:

"You do the hokey pokey."

They shake their arms above their head and turn around and sing. If there are couples, the boy turns the girl on his left once and a half with his right elbow and progresses one position clockwise:

"And you turn yourself around."

The children clap their hands four times and sing:

"That's what it's all about."

They repeat these calls, substituting the following parts of the body: left foot, right arm, left arm, right elbow, head, whole self, and back side.

Then they raise their arms above their head and lower their arms and head in a bowing motion and sing:

"You do the hokey pokey
You do the hokey pokey."

They kneel on both knees and raise their arms above their head and lower their arms and head in a bowing motion and sing:

"You do the hokey pokey."

Then they slap the floor six times and sing:

"That's what it's all about."

SKIP TO MY LOU

Formation: The children form a double circle, with boys in the inside circle. Partners face to the right and join hands.

Music: Folkraft 1192, Pioneer 3003, and Folk Dancers record MH 111

Procedure: All the children sing as the partners skip to the right around the circle:

"Flies in the buttermilk, skip to my Lou,
Flies in the buttermilk, skip to my Lou,
Flies in the buttermilk, skip to my Lou,
Skip to my Lou, my darling."

The girls continue skipping while the boys stand and sing:

"My partner's gone, what'll I do," etc.

The boys sing and skip around the inside circle, and the girls stand still:

"I'll find another one, prettier than you," etc.

On "skip to my Lou my darling," the boys take a partner nearest to them and repeat the dance with a new partner.

For variation, extra boys may be in the center of the circle. At the end of the third verse, they all try to get partners. The boys failing to get a partner go to the center and wait for a turn when the dance is repeated.

A-HUNTING WE WILL GO

Formation: The children form couples and stand in two lines, partners facing. There should be no more than six couples to a set.

Music: Folkraft 1191, RCA Victor 45-5064, and Childhood Rhythms, series 7, no. 705

Procedure: All the children sing as the head couple joins both hands and slides down between the lines and back:

"A-hunting we will go, a-hunting we will go,
We'll catch a fox, and put him in a box, and
then we'll let him go."

All partners sing and join hands and skip around in a circle counterclockwise, following the head couple:

Chorus:
"Tra la, la, la, la, la, la," etc.

When the children who are the head couple reach the foot of the line, they form an arch by joining both hands, and all the other couples pass through. The second couple then becomes the head couple to repeat the dance. The dance is repeated until each couple has been head couple.

CHIMES OF DUNKIRK

Formation: The children form a single circle with boys and girls alternating. Partners face each other with their hands on their own hips.

Music: RCA Victor LPM-1624, 45-6176, and 21618

Procedure

MEASURES 1-2: All the children stamp their feet (not too heavily) left, right, left.

MEASURES 3-4: They raise their arms overhead so that their faces can be seen between their arms and bend their bodies sharply to the left and clap their hands overhead and then to the right and clap, alternately. This represents the ringing of the town's bells.

MEASURES 5-7: The partners take each other's hands with their arms extended sideways. Starting with the left foot, they run in a small circle while turning their partners once around.

MEASURE 8: The children run forward on the last measure and secure new partners. The dance is continued until the music ends.

SEVEN JUMPS

Formation: The children form one large single circle, with boys and girls alternating, and join hands. A number of smaller circles may be used.

Music: RCA Victor 21617, 41-6172, and LPM-1623 and World of Fun M-108

Procedure

First jump

MEASURES 1-8: The children move in a circle to the right with step-hops, one to a measure (step on beat one and hop on beat two).

MEASURES 9-16: They all jump up high from the ground and come down with a stamp on both feet on the first beat of measure 9. Then they step-hop around the circle to the left.

MEASURE 17: They drop their hands and place them on their hips and bend the right knee upward.

MEASURE 18: They stamp their right foot to the ground on the first beat and join hands on the second beat.

Second jump

MEASURES 1-16: They repeat measures 1-16 of the first jump.

MEASURE 17: They all raise the right knee as before.

MEASURES 18-19: On the first beat, they stamp down right foot; on the second beat, lift left knee; on the third beat, stamp left foot; and on the fourth beat, join hands.

Third jump

MEASURES 1-17: They repeat measures 1-17 of the first and and second jumps.

MEASURES 18-20: They all stamp right foot, lift left knee, stamp left foot, place right toe backward on the floor, kneel on left knee, and then stand and join hands (one action to each beat).

Fourth jump

MEASURES 1-17: They repeat measures 1-17 as before.

MEASURES 18-21: They stamp right foot, lift left knee, stamp left foot, place right toe backward, kneel on left knee, pause, kneel on right knee (both knees down), and on the last beat, stand and join hands.

Fifth jump

MEASURES 1-17: They all repeat measures 1-17.

MEASURES 18-22: They stamp right foot; lift left knee; stamp left foot; place right toe backward; kneel on left knee; pause; kneel on right knee; put right fist to cheek, raising elbow; put right elbow on the floor, with cheek resting on fist; and on the last beat, stand and join hands.

Sixth jump

MEASURES 1-17: They repeat measures 1-17.

MEASURES 18-23: They stamp right foot; lift left knee; stamp left foot; place right toe backward; kneel on left knee; pause; kneel on right knee; put right fist to cheek, raising elbow; put right elbow on the floor, with cheek resting on fist; put left fist to cheek, raising elbow; put left elbow on floor, with cheek resting on fist; and on the last beat, stand and join hands.

Seventh jump

MEASURES 1-17: They repeat measures 1-17.

MEASURES 18-24: They stamp right foot; lift left knee; stamp left foot; place right toe backward; kneel on left knee; pause; kneel on right knee; put right fist to cheek, raising elbow; put right elbow on the floor, with cheek resting on fist; put left fist to cheek, raising elbow; put left elbow on floor, with cheek resting on fist; push body forward; touch forehead to floor; and on the last beat, stand and join hands.

BLEKING

Formation: The children form a single circle, and partners face each other and join both hands.

Music: RCA Victor LPM-1622 and 41-6169; Folkraft 1188; and Pioneer 3016

Procedure

MEASURE 1: the children hop on left foot, place right heel forward, and extend right arm and then hop on right foot and extend left foot and arm (bleking step).

MEASURE 2: They repeat the step with three quick changes, hopping left, right, left.

MEASURES 3-8: They repeat measures 1 and 2 three times.

MEASURES 9-16: With hands joined and arms extended to the side at shoulder level, the partners turn in place with step-hops. The boy starts on his right foot, and the girl starts on her left foot. They move their arms up and down in windmill fashion.

NORWEGIAN MOUNTAIN MARCH

Formation: The children form sets of three. Each set forms a triangle; for example, a boy in front holds the outside hands of two girls standing behind him, and the two girls join inside hands. The dance represents a guide pulling two others up and down a mountain.

Music: Folkraft 1177 and RCA Victor 45-6173

Procedure

MEASURES 1-8: All the children take eight step-hops (or stamp-step-steps) forward, starting on the right foot, accenting the first beat of each measure.

MEASURES 9-10: The boy takes four step-hops backward under the arms of the two girls.

MEASURES 11-12: The girl on the right turns under the boy's left arm with four step-hops.

MEASURES 13-14: The girl on the left turns under the boy's right arm with four step-hops.

MEASURES 15-16: The boy turns under his own left arm with four step-hops. Then they all face forward.

They repeat measures 9-16.

VIRGINIA REEL

Formation: Six couples form two parallel lines with the girls on the right and the boys on the left, facing each other.

Music: Folkraft 1249 and RCA Victor 45-6180 and LPM-1623

Procedure: The children follow the instructions as they are given.

"Forward and back":

Partners take four steps to the center, bow, and take four steps back to their places.

"Right hands around":

Partners meet, join right hands, swing around once, and return to their places.

"Left hands around":

They meet, join left hands, swing around once, and return to their places.

"Both hands around":

They meet, join both hands, swing around once, and return to their places.

"Do-si-do":

Partners walk forward, pass right shoulders, slide back to back, and walk backward to their places, passing left shoulders.

"Head couple down and back":

The children who are the head couple join both hands and slide down the set and back.

"Reel the set":

The children who are the head couple hook right elbows, turn around one and a half times, and then separate and go to the opposite line. The head boy turns the second girl around once with a left-elbow turn, and the head girl does the same with the second boy. Then the head couple meet in the center for a right-elbow turn and continue down the line, turning someone in the set with the left elbow and turning the partner with the right elbow, until they have reeled the entire set. On reaching the foot of the set, they swing halfway around so that the boy and girl are on the correct side, join hands, and slide back to their places.

"Cast off":

The lines face the front, and at the change of music, the head couple leads to the outside (boy to his left, girl to her right) and marches to the foot of the set, the two lines following.

"Form the arch":

On reaching the foot of the set, the children who are the head couple join hands to form an arch. The other couples meet and skip under the arch and return to their places. The second couple then becomes the head couple for the next figure, and the original head couple becomes the foot couple. The dance continues until all have been head couple.

SUPPLEMENTARY RECORDS LEVEL 3

1. Around the World in Dance, Glass, AR 542
2. Folk Dance Funfest, Kraus, Educational Recordings FD 1
3. From Singing Games to Folk Dancing, vol. 4, CM 1160
4. Lummi Stick Fun, Johnson, Kim 2000
5. Perceptual Motor Rhythm Games, Capon, A1
6. Rhythmic Parachute Play, Seker, KEA 6020
7. Streamer and Rhythm Activities, Glass, AR 578

16

Level 4: Refining

Level 4 activities are individual and team activities that require a high degree of skill. Successful performance in these activities is based on the motor skills developed at the lower levels. Participation at this level challenges the well-skilled child to employ individual and team strategy in competitive sport activities.

The games in level 4 can be organized for tournament play, and one class can challenge another in competition. Children who are not capable of successfully performing the skills necessary for level 4 activities should be given individual help to improve their skills before they are selected as full-fledged team members. For those children who have not achieved proper motor development for their particular maturational level, activities should be taken from levels 2 and 3 and administered on an individual or small group basis.

BALL ACTIVITIES

NATIONBALL

Behavioral objective: To dodge, catch, or throw a ball accurately

Developmental goal: Endurance, strategy, and agility

Space and equipment: Rectangular court with a center line (volleyball court) and a playground ball

Number of players: Entire class

Test reference: II and V

Procedure: The children divide into two equal teams. Each team chooses two goalies (usu-

ally the best dodgers and throwers). The players take positions as indicated in Fig. 16-1. The team 1 goalies throw the ball at the team 2 players in the center, and the team 2 goalies throw at the team 1 players. If a player is hit, he or she must go out. The person who is hit has the next throw after going out. Players are out of the game only if they drop the ball or are hit. If a team 2 player catches the ball without dropping it, he or she may then turn and throw it at the team 1 players in the next square. The goalies may throw the ball to their own team members, who work the ball back and forth and have the privilege of throwing at the opposite team from the center. Once a person is hit without catching the ball, he or she is out and must join the goalie and assist in catching the ball and throwing it at the players on the opposite team. When one person is left on a team, the goalies may go in, usually one at a time. The last team to have all its players put out wins.

Soccer activities

CIRCLE SOCCER

Behavioral objective: To learn kicking skills as lead-up skills to soccer

Developmental goal: Eye-foot coordination

Space and equipment: Multipurpose play area and soccer ball

Number of players: 20 to 30

Test reference: IV, V, and VI

Procedure: The children divide into two teams and form a circle, each team making up half the circle. The members of each team try to kick the ball with the inside of the foot through the members of the other team and

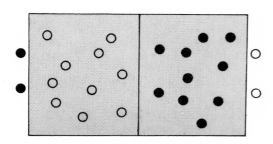

Fig. 16-1. Nationball court.

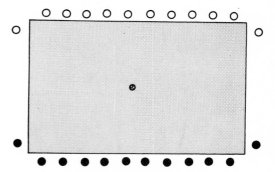

Fig. 16-2. Line soccer field.

out of the circle. The players may block the ball with their body or legs or may trap it with their feet or knees, but they may not use their hands and arms. The ball should be momentarily stopped before it is kicked back across the circle. One point is given to a team when its members kick the ball through the members of the other team, at shoulder level or below. If a player kicks the ball beyond his or her own team's circle, one point is given to the opposing team. If a ball is kicked through the members of the defending team above shoulder level, one point is given to the defending team. The first team to reach ten points wins. The game also may be played for a specified time period.

LINE SOCCER

Behavioral objective: To develop skill in maneuvering around an opponent

Developmental goal: Large-muscle development, eye-foot coordination, and agility

Space and equipment: Multipurpose play area and soccer ball

Number of players: 10 on a team

Test reference: IV and V

Procedure: The children divide into teams, and the teams line up opposite each other as indicated in Fig. 16-2. On a signal, the runner at the right end of each line runs to the center and attempts to take possession of the ball in the center by pulling it back or to one side before dribbling it with the foot. The runner advances the ball by dribbling it up close to the opposing team's goal line in order to kick it through. The opposing runner tries to take the ball from the runner in possession. The team members along the line defend their goal line, blocking the ball

with any part of their body except their hands; they may use their hands and arms when they are held in contact with the body, but only to stop the ball, not to advance it. When the ball goes out over the sidelines, it is kicked in at the point where it left the field, by the nearest sideline guard of the team opposite the one that sent it out. A point is scored each time a runner kicks the ball through the opposing team's goal line. Even if the ball touches the body of a defending player, a point is scored. After each goal or on the teacher's command, the players rotate as follows: the runner becomes right guard, right guard becomes left guard, left guard moves into the space at the left end of the goal, and all the players on the line move one space to their right, that is, counterclockwise, or toward the position of the runner.

Fouls

1. The player touches the ball with the hands or arms above shoulder height.
2. The player advances the ball with the hands or arms.
3. A line player or side guard plays in the center territory.
4. The player kicks the ball above shoulder height of the opponents. This is not a foul on a penalty kick, but no score is made. The players rotate, and the ball is put into play at the center.
5. The player pushes or holds another player or plays roughly.
6. On the initial play, the player fails to pull the ball back or to one side and dribble it before kicking for a goal.
7. A line player or guard kicks the ball through the opposing team's goal line.

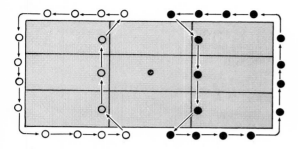
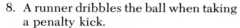

Fig. 16-3. Alley soccer field.

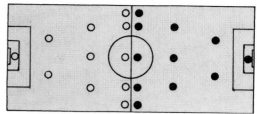

Fig. 16-4. Soccer field.

8. A runner dribbles the ball when taking a penalty kick.
9. An opposing runner crosses into the field of play before the ball reaches the goal line after a penalty kick.

The penalty for fouls is as follows: The runner on the opposing team is given a penalty kick from a mark 12 feet from the goal line. The free kick is a place kick, and the ball may not be dribbled. The runner of the offending team must go behind the goal line and remain there until the ball reaches the opposing goal line. If no score is made, the offending runner goes back into the field and the ball is put into play. If the runner of the offending team fails to stay behind that team's goal line until the ball reaches the goal line and a goal is made, it is counted and the players rotate and the ball is put into play at the center as it is at the beginning of the game; if the runner fails to stay behind the line and the goal is missed, another penalty kick is awarded to the same player.

ALLEY SOCCER

Behavioral objective: To develop skill in maneuvering a ball around an opponent
Developmental goal: Teamwork, sportsmanship, and eye-foot coordination
Space and equipment: Alley soccer field and soccer ball
Number of players: Two teams of 12 to 15 each
Test reference: IV and V
Procedure: The children divide into two teams. Each team has three forwards. The field is divided into three long alleys, and each forward must stay inside his or her team's alley at all times (Fig. 16-3). The other players on each team line up along the sidelines and the goal line of their own half of the field. No one may touch the ball

with the arms or hands. One of the center players starts the game by kicking the ball ahead at an angle to one of the team's forwards. They kick the ball to each other, trying to keep it away from their opponents, and move down the field. The forward or center player who gets control of the ball tries to kick it down the field and across the other team's goal line, below the heads of the players. If the forward kicks the ball across the goal line, the team scores a point. If the ball comes toward a player on the sidelines or goal line, the player tries to keep the ball in play by kicking it to a teammate. If the ball goes over the sideline, it is brought inside and kicked by the nearest player on the team that did not send it out.

This game is an excellent lead-up activity to soccer, since the players are required to stay in their alleys and thus to keep their distance to receive a ball.

Fouls

1. The player touches the ball with the arms or hands.
2. The player kicks the ball higher than a player's head.
3. A player other than a forward tries to score a goal.
4. The player pushes or trips another player or plays roughly.
5. The player tries to block a free kick.
6. A forward steps outside the alley.

When a foul is committed, a free kick is awarded to the opposing team.

SOCCER

Behavioral objective: To execute the skills of kicking, dribbling, trapping, and passing in a game situation
Developmental goal: Endurance and teamwork
Space and equipment: Soccer field and soccer ball

Number of players: Two teams of 11

Test reference: IV and V

Procedure: The game of soccer involves the skills of running and kicking in which the ball is controlled by the foot. The ball may not be touched with the hands or arms. The ball is advanced toward the opposing team's goal with the foot, body, or head.

At the start of the game, the players are positioned as indicated in the diagram in Fig. 16-4. Each team consists of the goalie, right fullback, left fullback, right halfback, center halfback, left halfback, outside right forward, inside right forward, center forward, inside left forward, and outside left forward. The forwards are primarily offensive players, and the halfbacks and fullbacks are primarily defensive players. It is decided which team will kick off. Then the center forward of the offensive, or kicking, team kicks the ball from the center circle toward a teammate. The ball must travel forward the length of its circumference. The opponents must remain outside the circle until the ball has been touched; then players on both teams may cross the center line and play the ball wherever it goes. They move the ball by dribbling it with the foot or passing it to another teammate. The team in possession of the ball tries to move it down the field and into the opposing team's goal. The defending players attempt to intercept the ball and reverse the direction of play (Fig. 16-5).

Rules of play: Soccer rules discourage any unnecessary roughness. When unnecessary roughness takes place, the offending team is penalized; a free kick is given to the other team.

A penalty kick is awarded to the offensive team when a foul is committed in the penalty area by the defensive team. The penalty area is the largest rectangular zone around the goal (Fig. 16-4). The offensive team takes the penalty kick from the penalty mark while all the players except the goalie stand outside the penalty area.

A free kick is awarded to the opposing team for any fouls committed outside the penalty area. It is kicked from the spot of the foul. The opponents must remain at least 10 yards away until the ball is kicked.

If the ball is kicked over the sideline, it is put into play by the opposite team. A halfback usually puts the ball into play from the sideline by throwing the ball in with two hands overhead.

When the ball is kicked over the goal

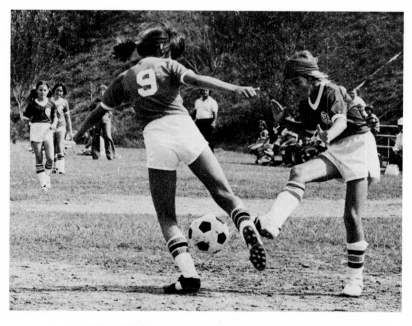

Fig. 16-5. Girls competing in a soccer game.

line but not through the goal by the offensive team, the goalie of the defensive team kicks the ball back into the game. The other team members must remain 10 yards away until the ball is kicked.

When the defensive team causes the ball to go over its own goal line, the offensive team gets a corner kick. This kick is taken by the outside forward from the corner of the field closest to the point where the ball went out of bounds.

Scoring: One point is awarded for each goal that is made. After a goal is scored, the team scored against kicks off.

Fouls

1. *Carrying.* The goalie takes more than two steps with the ball in the hands.
2. *Handling.* A player touches the ball with the hand or any part of the arm between the wrist and shoulder.
3. *Pushing.* A player moves an opponent away with the hands, arm, or body.

Privileges: Having the following privileges, the goalie:

1. May pick up the ball with the hands
2. May punt the ball away from the goal line
3. May throw the ball away from the goal
4. May take only two steps with the ball

The other players have the following privileges:

1. They may stop the ball with their feet.
2. They may dribble, pass, shoulder, or head the ball.
3. They may kick the ball to a teammate when trapped by an opponent.
4. They may stop the ball by blocking it with any part of the body except the hands or arms.

SPEEDBALL

Behavioral objective: To execute the skills of kicking, passing, dribbling, and trapping in a game situation

Developmental goal: Eye-hand and eye-foot coordination, teamwork, sportsmanship, and endurance

Space and equipment: Soccer field and soccer ball

Number of players: 6 to 11 on a team

Test reference: II, IV, and V

Procedure: The children divide into teams as in soccer. One team is awarded the kickoff to start the game. The forwards of that team take their positions on the line with the ball, which is placed in the center of the field, or they may stand in any part of the field between the ball and their own restraining line, which is halfway between the center of the field and the goal. The backfield players of the team kicking off must be behind their own restraining line at the time of the kickoff. All players on the defending team must be behind their restraining line until the ball has been touched by the offensive team. The penalty for any infraction of these kickoff rules made by the offensive team is loss of the kickoff. If the foul is made by the defending team, the offensive team takes the kickoff over again 5 yards nearer the goal of the defending team.

The duty of the forwards is to attempt to move the ball into scoring position. The backs play a defensive game chiefly, attempting to secure the ball from the opposing forwards and pass it to their own forwards. The goalies protect their own goals. The forwards may not play behind their own restraining line. The backfield players may not advance beyond the opposing team's restraining line. The penalty for any infraction of the rules concerning playing zones is a free kick for any opponent on the restraining line where the foul occurred. During the free kick, the members of the offending team must be at least 5 yards away from the ball.

The ball must be played as in soccer unless it comes directly off the foot of a player, in which case the ball may be caught and played as in basketball. However, a ball bouncing up from the ground cannot be played with the hands. Only a ball kicked into the air may be caught and played as an aerial ball. A ball going over the sidelines or over the end lines and not between the goal posts (except on a touchdown) is kicked in by an opponent at the spot where the ball crossed the line. The players on the team that sent the ball out must be at least 5 yards away from the ball when it is kicked.

Scoring: A goal made as in soccer earns two points. A touchdown earns one point. A touchdown is a completed forward pass like in football and must be made from a player in the goal area to a player in the end zone. If a pass is not completed, is caught by an opponent, or is made by a player not in the goal area, the ruling is the same as for an out-of-bounds play, with no score. After a team scores, the team scored against kicks off.

Fouls

1. The player travels with the ball in the hands.
2. The player holds the ball longer than 3 seconds.
3. The player catches or touches the ball when it is not kicked into the air.

Penalty: Except for violation of the kickoff rule, the penalty for a foul is a free kick for the opponents. A free kick is a place kick taken on the spot where the foul occurred. The ball must be passed to another player within the field of play. It may be lofted to another player on the free kick to convert the play into an aerial play. Players may not loft the ball to themselves on a free kick, nor may they score on a free kick. The players on the offending team must be at least 5 yards away from the ball when it is kicked.

Volleyball activities

TOSS-UP

Behavioral objective: To toss and catch quickly

Developmental goal: Throwing and catching skills

Space and equipment: Volleyball court and volleyball

Number of participants: 12 to 18

Test reference: II and V

Procedure: Players are divided into equal teams and numbered the same on each side. Teams line up in several lines, facing each other. Player number 1 starts the game by tossing to number 1 on the other side and going to the end of the line. After catching the ball, number 1 tosses over to number 2. Number 2 tosses back to the opposite side, and play continues with each player going to the end of the line after the toss (Fig. 16-6). The first team to score 25 catches wins.

SERVICE VOLLEYBALL

Behavioral objective: To serve a volleyball effectively

Developmental goal: Use of heel of hand and underhand swing with arm follow-through

Space and equipment: Volleyball court and one volleyball per squad

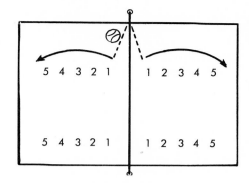

Fig. 16-6. Toss-up.

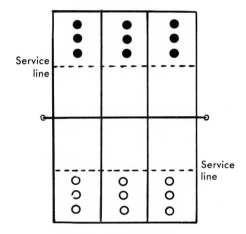

Fig. 16-7. Service volleyball.

Number of participants: 12 to 18

Test reference: II and VII

Procedure: The players line up as shown in Fig. 16-7. The first player in each line serves the ball over the net trying to place it in the opposite court. The server then goes to the end of the line. The first player on the opposite side catches the ball and serves it back to the other side and goes to the end of his or her line. Play continues in this manner. A game is 15 fair serves.

CIRCLE KEEP UP

Behavioral objective: To be able to volley successfully at least ten times

Developmental goal: Use of both hands and fingertips to volley

Space and equipment: One half volleyball court and one ball per squad

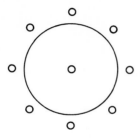

Fig. 16-8. Circle keep up.

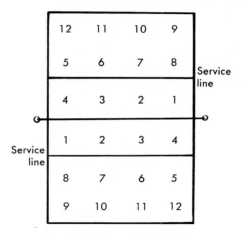

Fig. 16-10. One bounce volleyball.

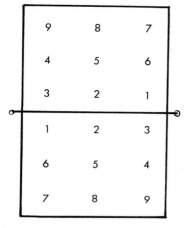

Fig. 16-9. One bounce keep up.

Number of players: 6 to 8

Test reference: II, V, and VII

Procedure: Each squad forms a circle with one player in the center (Fig. 16-8). The game consists of volleying the ball back and forth from center player to circle player trying to keep the ball in the air longer each time. In the beginning, the game works best when the teacher or a well-skilled player is in the center.

ONE BOUNCE KEEP UP

Behavioral objective: To hit the ball back and forth over the net

Developmental goal: To practice serving and volleying

Space and equipment: Volleyball court and two volleyballs

Number of players: 12 to 18

Test reference: II and V

Procedure: Each team fills up one side of the court (Fig. 16-9). A volleyball is served by

each team at the same time. The opposing team receives the ball after one bounce and attempts to keep the ball volleying on its side of the net. The team keeping the ball up the longest scores one point. Each player may hit the ball only once consecutively. Eleven points is a game. A ball served out of bounds or into the net scores one point for the opposing team.

ONE BOUNCE VOLLEYBALL

Behavioral objective: To serve the ball over the net and volley it back

Developmental goal: Rotation and use of both hands in volleying

Space and equipment: Volleyball court and volleyball

Number of players: 12 to 18

Test reference: II and V

Procedure: The players divide into two teams, one on each side of the court (Fig. 16-10). The ball is served over the net from a mid-court service line. The members of the team to which it was served must let the ball bounce once and hit the ball to a teammate and/or volley it over the net. The ball must bounce once before each player hits it. The third player must get the ball over the net. A point is scored or serve is lost when a player fails to return the ball over the net, hits the ball twice, hits the ball out of bounds, or fails to allow the ball to bounce after each volley. The team serving the ball is the only one to win the points. A game consists of 11 or 15 points.

VOLLEYBALL

Behavioral objective: To execute the skills of serving, receiving, passing, setting, and spiking in team play

Developmental goal: Eye-hand coordination, strategy, and teamwork

Space and equipment: Volleyball court and volleyball

Number of players: 12 to 24

Test reference: II and VI

Procedure: The children divide into two teams, and the teams stand on either side of a net. The player in the back right-hand corner on the serving team hits the ball from behind the back line over the net to the opposing team. If elementary school children do not have sufficient power to serve from the back line, the server may move up to an adjusted service line. The receiving team is allowed a maximum of three hits to return the ball. If the team members allow the ball to touch the ground, fail to return the ball over the net, hit the ball out of bounds, or catch, hold, push, or throw the ball, the serving team scores one point and the same person serves again. When the ball is returned to a server, it should be *rolled* under the net to avoid its being played. If the serving team members fail to get the serve over the net or hit the ball out of bounds or if they catch, hold, push, or throw the ball, they score no point and the serve goes to the opposing team. When the service returns to the other team, this team rotates positions as shown in the diagrams in Fig. 16-11. The game may be played for a specified length of time or until one team reaches 15 points.

Basketball activities

AROUND THE WORLD

Behavioral objective: To develop shooting skill as a lead-up skill to basketball

Developmental goal: Individual skill development, eye-hand coordination, and object management

Space and equipment: Basketball backboard and basketball

Number of players: 3 to 5

Test reference: II

Procedure: The children stand behind the basket as indicated in Fig. 16-12. They take turns shooting the ball at the basket from each position shown in Fig. 16-12. After

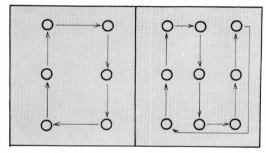

For six players   For nine players

Fig. 16-11. Volleyball rotations.

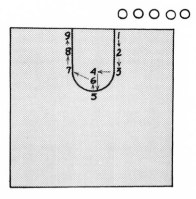

Fig. 16-12. Around the world. The open circles are children waiting to play. The numbers are the different positions from which the player shoots at the basket.

each shot, the waiting players retrieve the ball as the shooter moves to the next number. The player continues to shoot until he or she misses. After missing, the player goes to the end of the waiting line. The player's next turn begins at the spot where he or she last missed. The first player to succeed in scoring a basket from each position has traveled "around the world" and is declared the winner.

TWENTY-ONE

Behavioral objective: To develop shooting skill as a lead-up skill to basketball

Developmental goal: Eye-hand coordination and object management

Space and equipment: Basketball backboard and basketball

Number of players: 3 to 5

Test reference: II

Procedure: This is a basket-shooting game.

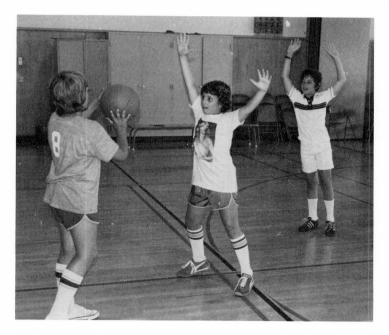

Fig. 16-13. Basketball keep away.

The players take turns shooting. Each player takes a long shot and then a short shot. The long shot distance can be adjusted to the skill level of the children. The short shot should be taken from where the shooter catches the rebound. A player earns two points for a basket on a long shot and one point for a basket on a short shot. The player who gets 21 points first wins.

BASKETBALL KEEP AWAY

Behavioral objective: To gain basketball control
Developmental goal: Dribbling, guarding, passing, and catching
Space and equipment: Half of a basketball court, basketball, and pinnies for one team
Number of players: 8 to 16
Test reference: II and V
Procedure: The players divide into two teams. The ball is tossed up at the center of the court. The team retrieving the ball tries to make 15 passes to teammates to score 1 point (Fig. 16-13). A player can dribble only three times to get a pass away. If the opponents secure the ball before 15 passes are made the count must start over when the ball is retrieved again. Violations occur if the ball is held more than 3 seconds, if there are more than three bounces made before a pass, and if overguarding or roughness is used. If any of these infractions occur the ball is awarded to the opponents.

BASKETBALL A GO-GO

Behavioral objective: To develop shooting and dribbling skills
Developmental goal: Dribbling, passing, and shooting
Space and equipment: Basketball court and basketball for each team
Number of players: 5 on a team
Test reference: II and VI
Procedure: Players line up as shown in Fig. 16-14. Player 1 dribbles around player 2 and toward the basket and shoots. A shooter is allowed two shots to make one basket. Player 1 passes to player 2 and player 2 passes to player 3 who repeats actions of player 1. Player 1 takes place of player 2 and player 2 goes to the end of the line. Player 3 dribbles around player 1. Game continues until one team scores ten baskets or a set time limit expires.

COUNT THE BASKETS

Behavioral objective: To shoot successfully into the basket

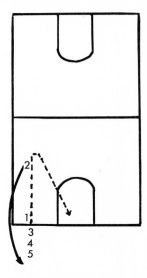

Fig. 16-14. Basketball a go-go.

Developmental goal: Accuracy and quickness in shooting skills

Space and equipment: Basketball court and basketballs

Number of players: 1 at each basket

Test reference: II and V

Procedure: Players may shoot from anywhere on the court and count the number of baskets made in 1 minute. Players must retrieve their own balls and count their scores out loud.

BASKETBALL

Behavioral objective: To effectively execute the skills of dribbling, passing, and shooting in a competitive situation

Developmental goal: Agility, endurance, and teamwork

Space and equipment: Basketball court and basketball

Number of players: 5 on a team

Test reference: II, V, and VI

Procedure: The children divide into two teams. Each team consists of two forwards, two guards, and a center. The forwards on the offensive team play near the opposing team's basket, the center plays in the center lane, and the guards play toward the center line. On the defensive team, the guards play near their own basket, the center plays in the center lane, and the forwards play toward the center line, ready to move toward the opposing team's basket. The game begins when the referee puts the ball into play by tossing it up between the two centers. Each center tries to tap it to one of his own teammates. The team that gets the ball passes or dribbles it among its players in an attempt to move it down the court toward the opposing team's goal (Fig. 16-15). Play continues until a basket is made or a foul is called. Any player may shoot for the basket. When a basket is made, the team scores two points. After each basket is made, the ball is given to one of the guards of the team scored against, who throws it in to a teammate, who moves it down the court in an attempt to score. When two or more opposing players have a firm hold on the ball with one or both hands, a held ball is called. The referee tosses the ball up between two of the opposing players involved as at the start of the game. A game consists of four 6-minute periods with 2 minutes between quarters and 10 minutes between halves.

Fouls: The breaking of a rule constitutes a foul if it is flagrant. Personal fouls are blocking, pushing, holding, tripping, or charging an opponent. Five personal fouls put a player out of the game. The penalty for a foul is a free throw for the opposite team; if a foul occurs while a player is shooting, two free throws are given to the player attempting the shot. A free throw that results in a basket counts one point.

Violations: The breaking of a rule constitutes a violation if it is of a lesser degree. Violations are stepping over the line on a free throw, throwing the ball out of bounds, taking steps with the ball, and beginning a second dribble before shooting or passing. A violation results in the ball's being given to the other team out of bounds.

Handball activity

ONE-WALL HANDBALL

Behavioral objective: To execute serving and striking skills in a game situation

Developmental goal: Eye-hand coordination and agility

Space and equipment: Handball courts or building wall

Number of players: 2 to 4

Test reference: II and VI

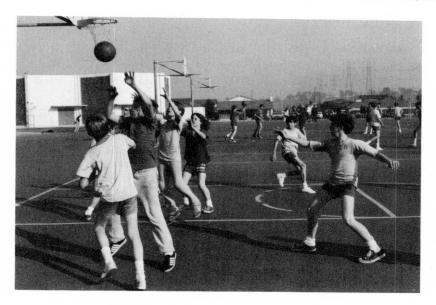

Fig. 16-15. Team competition in basketball.

Procedure: The children divide into teams. To begin the game, the serving team strikes the ball so that it hits anywhere on the front wall and then returns to the serving line. The receiving team may hit the ball on the fly or after it has bounced once. All the players must hit the ball with their hands. The players may not catch the ball and then hit it nor may they strike it with two hands simultaneously. Points are scored only by the serving team. The server continues to serve until the ball is missed. After each member of the team has lost the serve, the other team serves. The game may be played for a specified length of time or until one team reaches 21 points. Any building wall with a suitable playing surface may be used.

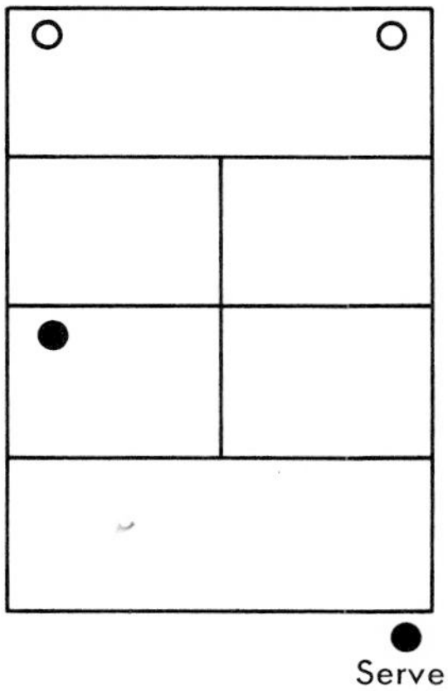

Tennis activity

PADDLE TENNIS

Behavioral objective: To strike a ball successfully over the net
Developmental goal: Eye-hand coordination
Space and equipment: Volleyball court, low net, paddles, and tennis balls
Number of players: 4 on each court
Test reference: II
Procedure: Paddle tennis is an excellent lead-up to tennis and can be played on a volley-ball court with the net lowered to a height of 3 feet (Fig. 16-16). The game is played identically to tennis except that an under-hand serve is required. Scoring is like that of tennis. When the score is deuce, one side must make two points in a row to win. One player serves the entire game beginning in the right service area and alternating diagonal serves throughout the game.

Receiver

Server

Fig. 16-16. Paddle tennis court.

Racquetball activity

RACQUETBALL

Behavioral objective: To effectively execute striking skills with an implement

Developmental goal: Eye-hand coordination

Space and equipment: Single- or three-wall courts, racquets, and balls

Number of players: 4 on each court

Test reference: II and V

Procedure: Racquetball is a fast-paced game using eye-hand coordination; it is easily learned by upper level elementary school children. The game may be played on a single-wall or three-wall court, 20 feet wide and 34 feet long, with the short line 16 feet from the wall and the service line 25 feet from the wall (Fig. 16-17). The game is started when one player serves the ball by dropping it in the service area and hitting it to the front wall first. The ball must rebound past the short line before the serve is legal. Two tries are allowed for each serve. Points are scored only by the serving player. The receiving player only wins the opportunity to serve. A game is 11 points. When doubles are played each team member has an opportunity to serve before the team loses the serve. Players serve until they lose a point.

Football activities

PUNT-PASS-KICK

Behavioral objective: To develop punting, passing, and kicking skills as lead-up skills to flag football

Developmental goal: Eye-hand and eye-foot coordination, object management, and strategy

Space and equipment: Football field and football

Number of players: 2 to 30

Test reference: II and IV

Procedure: The children divide into two teams and space themselves evenly on opposite ends of the field. The object of the game is to drive the opposing team back and to score by punting, passing, or kicking the ball over the opposing team's goal line without it being caught. The game is begun by one team kicking the ball from the 40-yard line. The ball is then played from the place where it is caught or first touched and by the person who catches or touches it. Passing the ball over the goal line counts one point, punting it over the goal line counts two points, and place kicking it over the goal line counts three points. This game is excellent for developing football skills (Fig. 16-18). To vary the game, the players can be given giant steps toward the opponents' goal for catching a ball—five for a punt, three for a place kick, and one for a pass. The players may save these steps and take them at any time during the game. This modification adds suspense and activity to the game, since the players take the steps prior to a kick in a attempt to catch the opponents off guard and move closer to scoring territory.

END ZONE BALL

Behavioral objective: To successfully throw a football to a teammate in the end zone

Developmental goal: Throwing and catching skills

Space and equipment: Basketball court with end zone marked in chalk and football

Number of players: 12 to 30

Test reference: II, IV, and V

Procedure: The players divide into two teams. Each team has four types of players: (1) quarterbacks, (2) ends, (3) defensive halfbacks, and (4) guards. Each team is assigned one half of the playing court to defend and one half in which to score touchdowns (Fig. 16-19). The game starts with a guard in possession of the football. The guard attempts to pass the football to one of the teammates in the field, either another guard or a quarterback. The player catching the ball must pass it from the spot where it was caught. The ball cannot be held for more then 5 seconds without being passed. Once the quarterbacks receive the ball they attempt to pass it for a touchdown to one of their ends who are assigned to play in the end zone. A touchdown counts as one point. Once a score is made the ball is put in play by a guard on the team who was scored against. A game consists of 11 points, or a time limit may be set. Rules that should be carefully enforced are:

1. Each player must stay in his or her assigned zone.
2. All passes for a score must be overhand forward passes, although players may pass laterally to other teammates.

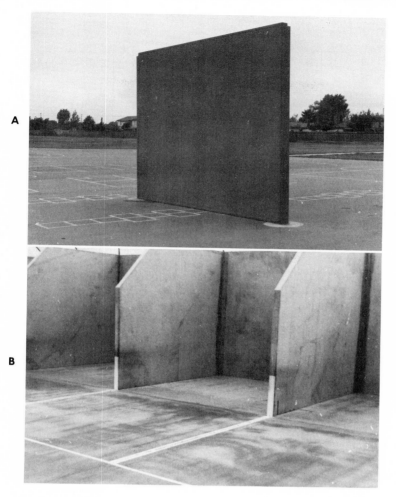

Fig. 16-17. A, Single-wall racquetball court. **B,** Three-wall racquetball court.

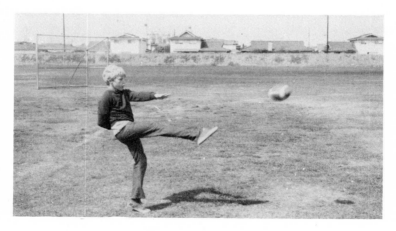

Fig. 16-18. Punting a football.

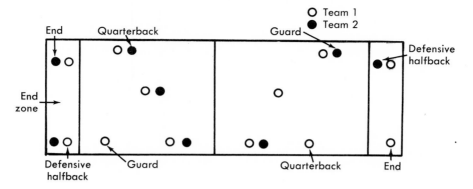

Fig. 16-19. End zone ball.

3. Any time a ball is dropped or goes out of bounds it is given to a player on the team opposite the team of the player who last touched it.
4. Players may attempt to block or intercept passes, but they cannot steal the ball.
5. When a rule is violated, the ball is given to the nearest member of the team that did not violate the rule to put into play.

The teacher should emphasize quick passing to keep the game moving and rotate players every three points or every 5 minutes. If one player is dominating the play, a rule can be made that the same player cannot pass for a touchdown twice in succession.

FLAG FOOTBALL

Behavioral objective: To execute passing, punting, running, receiving, and blocking skills in a game situation

Developmental goal: Large-muscle coordination, teamwork, and strategy

Space and equipment: Football field and football

Number of players: Two teams of 7 each

Test reference: II and V

Procedure: Each team tries to retain possession of the ball and advance it across the opposing team's goal line. The game involves most of the basic skills, strategies, and elements of team play found in American football but eliminates the hazards of blocking and tackling. The offensive team may advance the ball forward by running, passing, or kicking (Fig. 16-20). The center

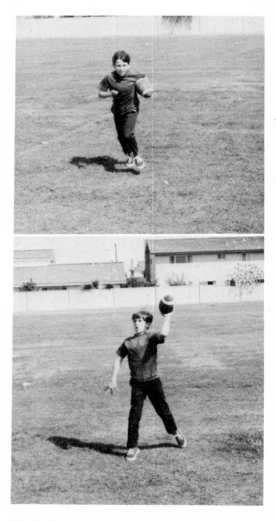

Fig. 16-20. Correct ball handling while running and passing.

must snap the ball backward to a teammate in the backfield before any other player may advance the ball beyond the line of scrimmage. The defensive team has the right to intercept passes and return kicks. Blocking of punts and recovering of fumbles are not allowed.

Formation: The game begins with a kickoff. The players of each team stand in their own half of the field with their backs toward their own goal until the ball is kicked. The players on each team are the left end, center, right end, left halfback, fullback, right halfback, and quarterback. The players of the receiving team may line up in any formation they wish, provided they form no group interference and are behind a line 20 yards away from where the ball is put into play. On scrimmage plays, the offensive team must have at least three players on the line of scrimmage and four or less players at least 1 yard behind the line of scrimmage when the ball is put into play. The defensive team is allowed to use any formation.

Rules of play: The game is started with a kickoff from any point on the 20-yard line. The ball may be place kicked or punted. It must travel at least 20 yards before it is in play. If the ball goes out of bounds between the goal lines without being in the possession and control of a player on the receiving team, it must be kicked over again.

The receiving team is allowed four downs, or tries, to advance the ball from the point of possession to, or beyond, the next first-down zone in the direction of the opposing team's goal. If in four downs this is not accomplished, the ball goes over to the opponents.

The offensive team may elect to kick the ball from the line of scrimmage rather than to run with it or pass it. This option is used by a team on the fourth down when they are not in scoring territory or on an earlier down as a surprise tactic.

If a kicked ball is muffed, fumbled, or touched, it is dead where it first touches the ground and is awarded to the receiving team at that spot.

Scoring: The scoring is the same as in football. A running play or forward pass play that results in the ball's being carried over the goal line is a touchdown and scores six points. The team scoring a touchdown may

receive an additional point by successfully carrying or passing the ball across the goal line from the 3-yard line. After each touchdown is made, the team that scored kicks off. A safety occurs when the ball carrier is tagged behind the team's own goal line. A safety scores 2 points. After a safety occurs, the ball is put into play by a place kick or punt from the 20-yard line by the team scored against.

Fouls and penalties: The fouls are tripping, clipping, body tackling, leaving the ground with the feet when blocking or pulling the flag, rough play, and unsportsman-like conduct. The team that is fouled is awarded 5 yards from the spot of the foul. The captain of the team who is fouled has the option of accepting or declining the yardage, the decision being governed by whether or not the yardage gained on the play is greater than that awarded because of the foul. It is also a foul for a player to be offside. The play is not called back until the ball is dead. A 5-yard penalty is assessed against the offending team from the position of the snap that put the ball into play. All fouls committed by the defensive team result in the down's becoming the first one for the opponents except for offside, in which case the down remains the same and a 5-yard penalty is assessed against the defensive team.

Playing terminology and rules

BLOCKING: Players on the offensive team may interpose their bodies between an opponent and the ball carrier. Players must have both feet on the ground while executing the block. They should hold their forearms against their chests when they make contact with a defensive player.

DEFENSIVE TEAM: The team that does not have the ball is the defensive team.

FLAGS: The flags are 18 inches long and 2 inches wide. Two flags are worn by all players and are located on each side of the waist.

FORWARD PASS: A pass made by the offensive team forward from any point behind the line of scrimmage is a forward pass. Any player of either team may receive or intercept a forward pass. Forward passes are allowed only on a scrimmage play. A forward pass caught by a player before the ball touches the ground is a completed pass. If a forward pass is not completed, the ball is put into play at the position of the previous down.

FUMBLE: Loss of possession of the ball after it has been received is a fumble. The ball is dead at the spot where it touches the ground and belongs to the team in possession of the ball when the fumble occurred.

HUDDLE: The group of players gathered together to call offensive and defensive plays is the huddle.

LINE OF SCRIMMAGE: An imaginary line extending across the field where the ball is to be put into play is the line of scrimmage.

OFFENSIVE TEAM: The team with the ball is the offensive team.

OFFSIDE: An infraction in which any part of a player's body is ahead of the near end of the ball when it is put into play is offside.

OUT OF BOUNDS: A ball is out of bounds when the ball carrier steps on or outside a sideline or when the ball hits the ground on or outside the sideline.

RUNNING PLAY: An attempt to carry the ball through or around the defensive team is a running play.

SAFETY: An action in which a player attempting to advance the ball is downed behind the team's goal line with the ball in his or her possession is a safety. The team scored against puts the ball into play by a free kick at the 20-yard line.

SNAP: The action of a center passing the ball between the legs to a player in the backfield is a snap.

TACKLING: An action in which the flag of the ball carrier is pulled and thrown to the ground is tackling. The ball is declared dead at the point where the flag was pulled. Pushing or striking the ball carrier is penalized as unnecessary roughness. The defensive player must make a direct attempt to pull the flag.

TOUCHBACK: An action in which a player who receives a ball behind the team's goal, with the impetus coming from the opponents, downs it in the end zone is a touchback. The ball is taken out to the 20-yard line, where the receiving team puts it into play.

USE OF HANDS: Defensive players may use their hands to protect themselves from offensive blockers and to get to the player with the ball. The use of their hands is restricted to touching the shoulders and body of attacking blockers. Offensive players may not use their hands in blocking defensive players.

Softball activities

THROW GOAL

Behavioral objective: To run all bases before the ball is thrown to the catcher

Developmental goal: Increase throwing accuracy and distance and quick base running

Space and equipment: Softball diamond and a softball

Number of players: 18 to 20

Test reference: II and IV

Procedure: The players divide into two teams. Team A is the fielding team; team B is the throwing team. Player B steps into the batter's box and throws the ball as far as possible. The team A fielder must get the ball and throw it home before player B gets there. Player B must run all the bases and is out when ball is held by the team A catcher (Fig. 16-21, A and B).

TEE SOFTBALL

Behavioral objective: To successfully strike a stationary ball

Developmental goal: To bat a ball for accuracy and distance, catch a fly ball, and field a ground ball

Space and equipment: Softball diamond, batting tee, softball, and bat

Number of players: 18 to 20

Test reference: II, IV

Procedure: The players divide into two teams. Team A is the fielding team; team B is the batting team. The batting tee is placed on home plate, and the first player on team B adjusts the tee to a desirable height. The batter calls "ready" and tries to hit the ball off the tee. If the batter misses the ball, a strike is called. If a fair ball is hit, bases are run as in regular softball. When team B has made three outs, the teams exchange places. So that all may have practice batting, each member of an entire team may have a turn before going out in the field.

SLO-PITCH SOFTBALL

Behavioral objective: To hit a pitched ball

Developmental goal: Striking and catching skills

Space and equipment: Softball diamond, a bat, and a ball

Number of players: 2 teams of 10 each

Test reference: II and IV

Procedure: The ball must be thrown to the batter so that the path of the pitch forms an arc between the pitcher and home plate. If it

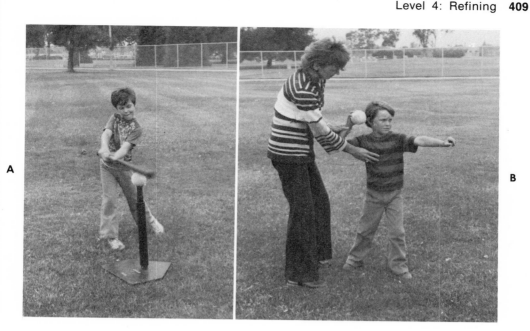

Fig. 16-21. Learning batting, **A**, and throwing, **B**, skills.

does not form an arc it is called a "ball." No bunting or chop hits are allowed. A base runner must maintain contact with the base until the ball has left the pitcher's hand. A base runner must be advanced by a hit by the batter.

LONG BALL

Behavioral objective: To develop throwing, running, catching, and batting skills as lead-up skills to softball

Developmental goal: Eye-hand coordination, object management, and teamwork

Space and equipment: Softball diamond, bats, softball, and catcher's mask

Number of players: 6 to 20

Test reference: II and IV

Procedure: The players divide into two teams, and the members are numbered. Each team elects a pitcher, catcher, and long baseman, or players may rotate to such positions with the change of innings; the remaining members of each team are fielders. The teams alternate as batters and fielders. A batting tee may be used instead of a pitcher for beginning players. Each member of the batting team tries to bat the ball and run to long base, which is a circle 5 yards past first base. A batter must continue to bat until the bat comes in contact with the ball. The contact may result in a foul tip, a foul ball, or a fair hit. The batter may not be put out on strikes.

The instant a batter contacts the ball, no matter how lightly and regardless of whether the ball is fair or foul, the batter must drop the bat and run to long base. If it is a fair hit, the base runners try to run back across the safety line at home plate before being put out by the fielding team; if it is a foul hit, the runners wait at long base until a succeeding batter makes a fair hit and then try to run to safety. The members of the fielding team move about as necessary, except for the long baseman, who remains near the long base. When runners are returning from long base, the fielders should go with them and be ready to receive a thrown ball so that they can tag out one or more runners before they can cross the safety line.

Foul ball: A ball that lands outside or behind one of the lines between home and first bases and home and third bases is a foul ball. When a batter hits a foul ball and reaches long base, he or she must remain there until a succeeding player of the team makes a fair hit.

Fair ball: A batted ball that lands inside the base lines is a fair ball. When a batter hits a fair ball, he or she should attempt to make a round trip to long base and back home across the safety line. At the same time, any players at long base should attempt to complete their run. To score a legal run, each runner must cross the safety line at some point between the two ends of the line without being tagged with the ball by a fielder who has it in his or her hand.

Outs: A team is out after each member has had a time at bat. Outs for individual players occur under the following conditions:

1. A fly ball hit by the player is caught.
2. A foul tip hit by the player is caught.
3. A runner is thrown out before reaching long base. Runners cannot be thrown out when trying to cross the safety line. They must be tagged with the ball by a fielder.
4. A runner going to long base or returning to the safety line is tagged with the ball by a fielder.
5. A runner at long base but not in contact with the base is tagged with the ball.
6. A batter throws the bat when starting for long base.

Scoring: Each time a runner reaches long base and on a fair hit returns successfully over the safety line, one point is scored. The team wins that has the higher number of points at the conclusion of the playing period.

WORK-UP

Behavioral objective: To execute the skills of batting, throwing, pitching, catching, and running in a game situation
Developmental goal: Eye-hand coordination, teamwork, and sportsmanship
Space and equipment: Softball diamond, bats, and softball
Number of players: 12 to 15
Test reference: II and V
Procedure: The children are numbered. Player 1 is the catcher; player 2, pitcher; player 3, first baseman; player 4, second baseman; and player 5, third baseman. Three players are batters, and the rest are fielders. The first batter hits a pitched ball and runs to first base or farther as in regular softball. The second batter then takes a turn at bat. Each batter continues at bat until put out as in softball and then takes the place of the last fielder, and all the players move up one position. A fielder who catches a fly ball may exchange places with the batter immediately. If all three batters are on the bases at one time, the first batter is put out and takes the last place in the field.

SOFTBALL

Behavioral objective: To execute the skills of throwing, catching, batting, and running in a game situation
Developmental goal: Object management, sportsmanship, and eye-hand coordination
Space and equipment: Softball diamond, softball, bats, and catcher's mask
Number of players: 18 to 20
Test reference: II and VII
Procedure: The players divide into two teams—one at bat and one in the field. The players on the fielding team take positions as indicated in Fig. 16-22. The members of the team at bat should stand or sit side by side behind the first-base line. No warm-up of the next batter is allowed unless a protected on-deck area is available. Play should not begin until the catcher has put on a protective mask. The pitcher throws the ball *underhand* to the batter, who tries to bat the ball and run to first base. The batter may take as many bases as safely possible or may stay at first and be advanced by the next batter. A runner may advance only one base on an overthrow at any base. No stealing or leading off bases is allowed. A run is scored when a runner successfully tags all three bases and home plate without being put out. After the team at bat makes three outs, the teams change positions. The game may be modified according to individual preferences, as follows:

1. Each batter is allowed only one to three pitches.
2. All the team members are permitted to bat before the positions are changed.
3. No fast pitching is allowed.
4. The batting team provides its own pitcher.

Outs: A runner is put out under the following conditions:

1. The ball the batter hit reaches first base before the batter does. (The batter does not have to be tagged.)
2. A fly ball hit by the batter is caught and held by a fielder.
3. The runner is tagged with the ball by a fielder when running to second, third, or home base.
4. The runner fails to return to the base before the ball does when a fly ball is caught.
5. The batter strikes and misses three times, or three strikes are called. Fouls

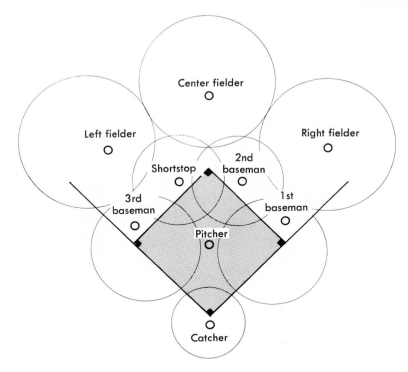

Fig. 16-22. Softball field positions.

count as strikes on the first two strikes.

6. For safety reasons, throwing of a bat constitutes an out for elementary school children.

Forced out play: If there is a runner on first base, if there are runners on first and second bases, or if the bases are loaded, the runner must advance to the next base when the next batter hits a fair ball. If a fly ball is hit and caught, a runner advancing a base must return and tag the base previously left before the ball is thrown to the base or an out occurs. On a fair hit in a force play, the base may be tagged instead of the runner.

TRACK AND FIELD

Track and field affords children opportunities to test their speed, endurance, and explosive power. However, boys and girls must be instructed in the need for adequate warm-up before participating in an all-out effort in any event. Children like to record their progress, and track and field events offer a perfect chance for this. Charts and graphs not only can be used as motivational aids but also can be shared with the parents and kept as mementos by the students.

Track and field activities

STARTING

Procedure: The start is an important phase of the sprint race. On the command, "Take your marks," the runner should back into the starting blocks and place the hands behind the starting line. When the runner hears the command, "Set," the hips should be raised slightly above shoulder height and the weight shifted forward. The head should be pointed straight ahead in a relaxed position (Fig. 16-23). On the command, "Go," one arm is thrust forward and the other back. Both legs push against the blocks simultaneously. As the back leg is brought forward for the first stride, the forward leg continues to drive. The body should be driven out of the blocks in a low forward and upward movement for 5 to 8 yards.

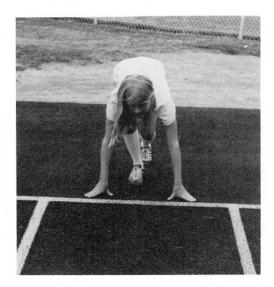

Fig. 16-23. Proper starting position.

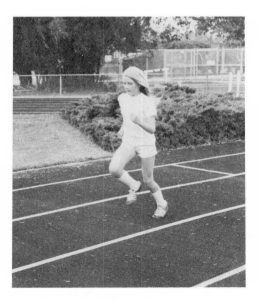

Fig. 16-24. Correct sprinting form, pushing off toes.

SPRINTING

Behavioral objective: To start quickly and run at top speed

Developmental goal: Explosive power and speed

Space and equipment: Running track and starting blocks

Number of players: Entire class

Test reference: IV and VI

Procedure: Sprinting is running high on the toes and driving for maximum speed with the body leaning forward. The knees should be lifted high and the arms bent at approximately a 90 degree angle (Fig. 16-24). All arm and leg movements should be parallel to the running direction. Lateral arm or leg movements will tend to interfere with maximum speed. The eyes should be focused on the track about 10 yards in front of the runner.

DISTANCE RUNNING

Behavioral objective: To be able to run continuously over long distances

Developmental goal: Cardiovascular fitness

Space and equipment: Running track

Number of players: Entire class

Test reference: IV

Procedure: The distance runner runs lower on the balls of the feet than the sprinter, drops down on the heel, and then pushes off with the toes. This more relaxed action enables a runner to develop a rhythm that can be maintained over long periods of time. Distance runners have a lower knee action than sprinters, with a greater variety of individual styles. The most important phase of distance running is comfort and relaxation.

HIGH JUMP

Behavioral objective: To jump as high as possible over the cross bar

Developmental goal: Explosive power

Space and equipment: High jump pit and cross bar

Number of players: Entire class

Test reference: IV

Procedure: High jump styles are determined by the approach and the position of the body as it passes over the bar. The common styles are the scissors, straddle, and flop. Most elementary children will use the scissors because it is easily learned. However, it limits the maximum height potential. Regardless of the style used, the jumper must have a smooth approach with an emphasis on acceleration rather than speed. The forward motion must be converted into an explosive vertical jump (Fig. 16-25). The takeoff point is determined by the distance needed for a runner to reach the highest point directly over the bar. This point is approximately an arm's length from the bar. Jumpers should practice and mark the correct starting and takeoff points for maximum results.

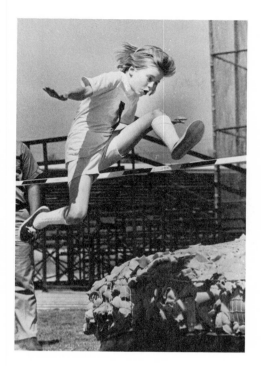

Fig. 16-25. High jump. (Courtesy Jim McCormick.)

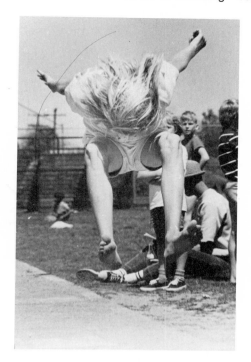

Fig. 16-26. Stretching for distance in the long jump. (Courtesy Jim McCormick.)

LONG JUMP

Behavioral objective: To jump as far as possible

Developmental goal: Explosive power and speed

Space and equipment: Long jump pit and runway

Number of players: Entire class

Test reference: IV

Procedure: The long jumper must combine speed with explosive power. The takeoff foot should hit the board with the heel touching slightly before the ball of the foot. The knee is bent and the toe pointed straight ahead. For maximum height, the center of gravity should be directly over the foot at the time of the jump. As the take-off leg is extended, the free leg is raised along with the arms and head. At the point of landing, the legs are extended forward for maximum distance (Fig. 16-26).

WEIGHT TRAINING

Many upper-grade elementary school children can feel the exhilaration result-ing from participation in a weight training program. Boys and girls should start with weights that can be handled with ease without placing undue strain on any part of the body. Many exercises can be conducted with homemade weights such as plastic bottles filled with sand. For those children to whom regular barbells are available for exercise programs, the following starting guidelines are suggested:

1. Press approximately one fourth of your body weight.
2. Curl 10 pounds less than you press.
3. Bench press one fourth of your body weight plus 10 pounds.
4. Squat one half of your body weight.

Begin with five repetitions of exercises for the arm and shoulders and ten repetitions for the back and legs. Weight can be increased commensurate with strength, development, and equipment control. Good posture should be maintained throughout all exercises and spotters used for all heavy weights (Fig. 16-27).

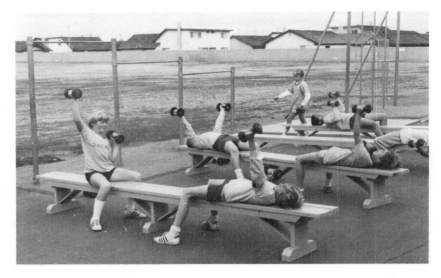

Fig. 16-27. Sixth-grade students participating in weight training unit.

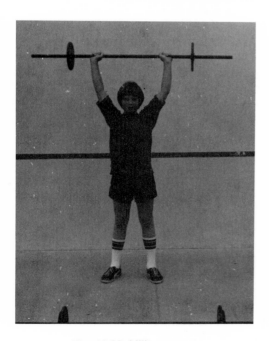

Fig. 16-28. Military press.

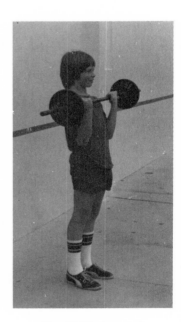

Fig. 16-29. Arm curl.

MILITARY PRESS

Behavioral objective: To lift weight overhead successfully

Developmental goal: Upper body strength

Space and equipment: Weight room and barbells

Number of players: Entire class

Test reference: VII

Procedure: When executing the military press, the child lifts the barbell to the chest, pushes it to the full extension of the arm overhead, and then lowers it back to the chest (Fig. 16-28). As the barbell passes the head, the child should maintain good balance, keeping the center of gravity over the feet. The barbell should be grasped slightly wider than shoulder width with the thumbs around the bar. The military press is a good shoulder and upper back developer.

ARM CURL

Behavioral objective: To lift barbell

Developmental goal: Upper body strength

Space and equipment: Weight room and barbells

Number of players: Entire class

Test reference: VII

Procedure: The child grasps the bar with the hands approximately a shoulder's width apart and the palms facing forward, keeps the elbows close to the side, brings the barbell up to the chest, and then lowers it back to the starting position (Fig. 16-29). When executing the curl, the child should keep the back straight, avoiding swaying or bending backward. The curl develops the biceps arm muscles.

HALF SQUAT

Behavioral objective: To support extra weight when executing a half squat

Developmental goal: Leg strength and balance

Space and equipment: Weight room and barbells

Number of players: Entire class

Test reference: IV and VI

Procedure: The bar should be gripped with the hands slightly wider apart than the shoulders and brought up to the chest as in preparation for the military press. With the bar in this position, the child straightens the arms and lifts the barbell over the head, lowering it to rest on the shoulders behind the head. From this position, the child should execute a half squat, keeping the heels flat on the ground, and then return to the normal standing position (Fig. 16-30). The back should be kept straight throughout the exercise. This exercise develops the upper leg muscles.

HEEL RAISE

Behavioral objective: To raise heels off ground carrying extra weight

Developmental goal: Lower leg strength

Space and equipment: Weight room and barbells

Number of players: Entire class

Test reference: IV and VI

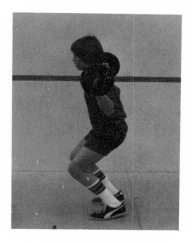

Fig. 16-30. Half squat.

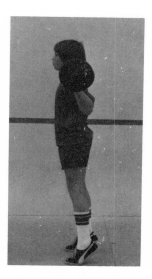

Fig. 16-31. Heel raise.

Procedure: To begin the heel raise, the child places the barbell on the back of the shoulders in the same manner as in the half squat. With the barbell in this position, the child raises the heels as far off the ground as possible and then returns them to the flat position (Fig. 16-31). The heel raise develops the lower leg muscles.

BENCH PRESS

Behavioral objective: To lift weight with arms while in supine position

Developmental goal: Upper body strength

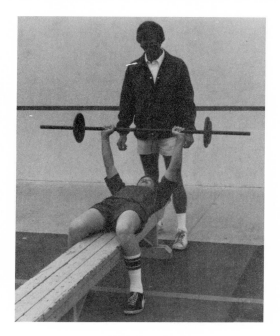

Fig. 16-32. Bench press.

Space and equipment: Weight room and barbells with bench

Number of players: Entire class

Test reference: VII

Procedure: Gripping the bar slightly wider than shoulder width, the child lies back on the bench with the barbell at chest level. The barbell is pushed to arms' length and then returned to the chest (Fig. 16-32). This exercise is best accomplished with a bench designed to support the barbell prior to the exercise.

AEROBIC DANCE

Another fitness activity that develops rhythm and fitness is aerobic dance. The word "aerobic" refers to the ability of a given activity to train and strengthen the heart, lungs, and vascular system. Aerobic dances can be choreographed to contain predetermined amounts of simple, vigorous dance steps to improve aerobic capacity, stretching and other movements to improve flexibility, and muscle toning movements to increase strength. Movements, such as running, rocking, hopping, and jumping, in various rhythms can be developed specifically for aerobic dancing.

Aerobic dance is fun and can be choreographed to be simple enough for the elementary child. Aerobic dancing is built on the principle of continuous rhythmical movement and its goal is fun and fitness. Fitness programs are more enjoyable when fun, variety, and novelty encourage development of cardiovascular endurance. The activity is most satisfying when teachers and children create their own routines. The following aerobic dance is designed for elementary children and was choreographed by Jacki Sorensen for the President's Council for Physical Fitness and Sport.

JOY TO THE WORLD

On formation: Even number of squads

Music: "Joy to the World" from the album *Class of '71*, Floyd Cramer, RCA Victor, LSP 4590 Stereo

Procedure

Introduction: 2 counts of 8
1. Knee lifts (can be hopping)—doubles; 4 fast singles
   Jumping Jacks—4 fast (can be in circle right)
   Knee lifts—4 fast singles
2. Jog in place—8.
3. *Chorus:*
   Run 4 into one line from two.
   Run 4 in a circle to the right.
   Run 4 crossing lines.
   Run 4 in a circle to the right.
   Break 4, moving backward into one line again.
   Run backward—8, ending facing forward in two lines.
4. *Repeat:*
   Repeat combination 1 as written.
   Repeat Chorus as written.
   Repeat combination 1 as written.
   Jog in place—8.
   Repeat Chorus as written.
5. Jump forward-bounce, jump back—2.
   Hop 8 on right foot in a circle to the right.
   Jump forward-bounce, jump back—2.
   Hop 8 on left foot in a circle to the left.
6. *Repeat:*
   Repeat Chorus as written.

Fitness contract

1. Name_____ Age_____ Sex_____

2. Strength fitness category:___0. Beginner ____III. Fair ____VI. Excellent

   ___I. Very poor ____ IV. Good

   ___II. Poor   ____ V. Very good

3. Body measurements: Weight_____ Waist_____   Chest_____

   Hips_____ Biceps: Right_____ Left_____

   Calf: Right_____ Left_____

4. Heart rate resting_____

5. Selected program: Weight training_____

   Cardiovascular_____

   Flexibility_____

6. Number of weeks for program_____

7. Individual goal_____

   _____

Student signature:_____

Contract approval date:_____ Approved by:_____

Reassessment check date:_____ Approved by:_____

Contract completion date:_____ Approved by:_____

Fig. 16-33. Sample fitness contract.

Repeat combination 5 as written.
Repeat Chorus, freezing on the seventh run backward.

FITNESS GAMES

Many traditional games can be modified to increase the fitness requirements. In touch football there can be multiple forward passes in which the ball is in play until a pass is dropped. In softball each batter can be required to run the bases whether he or she gets a hit or not before returning to the bench. Volleyball rotation can include a run around the court before changing positions. Push-ups, side straddle hops, and other exercises can be a part of any lull in the action of a number of games.

Teachers should create their own fitness games or variations to ensure adequate endurance challenges. Old fashioned games like tug of war and activities like log tosses can be incorporated into special events for fun and fitness.

FITNESS ACTIVITIES

Fitness activities for level 4 are similar to those for level 3, but with increased distances and more difficult challenges. Level 4 children are also ready to develop individual fitness programs in which goals are personalized to meet specific needs. Many children enjoy contracting for individual goals and are ready to accept the responsibility of self-motivation. A sample fitness contract is shown in Fig. 16-33. Refer to Chapter 10 for specific exercises.

Parcourse

Many children at this level enjoy distance running and conditioning exercises. The parcours system developed in Switzerland and mentioned in Chapter 15 is an excellent activity. The first course was opened in Zurich in 1968, and at last count, there were nearly 200 courses in Switzerland. Tourists from other countries have spread the idea, and the activity is becoming popular throughout Europe and the United States. In the United States the term has been changed to Parcourse. The Parcourse is usually a 1-mile jogging trail designed to blend into the natural contour of the area. The course is not designed solely for jogging; spotted along the way are a variety of exercise "stations" at which participants bend, stretch, and do push-ups, chin-ups, or other routines. The first stations consist of easy warm-up exercises, such as toe touching, arm circling, and torso stretching. The exercises in the middle section of the course are more strenuous, consisting of such activities as side vaults on bars, body circles on rings, and pull-ups. The last part of the course consists predominantly of relaxation exercises.

Instructions appear on the plaque located at each station, explaining the exercises and indicating the par (Fig. 16-34). The par, the number of times a person should repeat the exercise, varies according to the fitness level a person

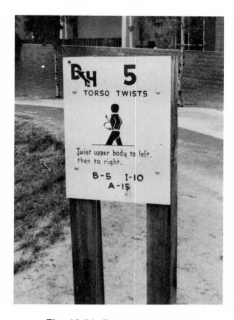

Fig. 16-34. Parcourse station.

wants to achieve—beginning, intermediate, or advanced. The value of the parcourse rests in the fitness benefits that can be derived and enjoyment of its natural environment. Business people, children, and senior citizens all can make use of the course at their own time and pace.

Sample Parcourse. The following course is suggested as a guide. Each school is encouraged to develop its own course in line with accepted principles of health and fitness.

Par levels:
B = Beginning
I = Intermediate
A = Advanced

Total distance: 1 mile
Number of stations: 18
Description of exercises and par repetitions

Station 1—Standing alternate toe touch

From a standing position with feet apart and arms out, bend down, keeping legs straight, and touch right hand to left toe. Alternate. B—5 I—10 A—15

Station 2—Up and back arm swings

From a standing position, swing both arms forward and up then down and back again. B—5 I—8 A—12

Station 3—360 degree waistline circles

From a standing position with hands on hips, bend forward at the waist and then move the upper body in a circular manner to the side, back, other side, and front. B—5 I—8 A—12

Station 4—Step ups

Step up with right foot and then left foot; step down with right foot and then left foot. Alternate. B—5 I—10 A—15

Station 5—Torso twist

Standing with hands on hips, twist upper body to the left and then to the right. B—5 I—10 A—15

Station 6—Log hops (Apparatus is used.)

Standing with feet together and with log to your right, jump over the log, keeping feet together. Alternate back and forth. B—5 I—10 A—15

Station 7—Arm circles

Standing with arms to your side, swing arms in a large circle alternating forward and backward directions. B—5 I—10 A—15

Station 8—Side vault on bars (Apparatus is used.)

Side vault over bar and crouch underneath to return. B—5 I—8 A—12

Station 9—Body circles on rings (Apparatus is used.)

With legs together hang from rings with toes barely touching the ground; form circles with your lower body, keeping your upper body still. B—5 I—8 A—12

Station 10—Sit-ups (Apparatus is used.)

Assume sitting position with knees bent and toes hooked under log; lie down, lock hands behind head; sit up until elbows touch knees; and return to back-lying position. B—8 I—12 A—15

Station 11—Pull-ups (Apparatus is used.)

With an overhand grip, hold bar and pull body up till chin is over bar and return to hanging position. Keep feet off ground throughout pull-ups. B—5 I—8 A—12

Station 12—Waist side-stretch

With arms at side, bend to the left at waist, moving left hand down leg; swing right arm over head to left side. Alternate. B—5 I—12 A—15

Station 13—Lying on side leg lifts

Lying on side with legs straight, lift top leg up, and lower again. Repeat on other side. B—8 I—12 A—15

Station 14—Standing knee lifts

In a standing position, bring right knee to chest and grasp knee with clasped hands. Repeat with other knee. B—8 I—12 A—15

Station 15—Elbow-knee sit-ups

Lying down with legs straight, clasp hands behind head, sit up, bring up left knee, and twist torso, enabling right elbow to touch left knee. Return to starting position and repeat with left elbow and right knee. B—5   I—10   A—15

Station 16—Shoulder bridge

Lying on back with knees bent, lift hips off ground until body is straight. B—8 I—12   A—15

Station 17—Push-ups (Apparatus is used.)

Assume push-up position with back straight and hands under shoulders. Beginning position: feet on ground and hands on log. Intermediate position: hands and feet on ground. Advanced position: feet on log and hands on ground. B—10   I—10   A—10

Station 18—Lying leg cross

Lying on back with arms out and legs straight, alternately raise legs straight up and swing them across body. B—5   I—10 A—15

FITNESS CLUBS

Elementary schools should develop fitness clubs that include activities such as jogging, hiking, biking, and rowing. The clubs may be general in nature, including a variety of activities or specific exercise groups. In order for children to become involved in fitness clubs, it is important that emphasis be placed on participation rather than competition. Although many children enjoy highly competitive activities, the purpose of the club would be to encourage as many as possible to become involved in some type of fitness activity.

A sample organizational structure would include a steering committee, involving boys and girls, usually with a teacher as an advisor. This steering committee would oversee any specialized fitness groups and could plan a number of fitness activities throughout the year. Allowing young children to have a voice in planning and organizing fitness activities gives leadership opportunities and responsibilities to a greater number of individuals. Award patches can be given for a 100 or 200 mile achievement, T-shirts can be sold to promote physical fitness activity, and the club in general

can become involved in fund raising by way of bake sales and other means to purchase equipment for the school. All students enjoy the values and benefits of belonging to a group, and one soon learns that fitness clubs attract students who are at varying levels of fitness.

Some activities that could be sponsored by the fitness club would be a "run-for-fun" day, encouraging everyone to come out and walk or run without any pressure of winning, or a "run-for-health" family activity that would involve children, teachers, and parents, all working together toward a common goal of better fitness.

Fitness clubs can do much to promote healthful activity and give recognition to outstanding performances by posting distances attained for all to view. Individuals will also have an opportunity to follow their progression in total miles jogged, bicycle miles ridden, or number of miles hiked. If conducted properly, fitness clubs will enjoy large enrollments and do much to promote unity and friendship throughout the school and community.

GYMNASTICS

Level 4 children have the strength and coordination necessary to successfully learn gymnastic routines. Determining which movements will follow each other tests the cognitive ability of each child as well as physical performance. Gymnastic activities are excellent for teaching posture, poise, and dedication to perfection. The challenge of gymnastics is exemplified by the many organized youth clubs throughout the nation. Being able to control the body in a variety of positions and in airborne activities does much to build not only a strong body but also a positive self-concept.

Spotting

Spotting serves primarily as a safety device but can be used to aid in teaching and to overcome the fear of some children. As a safety device, spotting is concerned with catching or supporting the performer or adjusting the performer's position to prevent a hard fall. In teaching, spotting is manual manipulation and aid to the performer in doing the stunt. Spotting hints are:

1. Remember that protection of the performer is the primary consideration.
2. Always be ready to move instantly.
3. Stand close to the performer, but do not interfere with the stunt.
4. When a performer falls, you may be able to check the fall by adjusting the head and shoulders so that the performer will land on the feet. The support should be near the head and shoulders.
5. Always know which stunt the performer is going to attempt, and determine the danger points.
6. Display confidence in yourself and instill confidence in the performer. Be aware of signs of fear and give special encouragement and help.
7. Don't divert your attention while the performer is attempting a stunt.

8. Always insist on a spotter before a child uses any equipment.

• • •

The following stunts can be put together to create routines in each gymnastic activity.

GYMNASTIC STUNTS

Behavioral objective: To execute controlled body movements utilizing strength, balance, and flexibility
Developmental goal: Coordination and activity routine development
Space and equipment: Gymnastic room, mats, and equipment
Number of players: Entire class
Test reference: III, VI, and VII

Tumbling stunts

FRONT ROLL (Fig. 16-35). Stay in a ball until on your feet.

BACKWARD ROLL (Fig 16-36). Push down with your hands to raise head from the floor.

HEADSTAND (Fig. 16-37). Form triangle with hands and head.

CARTWHEEL (Fig. 16-38). Stay in straight line with hands and feet.

NECK SPRING (Fig. 16-39). Push with hands while kicking feet up, out, and down.

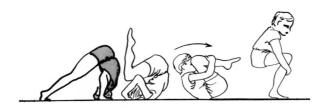

Fig. 16-35. Front roll.

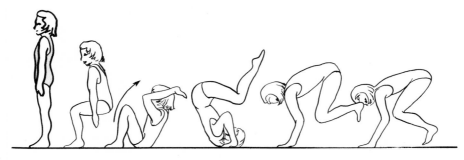

Fig. 16-36. Backward roll.

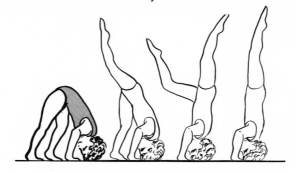

Fig. 16-37. Headstand.

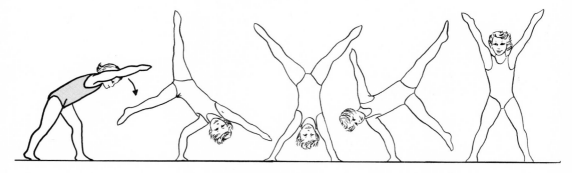

Fig. 16-38. Cartwheel.

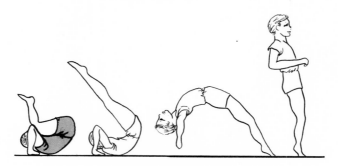

Fig. 16-39. Neck spring.

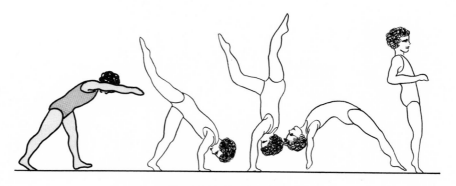

Fig. 16-40. Hand spring.

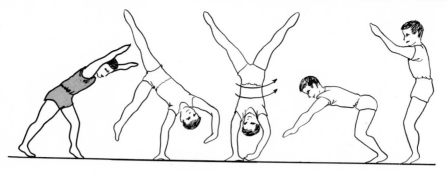

Fig. 16-41. Round-off.

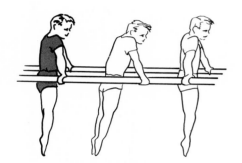

Fig. 16-42. Walk, travel.

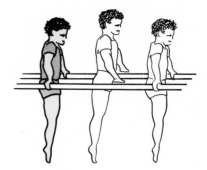

Fig. 16-43. Hop, travel.

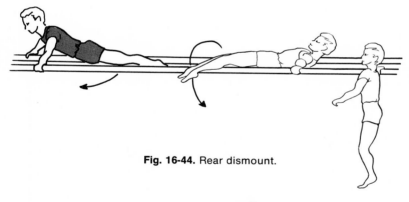

Fig. 16-44. Rear dismount.

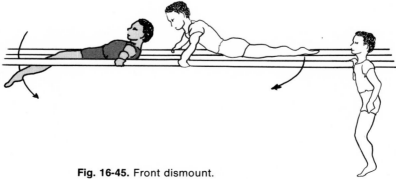

Fig. 16-45. Front dismount.

HAND SPRING (Fig. 16-40). Keep arms straight and head back.

ROUND-OFF (Fig. 16-41). Snap down, raising hands before feet land.

Parallel bars

WALK, TRAVEL (Fig. 16-42). Take small steps with hands.

HOP, TRAVEL (Fig. 16-43). Start with slight elbow bend and shoulder shrug.

REAR DISMOUNT (Fig. 16-44). Move sideways on front end of swing.

FRONT DISMOUNT (Fig. 16-45). Move sideways on rear end of swing.

SHOULDER STAND (Fig. 16-46). Keep elbows out, and stretch tall.

SCISSORS MOUNT (Fig. 16-47). Support left leg on right bar and right leg on left bar.

FORWARD ROLL (Fig. 16-48). Keep elbows out; shift hands quickly.

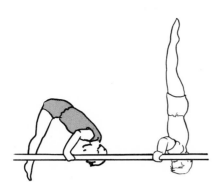

Fig. 16-46. Shoulder stand.

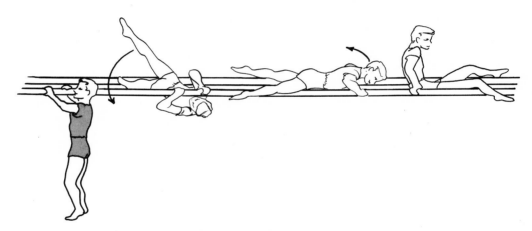

Fig. 16-47. Scissors mount.

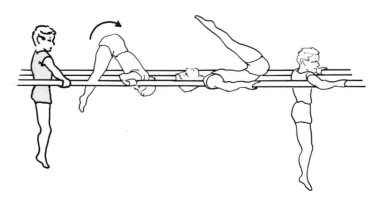

Fig. 16-48. Forward roll.

LAZY MAN'S KIP (Fig. 16-49). Push with feet to straight arm support.

END OF BAR KIP (Fig. 16-50). Initiate kick at rear end of swing.

Horizontal bar

SKIN THE CAT (Fig. 16-51). Bring legs overhead and under bar.

MONKEY HANG (Fig. 16-52). Skin the cat, release one hand, and turn.

PULL OVER (Fig. 16-53). Chin, and pull legs over bar.

SINGLE KNEE CIRCLE (Fig. 16-54). Lean backward, and throw head back as straight leg moves forward.

FORWARD CROTCH CIRCLE (Fig. 16-55). Reverse grip, take giant forward step to gain momentum.

BACKWARD HIP CIRCLE (Fig. 16-56). Swing leg up and back. Lean backward as body returns to bar.

KIP-UP (Fig. 16-57). Bring toes to bar, and kick up and out.

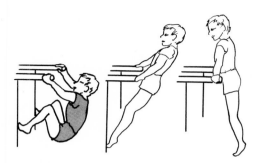

Fig. 16-49. Lazy man's kip.

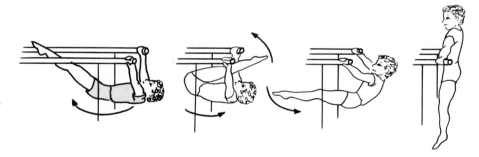

Fig. 16-50. End of bar kip.

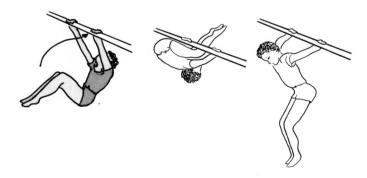

Fig. 16-51. Skin the cat.

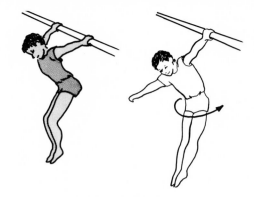

Fig. 16-52. Monkey hang.

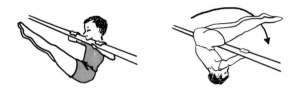

Fig. 16-53. Pull over.

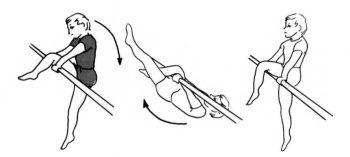

Fig. 16-54. Single knee circle.

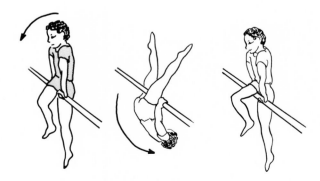

Fig. 16-55. Forward crotch circle.

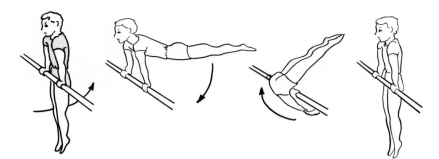

Fig. 16-56. Backward hip circle.

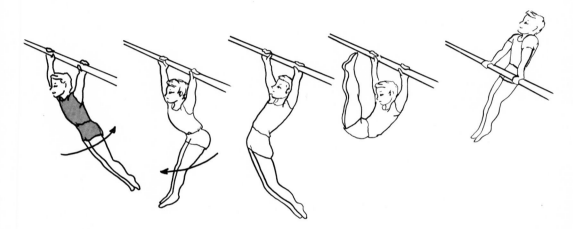

Fig. 16-57. Kip-up.

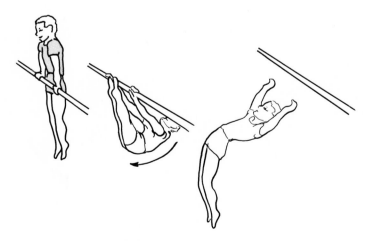

Fig. 16-58. Short underswing dismount.

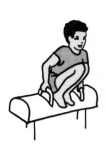

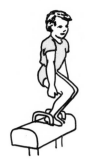

Fig. 16-59. Squat mount, jump dismount.

Fig. 16-60. Squat vault.

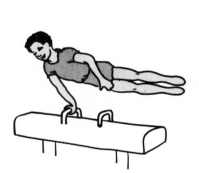

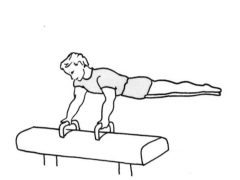

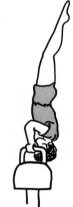

Fig. 16-61. Side vault.

Fig. 16-62. Front vault.

Fig. 16-63. Head spring.

SHORT UNDERSWING DISMOUNT (Fig. 16-58). Bring feet to bar, and cast up and out.

Side horse

SQUAT MOUNT, JUMP DISMOUNT (Fig. 16-59). Coordinate strong arm push with leg spring.

SQUAT VAULT (Fig. 16-60). Lift knees high to dismount.

SIDE VAULT (Fig. 16-61). Swing legs to side, keeping opposite supporting arm straight.

FRONT VAULT (Fig. 16-62). Vault with stomach facing horse, make quarter body turn.

HEAD SPRING (Fig. 16-63). Move to arched position after passing over the horse.

DANCE

Children in the upper elementary grades are ready to perform more complicated dance steps and enjoy the chal-

lenge of intricate rhythmical patterns. Participation in folk and square dance enhances the social objective of physical education. In some situations, children are ready to learn social dance in the form of contemporary dance steps appropriate to the time period and geographical location.

The square dances presented in Chapter 15 may also be applicable for level 4 children. If the children have had little exposure to simple square dance steps before reaching the fourth grade, it would be better to begin at the lower skill level. The primary difference between the levels is the ability of the children in level 4 to accomplish more sophisticated dance steps and routines.

Rather than separate dance steps and dance formations by level, we have elected to place them together in Chapter 15 for ease of reference (see pp. 388). See the record section at the end of this chapter for additional suggestions.

ROAD TO THE ISLES

Formation: Couples form a double circle facing counterclockwise in varsovienne position.
Music: Imperial 1005
Procedure: The dance has two parts, the second of which uses the schottische step.

Part 1

MEASURE 1: All the children point left toe forward slightly to the left and hold.

MEASURES 2-3: They take three steps, starting with the left foot, as follows: they place left foot slightly in back of the right foot on beat one, right foot to the right on beat two, and left foot forward in front of the right foot and hold on beats three and four.

MEASURE 4: They point right toe forward and slightly to the right and hold.

MEASURES 5-6: They take three steps, starting with the right foot, as follows: they place right foot slightly in back of the left foot on beat one, left foot to the left on beat two, and right foot forward in front of the left and hold on beats three and four.

MEASURE 7: They point left toe forward and hold.

MEASURE 8: They place left toe backward and hold.

Part 2

MEASURES 9-10: They all schottische forward slightly to the left, beginning with the left foot.

MEASURES 11-12: They schottische forward slightly to the right, beginning with the right foot. Then they hop on beat two of measure 12 and turn to the right and face the opposite direction, keeping their hands joined.

MEASURES 13-14: They schottische, beginning with the left foot. Then they hop and turn to the left and face the original direction

MEASURES 15-16: They step in place right, left, right, and hold.

PATTY CAKE POLKA

Formation: The children form a double circle, with the boys in the inside circle. Partners face each other and join hands.

Music: MGM S-4473 and Folkraft 1124
Procedure

MEASURES 1-2: The children perform the heel-and-toe twice, the boy starting with his left foot and the girl with her right foot.

MEASURES 3-4: They perform four slides counterclockwise.

MEASURES 5-8: They repeat measure 1-4 going clockwise, the boy starting with his right foot and the girl with her left foot.

MEASURE 9: They clap right hands with their partners three times.

MEASURE 10: They clap left hands with their partners three times.

MEASURE 11: They clap both hands with their partners three times.

MEASURE 12: They slap their own knees three times.

MEASURES 13-14: They swing their partners around once with their right elbows.

MEASURES 15-16: They walk to the left to new partners.

They repeat the dance with new partners.

CRESTED HEN

Formation: The children form sets composed of a boy and two girls, with the boy in the middle, or a girl and two boys. The sets are scattered about the room.
Music: RCA Victor LPM-1624 and 45-6176
Procedure

Figure 1

MEASURES 1-8: The children in each set join hands in a circle. Starting with a stamp of the foot, they move to their left, using a fast step-hop.

MEASURES 1-8, REPEATED: With a high jump, they reverse their direction and move to their right.

Figure 2

Throughout this figure, all the children perform the step-hop continuously. The girls release their hands from each other and dance on each side of the boy. They place their free hands on their hips.

MEASURES 9-10: The girl on the right step-hops under the arch formed by the boy and the girl on his left.

MEASURES 11-12: The boy then turns and step-hops under his own right arm.

MEASURES 13-14: The girl on the left step-hops under the arch made by the boy and the girl on his right.

MEASURES 15-16: The boy then turns under his own left arm.

They repeat measure 9-16 of figure 2. Then the entire pattern is repeated as often as desired.

LA RASPA

Formation: The children form couples and face in opposite directions, left shoulder to left shoulder. The boy puts his left hand in the girl's right hand in front of her chest, and his right hand in the girl's left hand in front of his chest.

Music: RCA Victor LPM-1623, 20-3189, and LPM-1072; Imperial 12207; and Monitor 82000

Procedure

Part 1

MEASURE 1: Both partners slide right foot forward and left foot back on beat one and slide foot forward and right foot back on beat two.

MEASURE 2: They both slide right foot forward and slide left foot back on beat one and hold on beat two.

MEASURES 3-4: They repeat measures 1-2, sliding left foot forward first.

MEASURES 5-8: Keeping their hands joined, they turn toward their partners and face in the opposite direction, right shoulder to right shoulder, and they repeat measures 1-4.

MEASURES 9-16: They repeat measures 1-8.

Part 2

MEASURES 1-4: With right elbows hooked and left hands held high, partners turn with eight running steps (two to a measure).

MEASURES 5-8: Reversing direction, with left elbows linked, the partners turn with eight running steps, clapping hands on measure 8.

MEASURES 9-12: Reversing direction again, the partners repeat the running steps. It is characteristic of this step to continue running without pause on changes of direction.

HEEL-AND-TOE POLKA

Formation: Couples are arranged informally around the room. Partners stand side by side with their inside hands joined, with the girl on the right of her partner. The couples face to the right around the room.

Music: Folkraft 1166 and MacGregor 4005 (45) and 400 (78)

Procedure

MEASURES 1-2: The children perform the heel-and-toe and then step, slide, step, starting with the outside foot.

MEASURES 3-4: They perform the heel-and-toe and then step, slide, step, starting with the inside foot.

MEASURES 5-8: They repeat measures 1-4.

MEASURES 9-16: They perform eight polka steps around the room, the partners facing each other on one polka step and turning away on the next polka step, alternately.

ACE OF DIAMONDS

Formation: The children form a double circle, with the boys in the inside circle, and face their partners.

Music: Folkraft 1176 and RCA Victor 41-6169 and LPM-1622

Procedure

MEASURES 1-8: The children clap their hands, stamp their right feet, and join their partners in right-elbow swings for six skips.

MEASURES 9-16: They clap their hands, stamp their left feet, and join their partners in left-elbow swings for six skips.

MEASURES 17-24: They perform two change-steps: they hop on the left foot, placing the right foot forward, and then hop on the right foot, placing the left foot forward. They do four more change-steps rapidly. Then they repeat the two slow and four fast change-steps.

MEASURES 25-32: The partners do the polka step around the room side by side, facing each other and then turning away from each other, or in closed dance position.

VARSOVIENNE

Formation: The children take the varsovienne position, with the boy slightly behind and to the left of the girl. The partners hold their hands high, right hand in right hand, left hand in left hand. The boy places his right arm behind the girl's shoulder. The waltz position may be used, with both partners moving sideward.

Music: Windsor 7516, Folkraft 1034, and MacGregor CPM 10-398-3

Procedure

Part 1

MEASURES 1-4: Both partners start with the left foot and perform the steps as follows: slide left foot to the left, close right foot to the left, raise left foot (swing foot out and in over supporting foot in a "cut step"); slide left foot to the left, close right foot to the left, and raise left foot; slide left foot to the left, close right foot to the left, and step with the left foot; and then turn and point right foot to the right side. They make a half turn on the last step.

MEASURES 5-8: They repeat measures 1-4, both moving to the right.

Part 2

MEASURES 9-10: Starting with the left foot raised to the left side, both partners make a half turn with the following steps: swing left foot over the right supporting foot, slide it left, close right foot to the left, step with the left foot, and point right foot and hold.

MEASURES 11-12: They repeat measures 9-10, starting with the right foot and moving back into position.

MEASURES 13-16: They repeat measures 9-12.

COTTON-EYED JOE

Formation: The children form a double circle, with the boys in the inside circle. They use the elbow grasp or social dancing position.
Music: RCA Victor LPM-1621 and EPA-4134
Procedure

MEASURE 1: The boy starts with his left foot and the girl with her right foot. They both take one heel-and-toe and three steps (the boy: left, right, left; the girl: right, left, right).

MEASURE 2: They repeat measure 1, the boy starting with the right foot and the girl starting with the left foot. (Many groups dance this step in the following manner: toe, toe, step together, step to side, and repeat to other side.)

MEASURES 3-4: Turning away from their partners, the boy to his left and the girl to her right, each takes four polka steps alone in a small circle. They end facing each other.

MEASURES 5-6: While facing each other, the partners take four push-steps counterclockwise and four back to place. The push-step is done as follows: the boy steps sideways on his left foot and then pushes away from the left foot with his right foot; then he takes another step sideways and gives a push with the right foot. The girl does the same, starting with her right foot.

MEASURES 7-8: In the elbow grasp or social dancing position, the partners take four polka steps in line of direction.

RYE WALTZ

Formation: Partners take the social dancing position or elbow grasp position.
Music: Folkraft 1103, Imperial 1044, MacGregor CPM 10-399-2, and Decca DLA 1420 (25058)
Procedure

MEASURE 1: The boy extends his left foot to the side and touches his toe to the floor on beat one, brings his left foot just behind his right heel and touches the floor with his toe on beat two, touches his left toe to the side again on beat three, and touches his left toe in front of his right toe on beat four. The girl does the same step simultaneously, with the right foot.

MEASURE 2: The partners take four slides to the boy's left.

MEASURES 3-4: They repeat measures 1 and 2, the boy starting with the right foot and the girl with the left foot and sliding to the boy's right.

MEASURES 5-8: They repeat measures 1-4.

MEASURES 9-24: They waltz around the room, moving counterclockwise.

LITTLE MAN IN A FIX

Formation: Two couples dancing together form a set. The boys hook left elbows, so that they will face in opposite directions. Their partners stand beside them. Each boy places his right arm around his partner's waist; each girl places her left hand on her partner's right shoulder and her right hand on her hip.
Music: RCA Victor 20449
Procedure

MEASURES 1-8: In the above position, the members of each set run forward in a circle, using small steps. The girls may have to lean backward if the tempo becomes too fast.

MEASURES 1-8, REPEATED: Without pausing in their run, the players begin to spread apart until the boys have their left hands joined and at the same time have their partner's left hand in their right hand. Simultaneously, the girls increase their speed and run under the boys' joined hands; then they turn left toward their partners, and the partners face each other. The girls extend their right hands, joining them above the boys' joined left hands, and they all run until the finish of measure 8.

MEASURES 9-10: Each boy takes the opposite girl's left hand in his right hand, and standing side by side, they dance the Tyroler waltz step, which is as follows: the boy begins with his left foot and the girl with her right foot, and doing the balance step, they move away from each other for three beats and toward each other for three beats.

MEASURES 11-12: They repeat the Tyroler waltz step.

MEASURES 13-16: In the social dancing position, the couples perform four waltz steps, turning.

MEASURES 9-16, REPEATED: The players may waltz continuously if desired.

At the end of the figure, each couple seeks a new couple with whom to repeat the pattern. If there is an odd number of couples, one will be unable to find another to dance with, so that with each repetition there will be one "little man in a fix," who dances alone with his partner. There is no pause in the music as new lines of four children are organized.

Square dances

Square dancing is native to the United States and fun for all ages. In square dancing, partners change often, and each individual has a chance to dance with many

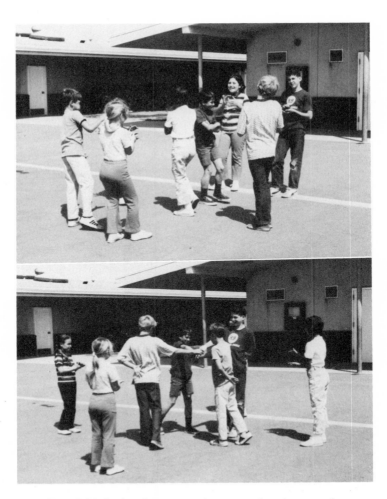

Fig. 16-64. Performing square dances on the playground.

different partners. Square dancing is not difficult to teach and even a novice teacher can have fun calling some of the more simple dances. Although the teacher may use records with calls on them, it is easier to teach the dance when the teacher makes the calls in relation to the children's learning speed in the activity. Some of the more simple square dances can be introduced as early as the first grade. Dances that involve some of the more sophisticated movements are usually more successful in the fourth and fifth grades (Fig. 16-64).

In teaching square dancing, it is best for the teacher to have the students listen to the music and then walk through the dance in response to the verbal calls. If a record player is used, the tempo should be slowed until the children learn all movements thoroughly.

Forming the square. A square is composed of four couples, each couple standing on one side of the square, with the girl to the right side of her partner. Caution should be taken not to get the square too large. If the couples extend their outside arms and touch fingertips they will be able to maintain the approximate correct distance for the square. The head couple is the couple toward the music. The couple to the right of the head couple is couple number two, the couple directly opposite is couple number three, and the couple to the left of the head couple is couple number four. The original positions of the couples are their home positions. The boy's corner girl is the one to his left. The girl's corner boy is the one to her right. Couples one and three are the head couples. Couples two and four are the side couples. The couples standing directly opposite are the opposite couples.

Basic step. The basic step in beginning square dancing is a short walking step in which the weight is kept on the balls of the feet.

Balance step. In the balance step, partners face each other, step backward,

join right hands and swing their right feet forward in a balancing action, and then return quickly to their original position.

Swing. Partners place their right sides together in a regular dance position and turn once in place, using the buzz step.

Grand right and left. Partners face each other and join right hands. Each person then advances forward to the next person, giving the left hand, and continues around the circle, alternating right and left hands, until he or she meets the original partner.

Promenade. Partners progress counter-clockwise around the square, the boy holding his partner in the skating position.

Allemande left. The boy turns to his corner girl and joins his left hand to hers, and they move around each other and then return to their home positions.

Do-sa-do. Partners move forward, passing each other with their right shoulders and stepping sideward back to back. They fold their arms across their chests as they execute the move without turning around.

Elbow swing. Dancer hooks right or left elbows with person indicated and swings around once.

Specific dances

OH JOHNNY

Formation: Couples may dance in square formation or in one large single circle, facing the center. The latter formation makes the dance a good mixer.

Music: MacGregor 6525 and 007-3, Folkraft 1037, and Imperial 1099-XR-239

Procedure

"Oh, you all join hands and circle the ring":

The children move clockwise in a circle.

"Stop where you are and give her a swing":

The boys swing their partners.

"Now swing that girl behind you":

The boys swing the corner girls.

"Go back home and swing your own if you have time":

The boys swing with their partners.

"Allemande left with your corner girl":

The boys do the allemande left with their corner girls.

"Do-sa 'round your own":

The children do-sa-do (sashay) around their partners.

"Now you all run away with your sweet corner maid":

The boys promenade counterclockwide with their corner ladies who become their new partners.

"Singing, oh, Johnny, oh, Johnny, oh!"

The teacher repeats the calls to the end of the recorded music.

SPLIT THE RING

Formation: Four couples dance as a set in the square formation.
Music: Decca Du-40080 and Du-720 (album)
Procedure

"First couple out balance and swing,
Down center and split the ring":

Couple one walks across the set and between (splits) couple three.

"Lady go right and the gent go left":

Girl one goes right and boy one goes left around the outside of the set, and then they go back home.

"Swing when you meet as you did before,
Down the center and cast off four":

Couple one walks across the set. Boy one goes left between girl three and boy four. Girl one goes right between boy three and girl two. They walk outside the set and go back home.

"Swing your honey and she'll swing you,
Down the center and cast off two":

Couple one moves forward to the center of the set. The boy goes left and between (splits) couple four. The girl goes right between (splits) couple two. They walk outside the set and go back home.

"Swing when you meet.
Swing at the head and swing at the feet":

Couples one and three swing.

"Side four the same":

Couples two and four swing.
The teacher repeats the call for couples two, three, and four.

HOT TIME

Formation: Four couples dance as a set in the square formation.
Music: Folkraft F-1037, Imperial 1096, Decca 9-28905, MacGregor 001-4 (album), and Windsor 7115
Procedure

"First couple out, and circle four around":

Couples one and two circle around.

"Pick up two, and circle six around":

Boy one breaks the circle by unclasping his left hand. They pick up couple three to form a circle of six.

"Pick up two, and circle eight around":

Boy one breaks the circle again. They pick up couple four, and the eight circle around.

"There'll be a hot time in the old town tonight.
Allemande left with the lady on the left":

The boys turn their corner girls with their left hands.

"Allemande right with the lady on the right":

The boys pass their partners on the inside of the set and turn the right-hand ladies with their hands.

"Allemande left with the lady on the left":

The boys pass their partners on the inside of the set and turn their corner girls with their left hands.

"And grand right and left all around":

The partners swing.

"When you meet your partner, sashay once around":

The children either sashay or do the do-sa-do around once with their partners.

"Take her in your arms and swing her 'round and 'round.
Promenade around with the prettiest girl in town.
There'll be a hot time in the old town tonight."

The teacher repeats the calls for couples two, three, and four.

BIRD IN THE CAGE

Formation: Four couples dance as a set in the square formation.
Music: Burns 895 and 896
Procedure

"First couple out, balance and swing,
Lead to the right, and form a ring
With four hands around.
Cage the bird with three hands 'round":

Girl one steps into the center. Couple two and boy one join hands and circle around girl one.

"Bird hops out, crow hops in":

Boy one steps into the center as girl one joins the circle with couple two.

"Ring up three and you're gone again.
Crow hops out with a right-hand cross":

Boy one steps out between the two girls, and all four form a right-hand star.

"Then back with the left and don't get lost":

They reverse the direction, forming a left-hand star.

"Form a ring and make it go":

They join hands and form a circle.

"Lead to the next."

The teacher may repeat the calls for couples two, three, and four.

TEXAS STAR

Formation: Four couples dance as a set in the square formation.
Music: MacGregor 001-1 and 12-392
Procedure

"Ladies to the center and back to the bar:"

The girls walk to the center and then back to their original positions.

"Gents to the center with a right-hand star
Right hands crossed":

The boys form a right-hand star in the center of the set by each grasping the wrist of the boy in front while walking forward in a circle.

"Back with the left right where you are":
The boys reverse the direction, forming a left-hand star.

"Wink at your honey as you go by":

The boys pass by their own partners.

"Pick up the next gal on the fly":

Each boy takes the next girl to be his partner. The girls hook onto the boys' right elbows with their left arms, or the boys may place their right arms around the ladies' waists. They continue the star counterclockwise.

"The gents swing out, ladies swing in
Form that Texas star again":

The boys break the star. The couples turn, moving counterclockwise, one and a half times. The girls then form a right-hand star in the center. The couples move in the star formation clockwise.

"Break in the center and everbody swing.
Promenade all around that ring.
Take your partner and promenade home."

The teacher repeats the calls three times until the ladies return to their original partners.

SALLY GOOD'IN

Formation: Four couples dance as a set in the square formation.
Music: World of Fun records M-117 and J80C-4415
Procedure

"First gent out and swing Sally Good'in":

Boy one swings the right-hand girl (Sally Good'in) around with his right hand.

"Now your taw":

Boy one swings his own partner around with his left hand.

"Swing the girl from Arkansas":

Boy one swings the opposite girl (Arkansas girl) around with his right hand.

"Then swing Sally Good'in":

Boy one again swings the right-hand girl around with his left hand.

"And then your taw":

Boy one swings his own partner around with his right hand.

"Now don't forget your old Grandma":

Boy one swings his corner girl (Grandma) around with his left hand.

"Home you go and everybody swing":

All the couples swing with a waist swing.

The teacher repeats the calls with boys one and two leading out simultaneously then repeats them again, with boys one, two, and three leading out simultaneously. When the teacher repeats the calls for the last time, all four boys lead out simultaneously.

The identity of the girls is the same for all boys; for example,. Sally Good'in is the right-hand girl, and Grandma is the corner girl. When more than one boy is called out, each reaches the opposite girl (Arkansas lady) by following the boy on the left.

ARKANSAS TRAVELER

Formation: Four couples dance as a set in the square formation.
Music: Burns 881 and 882 and Decca Du 40080 and Du 720 (album)
Procedure

"First four go forward and back":

Couples one and three go forward and back.

"Forward again in the same old track
Swing your opposite right hand around":

Boy one swings girl three and boy three swings girl one, using a forearm grasp.

"Partners left and left hand around":

All the boys swing their partners.

"Corners right and right hand around":

All the boys swing their corner girls.

"Partners left and left hand around":

All the boys swing their partners.

"And promenade your corners":

The boys promenade with their new partners to each boy's home position.

The teacher repeats the calls for couples two and four, and then repeats them from the beginning until the girls are returned to their original positions.

DIVE FOR THE OYSTER

Formation: Four couples dance as a set in the square formation.
Music: RCA Victor 20592
Procedure

"First couple out to the couple on the right,
and circle four":

Couple one walks to couple two, and they all join hands and circle around once to the left.

"Dive for the oyster, dive":

With both couples still holding hands, couple one dives under raised arms of couple two and steps back home.

"Dig for the clam, dig":

Couple two dives inder the raised arms of couple one and returns home, all four children still holding hands.

"Dive right through and on to the next":

Couple one dives under raised arms of couple two and walks on to couple three, releasing couple two's hands.

Couple one performs the figure with couple three and then with couple four. After diving under couple four's arms, couple one returns home.

"All swing partners and promenade":

All the children swing their partners and promenade.

They repeat the dance until all couples have had a turn.

COMPENSATORY ACTIVITIES

For those children in level 4 who have not achieved the proper development of motor skills, the teacher should individualize programs to include some of the basic movement activities described in levels 2 and 3. It is important that children be challenged and experience success at all levels. However, if the basic movement skills have not been learned, children will retreat to nonactivity because of their inability to perform effectively. Through observation and pre-activity testing, the teacher should identify those children falling below the norm and design compensatory programs in line with their developmental needs.

RECOMMENDED READINGS

Aitken, M. H.: Play environment for children: play space, improvised equipment and facilities, Bellingham, Washington, 1972, Educational Designs and Consultants.
Anderson, M. H., and others: Play with a purpose, New York, 1972, Harper and Row.

Bailie, S., and Bailie, A.: Elementary school gymnastics, St. Louis, 1969, Atlas Athletic Equipment Co.

Barlin, A., and Barlin, P.: The act of learning through movement, Los Angeles, 1971, Ward Ritchie Press.

Christian, Q. A.: The Beanbag Curriculum, Wolfe City, Texas, 1973, The University Press.

Cratty, B. J.: Developmental sequences of perceptual-motor tasks, Mountain View, California, 1970, Peep Publishing Co.

Dimondstein, G.: Children dance in the classroom, New York, 1971, The Macmillan Co.

Doray, M. B.: See what I can do! A book of creative movement, Englewood Cliffs, N.J., 1973, Prentice-Hall.

Fait, H. F.: Physical education for the elementary school child, ed. 3, Philadelphia, 1976, W. B. Saunders Company.

Fendeck, R.: Classroom capers: movement education in the class, Bellingham, Washington, 1971, Educational Designs and Consultants.

Fleming, G., editor: Children's dance, Washington, D.C., 1976, American Alliance for Health, Physical Education and Recreation.

Gallahue, D. L.: Motor development and movement experiences for young children, New York, 1976, John Wiley and Sons Incorporated.

Gilbert, A.: International folk dance at a glance, Minneapolis, 1974, Burgess Publishing Co.

Jensen, M. B., and Jensen, C. R.: Square dancing, Provo, Utah, 1973, Brigham Young University.

Joyce, M.: First steps in teaching creative dance, Palo Alto, California, 1973, National Press Books.

Los Angeles City Schools: Learning to move, moving to learn, 1968, Division of Instructional Planning and Services, Publication # EC 260.

North, M.: Body movement for children, Boston, 1971 Plays, Inc.

Orff-Schülwerk: A means or an end? The School Music News (New York School Music Association), vol. 31, Jan. 1968.

Portland Public Schools: Improving motor-perceptual skill, Corvallis, Oregon, 1970, Continuing Education Publications.

Schurr, E.: Movement experiences for children, New York, 1975, Appleton-Century-Crofts.

Vannier, F., and Gallahue, D. L.: Teaching physical education in elementary schools, Philadelphia, 1973, W. B. Saunders Co.

Vick, M.: A collection of dances for children, Minneapolis, 1970, Burgess Publishing Co.

Wagner, G., and others: Games and activities for early childhood education, New York, 1967, The Macmillan Co.

SUPPLEMENTARY RECORDS

1. Dances Without Partners, Glass 2 Volumes, AR 32, 33.
2. Disco and Soul Dance, Hallum, AR 569.
3. Elementary Floor Exercise Routines, Bramlish, KEA 9030.
4. Fundamentals of Square Dance, Ruff, Sets in Order, LP 6001.
5. Honor Your Partner, Durlacher, 4 volumes.

APPENDIXES

A

Source material

SELECTED FILMS

All the Self There Is. American Association for Health, Physical Education and Recreation, 1201 16th St., N.W., Washington, D.C. 20036. Color; 15 minutes.

Anyone Can. Rope skipping, ball handling, Stegel, and trampoline activities. Bradly Wright films, 309 N. Duane, San Gabriel, Calif. 91775. Color; 27 minutes; 1968.

A Time to Move. Early Childhood Productions, Box 352, Chatsworth, Calif. 91311. Color; 30 minutes.

Bridges to Learning. Perceptual physical education program K-6. Palmer Films Inc., 611 Howard St., San Francisco, Calif. Color; 30 minutes; 1970.

Creative Body Movements. Perceptual-motor and problem solving through movement activities K-3. Martin Moyer Productions, 900 Federal Ave., E. Seattle, Wash. 98102. Color; 11 minutes; 1969.

Discovering Rhythm. Basic motor concepts related to rhythm. Universal Education and Visual Arts, 221 Park Ave. S., New York, N.Y. 10003. Color; 11 minutes; 1968.

Every Child a Winner. American Association for Health, Physical Education and Recreation, 1201 16th St., N.W., Washington, D.C. 20036. Color; 15 minutes.

Fun with Parachutes. Locomotor, game, and rhythmic activities. Educational Activities, Inc., Freeport, N.Y. 11520. Color.

Innovations in Elementary Physical Education. Movement Activities K-6. Crown Films, 503 W. Indiana Ave., Box 890, Spokane, Wash. 99210. Color; 20 minutes.

Learning Through Movement. Creative expression from verbal and rhythmic cues. S and L Film Productions, 5126 Hartwick St., Los Angeles, Calif. 90041. Black and white; 32 minutes; 1966.

Movement Exploration. Movement activities K-6. Documentary Films, 3217 Trout Gulch Rd., Aptos, Calif. 95003. Color; 20 minutes.

Movement Exploration. Locomotor activities; Hula-Hoop, jump rope, and apparatus stations. Educational Activities, Inc., Freeport, N.Y. 11520. Color.

Perk! Pop! Sprinkle! Visual perception with motoric responses K-3. Martin Moyer Productions, 900 Federal Ave., E. Seattle, Wash. 98102. Color; 11 minutes; 1969.

Sensorimotor Training. Sensory-motor skills for preschool children. Valdhere Films, 3060 Valleywood Dr., Kettering, Ohio. Color; 24 minutes; 1968.

Sport Skills. Sport techniques for badminton, basketball, field hockey, football, golf, gymnastics, trampoline, ice hockey, volleyball, soccer, tennis, and track and field. The Athletic Institute, 705 Merchandise Mart, Chicago, Ill. 60654. Super 8 mm. loop cartridge films.

Thinking, Moving, Learning. Bradley Wright Films, 309 N. Duane, San Gabriel, Calif. 91775. Color; 30 minutes.

Up and Over—Exploring on the Stegel. Bradley Wright Films, 309 N. Duane, San Gabriel, Calif. 91775. Color; 12 minutes.

What Am I. Discovering how the body moves K-3. Film Associates, 11559 Santa Monica Blvd., Los Angeles, Calif. 90025. Color; 11 minutes; 1968.

EQUIPMENT AND MATERIAL SOURCES

Rhythm balls. AMF Voit catalog no. 672.

Physical activity charts. Balance beam skills, ball-handling skills, locomotor rhythms, striking skills, stunts, and tumbling. The Athletic Institute, 705 Merchandise Mart, Chicago, Ill. 60654.

Bulletin board charts. Football, basketball, baseball, gymnastics, soccer, golf, tennis, and volleyball. The General Tire and Rubber Company, Athletic Products Division, Jeannette, Pa. 15644.

Sensory-motor games and climbing apparatus. J. L. Hammatt Co., Physical Education Division, Hammatt Place, Braintree, Mass. 02184.

Table games. Gammatt and Sons, P.O. Box 2004, Anaheim, Calif. 92804.

Recreational games and nets. Catalog no. 971. Indian Head Recreational Products, Blue Mountain, Ala. 36201.

Mats, balance beams, net standards, and play-

ground equipment. J. E. Gregory Co., W. 922 First Ave., Spokane, Wash. 99204.

Plastic sport equipment and recreational games. Cosom Safe-T-Play Products, 6030 Wayzata Blvd., Minneapolis, Minn. 55416.

Records, filmstrips, cassettes, and instructional media. Educational Activities, Inc., Freeport, N.Y. 11520; Educational Record Sales, 157 Chambers St., New York, N.Y. 10007; and Kimbo Educational, Box 246, Deal, N.J. 07723.

Weight and exercise machines. Universal Athletic Saler Company, 1328 N. Sierra Vista, Fresno, Calif. 93703.

Athletic equipment. Mats, apparatus, and lockers. Gymnastic Supply Company, 247 W. 6th St., San Pedro, Calif. 90733; Sportime, 63 Plandome Road, Manhasset, N.Y. 11030; and G. S. C. Athletic Equipment Catalog, 600 N. Pacific Avenue, P.O. Box 1710, San Pedro, Calif. 90733.

Sports equipment, nets, and gymnasium apparatus. J. Ayfro Corporation, 1 Bridge St., P.O. Box 50, Montville, Conn. 06353.

Safety mats for indoor-outdoor equipment. Mallott and Peterson-Guindy, 2412 Harrison St., San Francisco, Calif. 94116.

Incline mats, spot trainers, and creative shapes. Skill Development Equipment Company, 1340 N. Jefferson, Anaheim, Calif. 92806.

Gymnastic equipment, trampolines, and tumbling mats. AMF American Athletic Equipment Division, Box 111, Jefferson, Iowa 50129.

Customized and all-purpose gym mats. Resilite, P.O. Box 764, Sunbury, Pa. 17801.

Field flags and obstacle markers. Flex-i-Flag Company, 2238 Buchanan St., N.E., Minneapolis, Minn. 55418.

Dance records and costumes. Pacific Dance Supplies, 1724 Taroval St., San Francisco, Calif. 94116.

B

Selected standards for AAHPER physical fitness profile

Table 1. Flexed-arm hang for girls*: percentile scores based on age/test scores in seconds

Percentile	Age					Percentile
	9-10	11	12	13	14	
100th	78	68	84	68	65	100th
95th	42	39	33	34	35	95th
90th	29	30	27	25	29	90th
85th	24	24	23	21	26	85th
80th	21	21	21	20	23	80th
75th	18	20	18	16	21	75th
70th	16	17	15	14	18	70th
65th	14	15	13	13	15	65th
60th	12	13	12	11	13	60th
55th	10	11	10	9	11	55th
50th	9	10	9	8	9	50th
45th	7	8	8	7	8	45th
40th	6	7	6	6	7	40th
35th	5	6	5	5	5	35th
30th	4	5	4	4	5	30th
25th	3	3	3	3	3	25th
20th	2	3	2	2	3	20th
15th	1	2	1	1	2	15th
10th	0	0	1	0	1	10th
5th	0	0	0	0	0	5th
0	0	0	0	0	0	0

*Procedures for conducting a flexed-arm hang test are described in Chapter 10.

Table 2. Pull-up for boys*: percentile scores based on age/test scores in number of pull-ups

Percentile	Age					Percentile
	9-10	11	12	13	14	
100th	19	16	18	17	27	100th
95th	9	8	9	10	12	95th
90th	7	6	7	9	10	90th
85th	5	5	6	7	9	85th
80th	4	5	5	6	8	80th
75th	3	4	4	5	7	75th
70th	3	4	4	5	7	70th
65th	2	3	3	4	6	65th
60th	2	3	3	4	5	60th
55th	1	2	2	3	5	55th
50th	1	2	2	3	4	50th
45th	1	1	1	2	4	45th
40th	1	1	1	2	3	40th
35th	1	1	1	2	3	35th
30th	0	1	0	1	2	30th
25th	0	0	0	1	2	25th
20th	0	0	0	0	1	20th
15th	0	0	0	0	1	15th
10th	0	0	0	0	0	10th
5th	0	0	0	0	0	5th
0	0	0	0	0	0	0

*Procedures for conducting a pull-up test are described in Chapter 10.

Table 3. Sit-up (flexed legs)*: percentile scores based on age/test scores in number of sit-ups

	Girls					Boys					
	Age					Age					
Percentile	9-10	11	12	13	14	9-10	11	12	13	14	Percentile
100th	56	60	55	57	52	70	60	62	60	73	100th
95th	45	43	44	45	45	47	48	50	53	55	95th
90th	40	40	40	41	43	44	45	48	50	52	90th
85th	38	38	38	40	41	42	43	45	48	50	85th
80th	35	36	37	38	39	40	41	43	47	48	80th
75th	34	35	36	36	37	38	40	42	45	47	75th
70th	33	33	35	35	35	36	39	40	43	45	70th
65th	31	32	33	33	35	36	38	39	42	44	65th
60th	30	31	32	32	33	35	37	38	41	43	60th
55th	29	30	30	31	32	33	35	37	40	41	55th
50th	27	29	29	30	30	31	34	35	38	41	50th
45th	25	28	28	29	30	30	33	34	37	40	45th
40th	24	26	27	27	29	29	31	33	35	38	40th
35th	23	25	26	26	27	28	30	32	34	37	35th
30th	22	24	25	25	25	27	28	30	32	35	30th
25th	21	22	24	23	24	25	26	30	30	34	25th
20th	20	20	22	22	22	23	24	28	29	32	20th
15th	17	18	20	20	20	21	22	26	27	21	15th
10th	14	15	17	18	18	19	19	23	24	27	10th
5th	10	9	13	15	16	13	15	18	20	24	5th
0	0	0	0	0	2	2	0	0	2	6	0

*Procedures for conducting the sit-up (flexed legs) test are described in Chapter 10.

Table 4. Shuttle run*: percentile scores based on age/test scores in seconds and tenths of seconds

	Girls					Boys					
	Age					Age					
Percentile	9-10	11	12	13	14	9-10	11	12	13	14	Percentile
100th	8.0	8.4	8.5	7.0	7.8	9.2	8.7	6.8	7.0	7.0	100th
95th	10.2	10.0	9.9	9.9	9.7	10.0	9.7	9.6	9.3	8.9	95th
90th	10.5	10.3	10.2	10.0	10.0	10.2	9.9	9.8	9.5	9.2	90th
85th	10.9	10.5	10.5	10.2	10.1	10.4	10.1	10.0	9.7	9.3	85th
80th	11.0	10.7	10.6	10.4	10.2	10.5	10.2	10.0	9.8	9.5	80th
75th	11.1	10.8	10.8	10.5	10.3	10.6	10.4	10.2	10.0	9.6	75th
70th	11.2	11.0	10.9	10.6	10.5	10.7	10.5	10.3	10.0	9.8	70th
65th	11.4	11.0	11.0	10.8	10.6	10.8	10.5	10.4	10.1	9.8	65th
60th	11.5	11.1	11.1	11.0	10.7	11.0	10.6	10.5	10.2	10.0	60th
55th	11.6	11.3	11.2	11.0	10.9	11.0	10.8	10.6	10.3	10.0	55th
50th	11.8	11.5	11.4	11.2	11.0	11.2	10.9	10.7	10.4	10.1	50th
45th	11.9	11.6	11.5	11.3	11.2	11.5	11.0	10.8	10.5	10.1	45th
40th	12.0	11.7	11.5	11.5	11.4	11.5	11.1	11.0	10.6	10.2	40th
35th	12.0	11.9	11.7	11.6	11.5	11.7	11.2	11.1	10.8	10.4	35th
30th	12.3	12.0	11.8	11.9	11.7	11.9	11.4	11.3	11.0	10.6	30th
25th	12.5	12.1	12.0	12.0	12.0	12.0	11.5	11.4	11.0	10.7	25th
20th	12.8	12.3	12.1	12.2	12.1	12.2	11.8	11.6	11.3	10.9	20th
15th	13.0	12.6	12.5	12.6	12.3	12.5	12.0	11.8	11.5	11.0	15th
10th	13.8	13.0	13.0	12.8	12.8	13.0	12.2	12.0	11.8	11.3	10th
5th	14.3	14.0	13.3	13.2	13.1	13.1	12.9	12.4	12.4	11.9	5th
0	18.0	20.0	15.3	16.5	19.2	17.0	20.0	22.0	16.0	18.6	0

*Procedures for conducting the shuttle run are described in Chapter 10.

Table 5. Standing long jump*: percentile scores based on age/test scores in feet and inches

| | Girls | | | | | Boys | | | | | |
| | Age | | | | | Age | | | | | |
Percentile	9-10	11	12	13	14	9-10	11	12	13	14	Percentile
100th	7'11"	7' 0"	7' 0"	8' 0"	7' 5"	6' 5"	8' 5"	7' 5"	8' 6"	9' 0"	100th
95th	5'10"	6' 0"	6' 2"	6' 5"	6' 8"	6' 0"	6' 2"	6' 6"	7' 1"	7' 6"	95th
90th	5' 8"	5' 9"	6' 0"	6' 2"	6' 5"	5'10"	6' 0"	6' 3"	6'10"	7' 2"	90th
85th	5' 5"	5' 7"	5' 9"	6' 0"	6' 3"	5' 8"	5'10"	6' 1"	6' 8"	6'11"	85th
80th	5' 2"	5' 5"	5' 8"	5'10"	6' 0"	5' 6"	5' 9"	6' 0"	6' 5"	6'10"	80th
75th	5' 2"	5' 4"	5' 6"	5' 9"	5'11"	5' 4"	5' 7"	5'11"	6' 3"	6' 8"	75th
70th	5' 0"	5' 3"	5' 5"	5' 7"	5'10"	5' 3"	5' 6"	5' 9"	6' 2"	6' 6"	70th
65th	5' 0"	5' 2"	5' 4"	5' 6"	5' 8"	5' 1"	5' 6"	5' 8"	6' 0"	6' 6"	65th
60th	4'10"	5' 1"	5' 2"	5' 5"	5' 7"	5' 1"	5' 5"	5' 7"	6' 0"	6' 4"	60th
55th	4' 9"	5' 0"	5' 1"	5' 4"	5' 6"	5' 0"	5' 4"	5' 6"	5'10"	6' 3"	55th
50th	4' 8"	4'11"	5' 0"	5' 3"	5' 4"	4'11"	5' 2"	5' 5"	5' 9"	6' 2"	50th
45th	4' 7"	4'10"	4'11"	5' 2"	5' 3"	4'10"	5' 2"	5' 4"	5' 7"	6' 1"	45th
40th	4' 6"	4' 8"	4'10"	5' 1"	5' 2"	4' 9"	5' 0"	5' 3"	5' 6"	5'11"	40th
35th	4' 5"	4' 7"	4' 9"	5' 0"	5' 1"	4' 8"	4'11"	5' 2"	5' 5"	5'10"	35th
30th	4' 3"	4' 6"	4' 8"	4'10"	4'11"	4' 7"	4'10"	5' 1"	5' 3"	5' 8"	30th
25th	4' 1"	4' 4"	4' 6"	4' 9"	4'10"	4' 6"	4' 8"	5' 0"	5' 2"	5' 6"	25th
20th	4' 0"	4' 3"	4' 5"	4' 8"	4' 9"	4' 5"	4' 7"	4'10"	5' 0"	5' 4"	20th
15th	3'11"	4' 2"	4' 3"	4' 6"	4' 6"	4' 2"	4' 5"	4' 9"	4'10"	5' 2"	15th
10th	3' 8"	4' 0"	4' 2"	4' 3"	4' 4"	4' 0"	4' 3"	4' 6"	4' 7"	5' 0"	10th
5th	3' 5"	3' 8"	3'10"	4' 0"	4' 0"	3'10"	4' 0"	4' 2"	4' 4"	4' 8"	5th
0	1' 8"	2'10"	3' 0"	3' 2"	3' 0"	3' 1"	3' 0"	3' 2"	3' 3"	2' 0"	0

*Procedures for conducting a standing long jump are described in Chapter 10.

Table 6. 50-yard dash*: percentile scores based on age/test scores in seconds and tenths of seconds

	Girls					Boys					
	Age					Age					
Percentile	9-10	11	12	13	14	9-10	11	12	13	14	Percentile
100th	7.0	6.9	6.0	6.0	6.0	7.0	6.3	6.3	5.8	5.9	100th
95th	7.4	7.3	7.0	6.9	6.8	7.3	7.1	6.8	6.5	6.2	95th
90th	7.5	7.5	7.2	7.0	7.0	7.5	7.2	7.0	6.7	6.4	90th
85th	7.8	7.5	7.4	7.2	7.1	7.7	7.4	7.1	6.9	6.5	85th
80th	8.0	7.8	7.5	7.3	7.2	7.8	7.5	7.3	7.0	6.6	80th
75th	8.0	7.9	7.6	7.4	7.3	7.8	7.6	7.4	7.0	6.8	75th
70th	8.1	7.9	7.7	7.5	7.4	7.9	7.7	7.5	7.1	6.9	70th
65th	8.3	8.0	7.9	7.6	7.5	8.0	7.9	7.5	7.2	7.0	65th
60th	8.4	8.1	8.0	7.7	7.6	8.0	7.9	7.6	7.3	7.0	60th
55th	8.5	8.2	8.0	7.9	7.6	8.1	8.0	7.7	7.4	7.1	55th
50th	8.6	8.3	8.1	8.0	7.8	8.2	8.0	7.8	7.5	7.2	50th
45th	8.8	8.4	8.2	8.0	7.9	8.4	8.2	7.9	7.5	7.3	45th
40th	8.9	8.5	8.3	8.1	8.0	8.6	8.3	8.0	7.6	7.4	40th
35th	9.0	8.6	8.4	8.2	8.0	8.7	8.4	8.1	7.7	7.5	35th
30th	9.0	8.8	8.5	8.3	8.2	8.8	8.5	8.2	7.9	7.6	30th
25th	9.1	9.0	8.7	8.5	8.3	8.9	8.6	8.3	8.0	7.7	25th
20th	9.4	9.1	8.9	8.7	8.5	9.0	8.7	8.5	8.1	7.9	20th
15th	9.6	9.3	9.1	8.9	8.8	9.2	9.0	8.6	8.3	8.0	15th
10th	9.9	9.6	9.4	9.2	9.0	9.5	9.1	9.0	8.7	8.2	10th
5th	10.3	10.0	10.0	10.0	9.6	9.9	9.5	9.5	9.0	8.8	5th
0	13.5	12.9	14.9	14.2	11.0	11.0	11.5	11.3	15.0	11.1	0

*Procedures for conducting the 50-yard dash are described in Chapter 10.

Table 7. 600-yard run*: percentile based on age/test scores in minutes and seconds

	Girls					Boys					
	Age					Age					
Percentile	9-10	11	12	13	14	9-10	11	12	13	14	Percentile
100th	2' 7"	1'52"	1'40"	1'43"	1'33"	1'52"	1'47"	1'38"	1'26"	1'27"	100th
95th	2'20"	2'14"	2' 6"	2' 4"	2' 2"	2' 5"	2' 2"	1'52"	1'45"	1'39"	95th
90th	2'26"	2'21"	2'14"	2'12"	2' 7"	2' 9"	2' 6"	1'57"	1'50"	1'44"	90th
85th	2'30"	2'25"	2'21"	2'16"	2'11"	2'11"	2' 9"	2' 0"	1'54"	1'47"	85th
80th	2'33"	2'30"	2'23"	2'20"	2'15"	2'15"	2'12"	2' 4"	1'57"	1'50"	80th
75th	2'39"	2'35"	2'26"	2'23"	2'19"	2'17"	2'15"	2' 6"	1'59"	1'52"	75th
70th	2'41"	2'39"	2'31"	2'27"	2'24"	2'20"	2'17"	2' 9"	2' 1"	1'55"	70th
65th	2'45"	2'42"	2'35"	2'30"	2'29"	2'27"	2'19"	2'11"	2' 3"	1'57"	65th
60th	2'48"	2'45"	2'39"	2'34"	2'32"	2'30"	2'22"	2'14"	2' 5"	1'58"	60th
55th	2'51"	2'48"	2'43"	2'37"	2'36"	2'31"	2'25"	2'16"	2' 7"	2' 0"	55th
50th	2'56"	2'53"	2'47"	2'41"	2'40"	2'33"	2'27"	2'19"	2'10"	2' 3"	50th
45th	2'59"	2'55"	2'51"	2'45"	2'44"	2'35"	2'30"	2'22"	2'13"	2' 5"	45th
40th	3' 1"	2'59"	2'56"	2'49"	2'47"	2'40"	2'34"	2'24"	2'15"	2' 7"	40th
35th	3' 8"	3' 4"	3' 0"	2'55"	2'51"	2'42"	2'37"	2'28"	2'20"	2'10"	35th
30th	3'11"	3'11"	3' 6"	2'59"	2'56"	2'49"	2'41"	2'32"	2'24"	2'12"	30th
25th	3'15"	3'16"	3'13"	3' 6"	3' 1"	2'53"	2'47"	2'37"	2'27"	2'16"	25th
20th	3'21"	3'24"	3'19"	3'12"	3' 8"	2'59"	2'54"	2'42"	2'32"	2'22"	20th
15th	3'25"	3'30"	3'27"	3'20"	3'16"	3' 7"	3' 2"	2'48"	2'37"	2'30"	15th
10th	3'38"	3'44"	3'36"	3'30"	3'27"	3'14"	3'14"	2'54"	2'45"	2'37"	10th
5th	4' 0"	4'15"	3'59"	3'49"	3'49"	3'22"	3'29"	3' 6"	3' 0"	2'51"	5th
0	5'48"	5'10"	6' 2"	5'10"	5' 0"	4'48"	6'20"	4'10"	4' 0"	6' 0"	0

*Procedures for conducting the 600-yard run are described in Chapter 10.

Index